D1629833

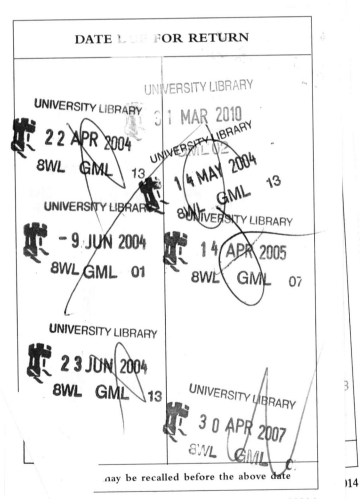

A Clinical Guide to
AIDS and HIV

A Clinical Guide to AIDS and HIV

Editor

Gary P. Wormser, M.D.

Professor of Medicine and Pharmacology
Chief, Division of Infectious Disease
New York Medical College
Westchester County Medical Center
Valhalla, New York

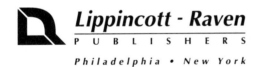

Lippincott - Raven
P U B L I S H E R S
Philadelphia • New York

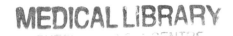
Printed in the United States of America

9 8 7 6 5 4 3 2 1

Library of Congress Cataloging-in-Publication Data

Clinical guide to AIDS and HIV / editor, Gary P. Wormser.
    p.   cm.
    Includes index.
    ISBN 0-7817-0304-2
    1. AIDS (Disease)—Handbooks, manuals, etc. I. Wormser, Gary P.
    [DNLM: 1. HIV Infections. 2. Acquired Immunodeficiency Syndrome.
WC 503 C641 1996]
RC607.A26C574   1996
616.97′92—dc20
DNLM/DLC   96-6049
For Library of Congress   CIP

To Joni Laden and to the memory
of my good friend, Dr. Zal Arlin.

Contents

Contributors

Donald I. Abrams, M.D.
Professor of Clinical Medicine
AIDS Program
San Francisco General Hospital
University of California at San Francisco
Ward 84, 995 Potrero Avenue
San Francisco, California 94110

Kathryn Anastos, M.D.
Associate Professor of Medicine
Montefiore Medical Center, and
Department of Medicine
Albert Einstein College of Medicine
3544 Jerome Avenue
Bronx, New York 10467

John G. Bartlett, M.D.
Professor of Medicine
Chief, Division of Infectious Diseases
The Johns Hopkins University School of
    Medicine
1159 Ross, 720 Rutland Avenue
Baltimore, Maryland 21205

William Breitbart, M.D.
Associate Professor of Psychiatry
Department of Psychiatry
Cornell University Medical College; and
Memorial Sloan-Kettering Cancer Center
Psychiatry Service Memorial Hospital
1275 York Avenue
New York, New York 10021

Richard E. Chaisson, M.D.
Associate Professor of Medicine,
    Epidemiology, and International Health
Department of Medicine
The Johns Hopkins University School of
    Medicine
Carnegie 292
600 North Wolfe Street
Baltimore, Maryland 21287-6220

Risa Denenberg, R.N, M.S.N.
Family Nurse Practitioner
Bronx, New York 10456

D. Peter Drotman, M.D., M.P.H.
Assistant Director for Public Health
Division of HIV/AIDS Prevention
National Center for Infectious Diseases
Centers for Disease Control and
    Prevention
1600 Clifton Road, North East; and
Clinical Assistant Professor
Department of Family and Preventive
    Medicine
Emory University School of Medicine
Atlanta, Georgia 30333

Emily J. Erbelding, M.D., M.P.H.
Senior Clinical Fellow, Infectious Diseases
Department of Medicine
The Johns Hopkins University School of
    Medicine
1159 Ross, 720 Rutland Avenue
Baltimore, Maryland 21205

Joel E. Gallant, M.D., M.P.H.
Assistant Professor of Medicine
Department of Medicine
Division of Infectious Diseases
The Johns Hopkins University School of
    Medicine
Carnegie 292
600 North Wolfe Street
Baltimore, Maryland 21287-6220

Parkash S. Gill, M.D.
Division of Hematology
Department of Internal Medicine
University of Southern California
School of Medicine
Los Angeles, California 90033

Samuel Grubman, M.D.

Associate Chairman, Department of
Pediatrics, and
Section Chief, Department of Pediatric
Allergy and Immunology
Saint Vincent's Hospital and Medical
Center
New York, New York 10011

Harold W. Horowitz, M.D.

Associate Professor of Medicine
Department of Internal Medicine
Division of Infectious Diseases
New York Medical College
Westchester County Medical Center
Macy Pavilion, Room 209
Valhalla, New York 10595

Barbara S. Koppel, M.D.

Professor of Clinical Neurology
Department of Neurology
New York Medical College
Valhalla, New York 10595; and
Metropolitan Hospital
1901 First Avenue
New York, New York 10029

Donald P. Kotler, M.D.

Associate Professor of Medicine
Department of Medicine, Division of
Gastroenterology
College of Physicians and Surgeons,
Columbia University
Saint Luke's Roosevelt Hospital Center
1111 Amsterdam Avenue
New York, New York 10025

Alexandra M. Levine, M.D.

Professor of Medicine
Chief, Division of Hematology
Department of Internal Medicine
University of Southern California
School of Medicine
1441 Eastlake Avenue
Los Angeles, California 90033

Arlene J. Lowenstein, R.N., Ph.D.

Professor and Chairperson
Department of Nursing Administration,
School of Nursing
Medical College of Georgia
997 Saint Sebastian Way
Augusta, Georgia 30912-4230

William J. Martone, M.S., M.D.

Senior Executive Director
National Foundation for Infectious
Diseases
4733 Bethesda Avenue
Bethesda, Maryland 20814

James Oleske, M.D., M.P.H.

François-Xavier Bagnaud Professor of
Pediatrics
Division of Allergy Immunology and
Infectious Diseases
University of Medicine and Dentistry of
New Jersey
New Jersey Medical School
185 South Orange Avenue
Newark, New Jersey 07103

Robert T. Schooley, M.D.

Professor of Medicine
Chief, Infectious Diseases Division
University of Colorado Health Sciences
Center
4200 East Ninth Avenue
Denver, Colorado 80134

Laurie Solomon, M.D.

Assistant Professor of Obstetrics and
Gynecology
Albert Einstein College of Medicine
Director of Ambulatory Obstetric and
Gynecologic Services
Bronx Lebanon Hospital Center
1275 Fulton Avenue
Bronx, New York 10461

Richard L. Sowell, Ph.D., R.N., F.A.A.N.
Associate Professor and Chair
Department of Administrative and Clinical
  Nursing
University of South Carolina
Greene and Pickens Streets
Columbia, South Carolina 29208

Troy Spicer, M.N., C.F.N.P.
Clinical Director
Early Intervention Program
AID Atlanta Inc.
1438 West Peachtree Street, Suite 100
Atlanta, Georgia 30309-2955

Jerome I. Tokars, M.D., M.P.H.
Medical Epidemiologist
Hospital Infections Program
Centers for Disease Control and
  Prevention
1600 Clifton Road MS E-69
Atlanta, Georgia 30333

Anil Tulpele, M.D.
Assistant Professor of Medicine
Department of Medicine
University of Southern California
Norris Cancer Hospital
1441 Eastlake Avenue, #162
Los Angeles, California 90033

John W. Ward, M.D.
Chief, Surveillance Branch
Division of HIV/AIDS Prevention
National Center for Infectious Diseases
Centers for Disease Control and
  Prevention
Atlanta, Georgia 30333

Gary P. Wormser, M.D.
Professor of Medicine and Pharmacology
Chief, Division of Infectious Disease
New York Medical College
Westchester County Medical Center
Macy Pavilion, Room 209, SE
Valhalla, New York 10595

Foreword

The care of patients with human immunodeficiency virus (HIV) infection and with the acquired immunodeficiency syndrome (AIDS) is exceedingly complicated. I know of no greater challenge in infectious diseases, indeed in all of medicine. *A Clinical Guide to AIDS and HIV* tackles this problem from a practical point of view for the practicing physician. From epidemiology through the clinical manifestations and treatment of HIV infection and AIDS in both adults and children, this book educates and guides the practitioner. It includes infection control and even alternative therapies, an area in which we all need more information. Unless we get to know our patients and keep an open mind about them, our patients will not reveal to us that they are taking various types of alternative therapy. The editor and authors of this volume skillfully share with the reader their wealth of experience. This book should be within easy reach of physicians caring for patients with HIV infection or AIDS. It will serve as a practical guide to the understanding of HIV infection and to the management and care of people with HIV infection and AIDS.

Donald Armstrong, M.D.

Preface

In 1981 when AIDS was first recognized, cases were rare and the disease was regarded mostly as a curiosity. By the mid 1980s, the etiologic agent, HIV, had been discovered and partially characterized, allowing the enormity of the pandemic to be appreciated. It has become accepted that HIV infection is a chronic illness whose natural history may span more than a decade, with symptoms arising transiently within the first 2 months for some, and during the last few years of life for almost all. The most common method of transmission is sexual, with populations who have traditionally been at greatest risk for sexually-transmitted diseases disproportionately affected. Because of this, it affects a much younger population than do most other chronic diseases.

In the early 1980s, management was relegated to the diagnosis and treatment of the late opportunistic infections. The clinical approach has changed dramatically with time. By 1996, HIV-infected persons were placed under medical supervision as soon as they were diagnosed, even though they may have been asymptomatic for years. Equipped with an expanding array of diagnostic tests (e.g., T cell subsets, *Pneumocystis carinii* direct fluorescent assays) and an even wider variety of new drugs (AZT, fluconazole, and many others), the health care practitioner has more to offer these patients than ever before. Objective but suboptimal improvements in quality and duration of life have resulted.

The purpose of this book is to assist the health care practitioner in providing the necessary primary care for HIV-infected patients. This care involves science, art, and a tremendous amount of compassion.

The road map to this volume is provided by the chapters, "Care of the Adult Patient with HIV Infection," and "HIV in Infants, Children, and Adolescents." These chapters give an overview of care from initial testing and counseling through treatment and prevention of the most opportunistic of the infections. These chapters represent a distinguishing and important feature of the book. Elaboration of the discussion of particular clinical issues is done on a system-by-system basis for the major systems involved. Particular emphasis is given to the emerging pharmacotherapy. For example, Chapter 11 provides a list of many important drugs with their actions, indications, pharmacokinetics, cost, availability, adverse effects, and drug interactions.

This book will provide a practical reference for practitioners directly involved in the care of patients. For further information regarding the basic science and clinical pathology of HIV infection, the reader is referred to the volume entitled *AIDS and Other Manifestations of HIV Infections*, also published by Lippincott-Raven Publishers.

Gary P. Wormser, M.D

Acknowledgments

Special thanks to Mrs. Eleanor Bramesco for her assistance with this project; to my Infectious Diseases colleagues, research team, office staff, and Fellows for their understanding; to Steven Gambert, Jack McGiff, Soldano Ferrone, Susan Kline, and Nadine Latterman for their general support; and to my special friends Edward Bottone and Rosalyn Stahl who helped lay the ground work.

A Clinical Guide to
AIDS and HIV

A Clinical Guide to AIDS and HIV,
edited by Gary P. Wormser.
Lippincott-Raven Publishers, Philadelphia 1996.

1

The Epidemiology of HIV and AIDS

John W. Ward and *D. Peter Drotman

*Division of HIV/AIDS, National Center for Infectious Diseases, Centers for Disease
Control and Prevention; and *Department of Family and Preventive Medicine,
Emory University School of Medicine, Atlanta, Georgia 30333*

The acquired immunodeficiency syndrome (AIDS) is characterized by the severe immunosuppression, wasting, dementia, opportunistic infections, and cancers that result from infection with the retrovirus human immunodeficiency virus (HIV). AIDS was first recognized in 1981 with the unexplained occurrence of clusters of cases of *Pneumocystis carinii* pneumonia (PCP) and Kaposi's sarcoma (KS) among young homosexual/bisexual men in California and New York City. Cases of these and other opportunistic infections associated with unexplained immunosuppression were subsequently reported among persons with hemophilia, recipients of blood and blood components, injecting drug users and their heterosexual partners, and children with similar opportunistic conditions. The occurrence of these conditions in epidemiologically distinct populations suggested that AIDS was caused by an infectious agent. In 1983, a previously unknown cytopathic retrovirus was isolated from persons at risk for AIDS. Subsequently, serologic tests to detect antibody to HIV were developed and became available in March 1985. The use of these serologic assays led to the observation that the number of persons infected with HIV was much larger than the number diagnosed with AIDS and that the period between infection with HIV and the development of AIDS is long.

Since the initial case reports of AIDS, the number of persons with HIV infection and AIDS has grown rapidly in the United States and globally. By 1995, the World Health Organization (WHO) estimated that 18 million persons were infected with HIV worldwide including approximately 1 million persons in the United States. As the epidemic has grown, the characteristics of populations affected by HIV have also changed. While the first cases of HIV were recognized among young adult homosexual/bisexual men in the 1980s, the epidemic was expanding most rapidly among persons at risk for heterosexual transmission both in the United States and in other areas by the 1990s. The development of antiretroviral therapies and the increasing use of pharmacologic agents to delay or prevent the opportunistic infections associated with HIV infection has altered the natural history of HIV disease and extended the survival of persons with AIDS. The growth of the HIV epidemic has also contributed to an increase in the number of persons with tuberculosis. An understanding of the epidemiology of HIV infection in the United States and abroad is necessary to properly target prevention and education efforts to where they are most needed, to counsel individuals about their risks for HIV infection, and to guide the diagnosis and medical management of HIV infection and related illnesses.

AIDS IN THE UNITED STATES

All 50 states, the District of Columbia, and all territories of the United States require AIDS cases to be reported to local health authorities. The reporting of AIDS is based on standard case definitions for adults and children developed by the Centers for Disease Control and Prevention (CDC) in collaboration with state and local health departments. One of the initial uses of AIDS surveillance was to investigate retrospectively physician and hospital records and death certificates to identify earlier cases of AIDS that had gone unrecognized or unreported. Investigators eventually located 125 cases diagnosed from 1977 to 1981. This provided evidence that AIDS was a relatively new disease in the United States. Although a few cases compatible with AIDS were retrospectively diagnosed in the 1950s and 1960s, the AIDS epidemic in the United States clearly started in the mid- to late 1970s.

The AIDS surveillance case definition was revised in 1985, 1987, and 1993 to incorporate additional severe illnesses found to be associated with HIV infection. Although not required for the diagnosis of all AIDS-related opportunistic infections (AIDS-OIs), a positive HIV antibody test result serves to improve the sensitivity and specificity of reporting of certain AIDS-OIs and was added in 1985. In 1987, the surveillance criteria were revised to include the presumptive diagnosis of some opportunistic infections to reflect changes in the diagnostic practices of physicians caring for persons with AIDS and to add HIV encephalopathy and wasting syndrome as reportable conditions. In 1993, to include all persons with severe HIV-related immunosuppression, the surveillance definition was expanded to include HIV-infected persons with a $CD4^+$ lymphocyte count of less than 200/μL or a percentage of total lymphocytes of less than 14 and three clinical conditions—pulmonary tuberculosis, recurrent pneumonia, and invasive cervical cancer. The $CD4^+$ lymphocyte is the primary target cell for HIV because of the affinity of the virus for the $CD4^+$ surface marker, and measures of $CD4^+$ lymphocytes are widely used to guide clinical and therapeutic management of HIV-infected patients. As the number of $CD4^+$ lymphocytes decreases, the risk and severity of opportunistic infections tends to increase. As a result, chemoprophylaxis against PCP, the most common serious opportunistic infection diagnosed in AIDS patients, is recommended for all persons with $CD4^+$ lymphocyte counts of less than 200/μL. The early use of specific antiretroviral therapy and PCP prophylaxis has influenced the national epidemiologic pattern of AIDS by delaying the onset of opportunistic illnesses included in the earlier surveillance case definitions.

Although all revisions to the AIDS surveillance definition have resulted in larger proportions of the HIV-infected population being defined as having AIDS, the 1993 expansion has had the largest impact on case reporting. In 1993, the number of AIDS cases reported increased by more than 100%, nearly all of which resulted from the expansion of surveillance criteria and the use of the $CD4^+$ cell count reporting criteria. Although the inclusion of the $CD4^+$ criteria provides a more complete description of all persons with severe HIV-related immunosuppression and results in the reporting of infected persons at an earlier stage of HIV infection, the large increase in case reporting has severely constrained the use of AIDS data based on year of report to monitor AIDS trends. Meaningful analysis of temporal trends is based on dates of diagnosis and statistical adjustments for delays in reporting. For analysis based on diagnosis dates, an additional step is needed to estimate the date of the development of AIDS-OIs for cases reported based only on the $CD4^+$ reporting criteria. This additional step is necessary so that temporal trends can be compared using a definition based on the diagnosis of AIDS-OIs as was done before the 1993 expansion of the definition.

AIDS case surveillance is conducted via a cooperative active system that provides complete and timely reporting. A national multicenter study of medical records found that 92% of persons with AIDS-defining conditions were reported to local health departments; 67% of these reports were received within 2 months of diagnosis. Another review based on death certificates found that 70–90% of HIV-related deaths among men and women 25 to 44 years of age occurred in cases previously included in the AIDS surveillance database. These rates of reporting for AIDS are as good as or better than surveillance for other reportable illnesses.

Concurrent with the expansion of the AIDS surveillance case definition, CDC revised the classification system for HIV disease in adults and adolescents (Table 1). The HIV classification system divides HIV-infected patients into three clinical categories and three ranges of $CD4^+$ lymphocyte cell counts or percentages to classify the symptomatology and degree of immunosuppression for HIV-infected adults. The HIV classification system should be particularly useful for the public health

TABLE 1. *1993 revised classification system for HIV infection and expanded AIDS surveillance case definition for adults and adolescents ≥ 13 years of age[a]*

	Clinical Categories		
CD4$^+$ T-cell categories	(A) Asymptomatic, acute (primary) HIV, or PGL	(B) Symptomatic, not (A) or (C) conditions	(C) AIDS-indicator conditions
≥ 500/μL	A1	B1	C1
200–499/μL	A2	B2	C2
< 200/μL	A3	B3	C3

[a]HIV-infected persons classified in A3, B3, or any C cell meet the 1993 AIDS surveillance case definition.

PGL, persistent generalized lymphadenopathy.

purposes of HIV infection reporting and AIDS surveillance as well as for research activities such as drug treatment trials where categorization of HIV-related illnesses may be necessary.

Trends in AIDS Case Surveillance

As of December 31, 1994, 441,528 cases of AIDS were reported to the CDC. Since 1981, the number of reported AIDS cases has increased rapidly. The first 100,000 cases were reported over an 8-year period, whereas the second 100,000 cases were reported in just over 2 years (1989–1991). Due in large part to the expansion of the AIDS surveillance case definition in 1993, 187,309 (42%) AIDS cases were reported in 1993 and 1994.

The rate of increase in the diagnosis of AIDS-defining conditions (slope of the epidemic curve) has varied over time. From January 1982 to December 1984, the number of cases increased by approximately 100–260% annually. The rate of growth in AIDS diagnoses slowed from the explosive rates of the early 1980s to annual increases of approximately 50–80% in 1985–1987, 15–25% in 1988–1989, and 10–15% in 1990–1992. In 1993, the incidence of AIDS-OIs was estimated to have been 62,000 cases, representing a 3% increase compared with the rate in 1992. A similar rate of increase was anticipated for 1994. Possible reasons for the decrease in the rate of growth of the AIDS epidemic include the decreased incidence of new HIV infections. Cohort studies of homosexual/bisexual men, the largest transmission category among persons with AIDS in the United States, have demonstrated this decreased incidence, and the rate of other sexually transmitted diseases has also fallen sharply among white homosexual/bisexual men. However, HIV infections continue to occur among some homosexual/bisexual men. A similar reduction in HIV seroprevalence has not been seen among injecting drug users or persons at risk for heterosexual transmission.

Since 1981, most persons with AIDS have had a history of homosexual male contact or injecting drug use. However, the distribution of these behaviors among persons reported with AIDS has changed over time (Fig. 1). About 43% of the AIDS cases reported in 1994 occurred in homosexual/bisexual men compared with 63% of cases reported in 1988. Over this same interval, the proportion of AIDS patients who reported a history of injecting drug use increased from 20% to 28%. The most rapidly growing population of AIDS patients in 1994 was heterosexually infected adults who represented more than 10% of persons reported with AIDS in 1994, compared with 5% of cases in 1988. From 1990 through 1993, diagnoses of AIDS-OIs increased 13% among homosexual/bisexual men, 46% among injecting drug users, and 114% among persons heterosexually infected with HIV.

The incidence of AIDS has begun to decrease in some HIV transmission categories. In 1994, there were 779 transfusion recipients reported with AIDS, down from the 935 reported in 1988 in this category; and transfusion recipients and persons with hemophilia represented 1.6% of cases in 1994 versus 3.9% of cases in 1988.

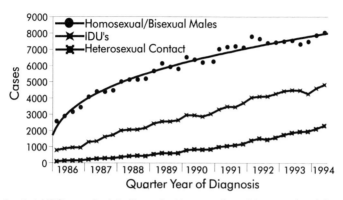

FIG. 1. Estimated AIDS-opportunistic illness incidence, adjusted for reporting delays, by transmission category, and quarter year of diagnosis, United States, 1986–1993.

Most persons with hemophilia and transfusion-associated AIDS were infected with HIV prior to 1985. In 1985, measures were adopted to protect the blood supply by instituting HIV antibody screening of blood and plasma donations and heat treatment to inactivate HIV in pooled plasma from which clotting factor concentrates are derived. Since the adoption of these measures, transmission of HIV through blood transfusion has become rare. As of the end of 1994, only 29 of the 6,866 cumulative transfusion-associated AIDS cases were ascribed to blood screened negative for HIV antibody.

Of the 441,528 AIDS cases reported through 1994, 26,370 (6%) were in persons who did not have a risk of HIV infection reported. When additional investigation is carried out, most of these persons will have risks for HIV infection identified and will be reclassified into the appropriate transmission category. Some persons with AIDS who do not have a risk identified on follow-up investigation represent unreported or unrecognized heterosexual transmission or other risk behavior for HIV. The small number of these cases suggests that HIV transmission is limited to the well-documented sexual, blood-contact, and perinatal routes that were identified in the 1980s. The often-repeated but unfounded fears of HIV transmission via air, food, water, and insects find no support in the pattern of AIDS case reporting. A very small number of cases reported without risks represent transmissions that occurred among workers or patients in health care settings, and laboratory employees. These generally are due to blood contacts traced to needle-stick or other injuries.

AIDS in Men

Nearly 87% (376,889) of the 435,319 adolescents and adults reported with AIDS through 1994 have been males and the rate of AIDS is high among men in many areas of the country (Fig. 2). The median age at diagnosis has been 36 years. Of the

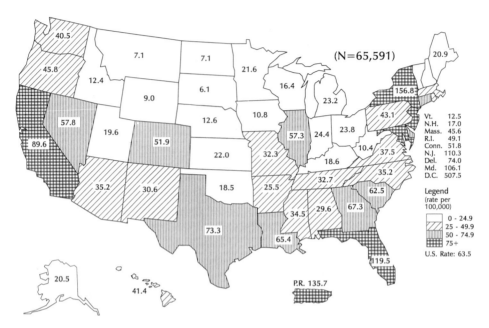

FIG. 2. Male AIDS annual rates per 100,000 population for cases reported in the United States, 1994.

65,591 men reported with AIDS in 1994, 34,974 (53%) reported homosexual/bisexual contact, 15,968 (24%) were injecting drug users, and 3,853 (6%) reported both of these activities. Another 483 (less than 1%) had hemophilia A or B or some other coagulation disorder, 432 (less than 1%) had only a history of a blood transfusion, and 2,946 (4%) had heterosexual contact with persons at risk for or known to have HIV infection.

AIDS in Women

As of December 31, 1994, 58,428 women were reported with AIDS, constituting more than 13% of the 435,319 adult and adolescent cases. States with the highest rate of AIDS among women tend to be in the eastern United States (Fig. 3). The proportion of persons with AIDS who are women has increased over time. Based on the year of diagnosis with adjustments for delays in reporting and for the inclusion of the CD4$^+$ criteria in the surveillance definition, from 1990 through 1993 the rate of AIDS-OIs increased by 72% among women compared with 27% among men. In 1994, 14,081 (18%) of persons reported with AIDS were women compared with 11% of persons reported with AIDS in 1988. Women with AIDS have a median age of about 35 and women aged 15 to 44 years account for 84% of cases. Of the

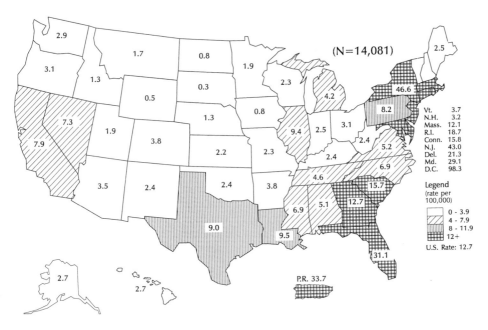

FIG. 3. Female AIDS annual rates per 100,000 population for cases reported in the United States, 1994.

women reported with AIDS in 1994, 5,749 (41%) reported injecting drug use, 5,353 (38%) reported heterosexual contact with persons with or at risk for HIV infection, and 337 (2%) have received blood transfusions or tissue transplants. Of women with AIDS whose HIV infections were ascribed to heterosexual contact, 2,032 (38%) were sex partners of injecting drug users, 363 (7%) were partners of bisexual men, and 2,839 (53%) were partners of HIV-infected men whose risk was not known or not reported. Women who have had sex with other women have been reported with AIDS, but most were injection drug users. Female-to-female sexual transmission can occur but is rare.

AIDS in Children

Through 1994, 6,209 children under 13 years of age have been reported with AIDS. In 1994, 1,017 children were reported with AIDS, an 80% increase from the 565 children reported with AIDS in 1988 (Fig. 4). Of the cases reported in 1994, 933 (92%) were infected perinatally, 506 (50%) were female, 631 (62%) were black, and 236 (23%) were Hispanic. In 1994, a regimen of zidovudine given to infected mothers before and at the time of birth and to infants following birth, was shown to reduce the risk of perinatal HIV transmission by approximately two-

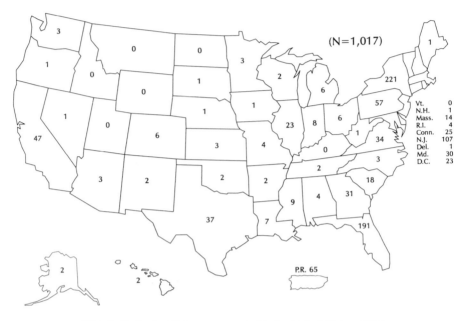

FIG. 4. Pediatric AIDS cases reported in the United States, 1994.

thirds. This finding represented one of the most significant advances in HIV prevention and recommendations have been published to guide the use of zidovudine by
pregnant women. If the use of zidovudine is widely adopted by pregnant women
and its effectiveness is generalizable outside the study population, the number of
children with AIDS should begin to decrease by the late 1990s.

AIDS Among Racial and Ethnic Minority Populations

Of the 80,691 persons reported with AIDS in 1994, 41% were white, 39% were
black, and 19% were Hispanic. In 1994, black and Hispanic men had the highest
annual rates per 100,000 population for AIDS, 208 and 110 cases, respectively,
followed by black women (63), white men (39), American Indian/Alaska Native
men (27), Hispanic women (26), and Asian/Pacific Island men (15). In 1994, the
rate of AIDS was 6.2 times higher among blacks and 3.3 times higher among Hispanics than among whites. Based on the year of diagnosis with adjustments for
delays in reporting and for the inclusion of the CD4$^+$ criteria in the surveillance
definition, the rate of AIDS-OIs increased from 1990 through 1993 by 58% for
blacks, 42% for Hispanics, 53% for Asian/Pacific Islanders, and 55% for American
Indian/Alaskan Natives, compared with only 14% for whites.

A much larger proportion of the 30,854 black (38%) and 14,830 Hispanic (37%)

persons reported with AIDS in 1994 had a history of injecting drug use than whites (14%) with AIDS, and 79% of the 21,717 heterosexual men and women with AIDS who reported injecting drug use were black or Hispanic. A history of heterosexual transmission is also more common for blacks (14%) and Hispanics (14%) compared with whites (5%). Of the 14,081 women reported with AIDS in 1994, 10,830 (77%) were black or Hispanic.

Different racial/ethnic minority communities have different rates of AIDS and different profiles of risks for HIV transmission. An analysis of AIDS trends in 1993 found that blacks and Hispanics in the Northeast and Florida had the highest rates of AIDS compared with other areas (49). Although injecting drug use was the most common mode of transmission among black men with AIDS nationally, male sexual contact was the most common mode of exposure for black men with AIDS in the District of Columbia and 32 (67%) of the 48 states that reported black men with AIDS.

The incidence of AIDS and the risks for HIV infection among Hispanics and Asian/Pacific Islanders varies by country of origin. For example, male homosexual contact was the risk for 60% of the 1,068 persons reported with AIDS in 1994 who were born in Mexico and for 58% of the 656 persons born in Cuba. In contrast, the most common transmission mode among the 3,921 persons with AIDS born in Puerto Rico was injection drug use (51%) and only 17% reported sexual contact with another man. These differences emphasize the need to consider differences in language, culture, and risk behavior when developing and implementing prevention programs and clinical services.

AIDS-Related Mortality

Of 435,319 adults and adolescents reported with AIDS through 1994, 267,479 (61%) were known to have died. The crude mortality rate among AIDS patients increases sharply over time following diagnosis, with 47% reported to have died within 2 years and 65% reported to have died within 3 years. A study of 1,622 HIV-infected persons who died in ten U.S. cities from January 1990 through August 1992 found that 1,578 (97%) were diagnosed with an AIDS-defining condition before death. Of persons diagnosed with AIDS in 1988 through 1990 in areas where AIDS surveillance records are cross-matched with the National Death Index, the median survival time for 34,425 homosexual/bisexual men was 19 months, which was longer than the median survival of 15 months for 16,913 injecting drug users and those infected heterosexually. Other studies have found that survival after AIDS diagnosis may also be influenced by older age at the time of diagnosis, the number and type of opportunistic illnesses, race/ethnicity, and the use of antiretroviral therapy and chemoprophylaxis against opportunistic illnesses.

Vital statistics provide an independent form of surveillance to track the course of the HIV epidemic in the United States. Provisional mortality data for 1993 showed that HIV was the eighth leading cause of death for persons of all ages. Because HIV infection and AIDS are most common among young adults, the increase in mortality has been most profound for this age group. For the first time, the 1993 data showed HIV to be the leading cause of death for Americans 25 to 44 years of age, accounting for 18% of deaths in this age group and a death rate of 34 per 100,000 population (Fig. 5). HIV was the leading cause of death for black men in this age group with a mortality rate of 157 per 100,000 population and triple that of white men (48 per 100,000).

HIV infection and AIDS has also emerged as an important cause of mortality in U.S. women aged 15 to 44 years. Deaths attributable to HIV infection and AIDS increased from 18 (0.03 per 100,000 women aged 25 to 44 years) in 1980 to 3,780 (9 per 100,000) in 1993. HIV infection was responsible for 8% of all deaths among women in this age group in 1993, but the HIV-related death rate among black women (40 per 100,000) was ten times greater than the rate among white women (4 per 100,000).

HIV mortality was a particular problem for certain metropolitan areas in the United States. An analysis of deaths in 1991 found that HIV was the leading cause of death for men 25 to 44 years of age in 79 U.S. cities and was responsible for 14% to 64% of deaths in these cities. For women of similar age, HIV was the leading cause of death in 15 cities and was responsible for 15% to 46% of deaths.

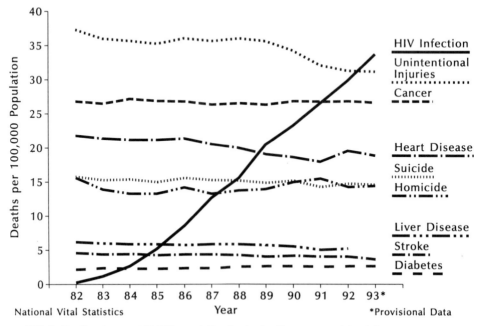

FIG. 5. Death rates per 100,000 population for the leading causes of death for persons 25–44 years of age, by year, United States, 1982–1993.

Geographic Distribution of AIDS Cases

The first cases of AIDS were reported from the largest cities on the east and west coasts of the United States. Since that time, AIDS cases have been reported from all 50 states, the District of Columbia, and all U.S. territories. However, the geographic distribution of these cases is uneven and changes over time. In 1994, the annual incidence rates by geographic areas varied from 2.6 cases per 100,000 persons in North Dakota to 245 in the District of Columbia.

The geographic distribution has changed gradually with time, but five states have consistently reported the largest numbers of cases. New York, New Jersey, and California have reported 42% (186,370 of 441,528) of all AIDS cases in the United States. However, this proportion has gradually decreased from 54% of the 50,316 cases reported before 1988 to 40% of the 80,691 cases reported in 1994. This decrease is due to the greater rate of increase of AIDS cases in Florida and Texas, which accounted for 14,496 (18%) of the AIDS cases reported in 1994 as well as other states, mainly in the south. From 1990 through 1993, the area of the country with the greatest rate of increase of AIDS-OI diagnosis was the South (41%) while the lowest was the West (18%).

AIDS has primarily been an urban disease, particularly clustered in inner-city communities. In 1994, 84% of the 80,691 cases were reported from metropolitan areas with more than 500,000 population. The AIDS rate in these metropolitan areas was 41 per 100,000 population but ranged from 44 in the central counties of the metropolitan areas to 9 in the outlying (suburban) counties. The per capita rate of AIDS found in these outlying counties is the same as the rate found in rural areas. The AIDS rate for metropolitan areas of 50,000 to 500,000 was 16 per 100,000. The AIDS epidemic has grown faster in medium-sized and smaller cities. In 1992, the number of reported cases increased by 32% for cities with populations of 500,000 or less compared with only a 5% increase for metropolitan areas of 1,000,000 population or more. Even so, most cases have occurred among residents of large cities.

SURVEILLANCE OF HIV INFECTION

Because of the long interval between infection with HIV and the development of AIDS, additional HIV serologic surveys are necessary to supplement the information obtained through AIDS surveillance. These serologic surveys are useful for ascertaining the rate of HIV infection in certain populations. Estimates of the prevalence and incidence of HIV infection have been made using various methods. In 1990, approximately 1 million persons were believed to be infected with HIV, with at least 40,000 new infections occurring annually. A study based on serologic surveys conducted from 1988 to 1991 in a random sample of U.S households found 29 HIV-infected persons and estimated that approximately 547,000 persons were infected with HIV in the United States. However, this study was limited in that it did not include populations such as homeless or incarcerated persons who are at higher risk for HIV infection.

HIV seroprevalence studies are useful to identify trends in HIV transmission, risk factors for infection, vulnerable populations, and communities in need of HIV-related prevention and health care services. Some HIV seroprevalence surveys have been performed on specimens not linked to the individual so as to reduce the likelihood of self-selection bias, which may result in an underestimate of the HIV seroprevalence rate. Other surveys collect only specimens linked to specific patients so that information on HIV-associated risk factors can be correlated with HIV seroprevalence. The CDC has conducted national HIV seroprevalence studies in populations at risk for HIV infection, women of reproductive age, persons in various clinical settings, and certain large groups that are subject to mandatory or routine testing such as blood donors or military recruits.

Homosexual/Bisexual Men

HIV-seroprevalence studies from 1984, when HIV antibody was first detected, to 1987 demonstrated that a large proportion of homosexual and bisexual men had already been infected with HIV. In the mid-1980s, the HIV seroprevalence among these men ranged from 36% (24/74) in New York City and 42% (38/90) in Los Angeles to 70% in San Francisco. In other cities, where studies were primarily conducted in sexually transmitted disease (STD) clinics, HIV seroprevalence ranged from 12% in Arizona to 58% in Seattle. In 1991–1992, the CDC conducted HIV seroprevalence surveys of anonymously obtained specimens from men who reported sex with men in 42 STD clinics in 29 metropolitan areas. Of the homosexual/bisexual men with a newly diagnosed STD in these clinics, 27% were HIV antibody positive. The median HIV seroprevalence rate decreased by almost 6% from surveys conducted in the same clinics in 1989–1990. This suggested a decrease in incidence of HIV infection. White homosexual/bisexual men had a lower HIV seroprevalence rate (20%) than black (43%) or Hispanic (31%) men with this sexual history, and the decrease in HIV seroprevalence from 1989–1990 to 1991–1992 was greater for whites compared with blacks and Hispanics, 6% vs. 2% and 3%, respectively.

The incidence of HIV infection among homosexual/bisexual men in some cohort studies dropped during the late 1980s. However, the prevalence of HIV infections among homosexual/bisexual men remained high and new HIV infections continued to occur. In San Francisco, the HIV seroprevalence was 12% among men 17 to 22 years of age recruited from public parks and bars and other congregating areas. In 1992–1993, a household survey of unmarried men 18 to 29 years of age in San Francisco found an HIV seroprevalence of 18% among the 380 men who reported sex with other men and an annual HIV seroincidence of 2.7% on repeat testing of those men who were initially seronegative. At this rate of new HIV infections the HIV seroprevalence will be 35% when this cohort of men reaches a median age of 34 years. This is lower than the 49% seroprevalence among a cohort with this median age recruited in a similar fashion in San Francisco in 1984. Thus, the rate of HIV transmission has slowed but a high proportion of homosexual/bisexual men continue to be infected with HIV.

Injecting Drug Users

In contrast to the epidemic among homosexual/bisexual men, HIV-infected injecting drug users are more tightly clustered geographically. The initial HIV seroprevalence studies demonstrated very high rates of HIV infection among injecting drug users in the northeastern U.S and the highest rates of HIV infection have continued to be observed among injecting drug users along the Atlantic coast. During 1991–1992, serologic surveys of persons entering drug treatment clinics in 35 cities had a HIV median seroprevalence of 7% with a range of 0.6% to 53%. In New York City and New Jersey, the median seroprevalence was 40% and 33%, respectively. In contrast, only 2% of injecting drug users tested entering drug treatment centers in Los Angeles, 7% in San Francisco, and 3% in Denver were HIV-seropositive. Although the highest rates of HIV infection were seen in the Northeast, other areas of the country have had appreciable rates of HIV infection among drug users. Studies in Baltimore and Atlanta drug treatment centers conducted in 1991–1992 revealed seroprevalence rates of 18% and 14%, respectively, and a study in Chicago during the same years found a HIV seroprevalence of 17%. Studies in sexually transmitted disease clinics have also shown higher rates of HIV infection among drug users compared with other heterosexual men and women. High rates of sexually transmitted diseases among injecting drug users suggest that their risky behavior has not been limited to drug use practices.

The rate of HIV infection among injecting drug users has been related to the frequency of sharing injection equipment with other persons, the number of needle-sharing partners, the use of "shooting galleries" where the sharing of equipment is common, and other factors. Black and Hispanic injecting drug users have had higher seroprevalence rates than white users. Although HIV infection is typically associated with the injection of heroin, in some areas a high proportion of persons with HIV infection and AIDS have more commonly reported injecting cocaine or amphetamines than heroin. Some studies have found a higher rate of HIV infection among cocaine injectors than heroin injectors, perhaps related to the increased frequency of injection among cocaine users.

Public health prevention programs have encouraged injecting drug users to stop using drugs, to seek treatment, not to share injection equipment, and to exchange used needles and syringes for sterile equipment. These efforts have been shown to be effective at reducing the rate of HIV infection among drug users.

Persons with Hemophilia

Many persons with coagulation abnormalities, primarily hemophilia, require clotting factor replacement derived from plasma pools donated by hundreds or even thousands of different individuals. Because clotting factor concentrate users were exposed to plasma of so many donors, the chance of having one or more exposures to HIV was enormous until 1985, when HIV antibody screening of donors and heat treatment of the lyophilized factor concentrate began. As a result, many persons with hemophilia A or B were infected with HIV. A study conducted by the National Hemophilia Foundation tested 9,496 patients between 1987 and 1992; 4,366 (46%) were HIV seropositive. Persons with hemophilia A, which is far more common than hemophilia B (also called Christmas disease), tend to require more clotting factor therapy than do persons with hemophilia B, and thus have higher rates of HIV infection; in the National Hemophilia Foundation study, 53% of patients who received factor VIII concentrate (hemophilia A) and 30% of patients who received factor IX concentrate (hemophilia B) were HIV infected. Because clotting factor concentrates are manufactured by a small number of suppliers for use throughout the country and internationally, HIV-infected persons with hemophilia have been found in all geographic areas. The classic epidemiologic paradigm for this aspect of the HIV epidemic was that of a point-source contamination with widespread distribution of a tragically tainted product. Although the HIV epidemic in persons with hemophilia essentially ended with the eradication of the contamination at its source, the AIDS epidemic that followed will be with us for years, and sexual and perinatal transmission prevention have become important priorities for persons with hemophilia and their loved ones.

Heterosexual Transmission

Studies of heterosexual partners of HIV-infected persons have shown varied but appreciable rates of transmission. What may be surprising to some is that the observed risk is far below 100%. Studies of heterosexual partners of infected persons conducted in the 1980s found 0% to 58% infected with a median of 24%. The risk of male-to-female transmission appears to be greater than for female-to-male transmission. Although all HIV-infected persons probably can transmit HIV during sexual contact, certain factors facilitate transmission. The likelihood of transmission from the infected partner seems to be large during acute HIV infection but rapidly declines and remains low as the infected person enters the long asymptomatic stage; transmission risk rises again as the immunosuppression worsens. This relationship is probably due to increasing viral concentration in plasma, and in semen and cervicovaginal secretions, that is associated with immune cellular destruction. The presence of genital ulcer diseases and nonulcerative sexually transmitted diseases among infected persons and their partners may also facilitate HIV transmission. In addition to sexually transmitted diseases, other conditions or sexual practices that disrupt mucosal surfaces increase the risk of transmission to sexual partners of infected persons. As with homosexual men, receptive anal intercourse increases the risk of heterosexual HIV transmission. The higher rate of penile inflammatory conditions among uncircumcised men may explain their increased risk of infection compared with circumcised men. Other potential host, agent, and environmental factors may play roles in as-yet-undetermined ways to influence risk of sexual transmission of HIV.

HIV Infection in Women of Reproductive Age

The rate of HIV infection among young women vary among different geographic areas and populations. Surveys of women in clinical settings in the late 1980s revealed HIV seroprevalence rates ranging from less than 1% to slightly greater than 2%. Most of the rates above 1% were from inner-city hospitals in the Northeast and Puerto Rico, the regions that have the highest incidence of AIDS in women. In a CDC survey of 254,828 specimens collected from women attending reproductive health clinics during 1991–1992, 0.2% were HIV seropositive with a range of 0 to 1% across clinic sites; the median seroprevalence rate among black women (0.4%, range 0–8.2%) was greater than for white (0%, range 0–8.2%) and Hispanic women (0%, 0–1.5%).

Prevalence of HIV infection in childbearing women can be determined by testing blood samples that are routinely collected from all newborn infants for early diagnosis of hereditary metabolic disorders. These samples are suitable for detection of HIV antibody, which is passively transferred to all infants of seropositive mothers. Thus, newborn screening yields direct information about maternal infection but indirect information about the infants, because less than half of such children acquire HIV infection. This technique was applied anonymously and in an unlinked fashion in many states and cities across the country in 1989. The initial results proved compelling and very useful to public health practitioners.

In 1993, the HIV seroprevalence among childbearing women was 0.17% which is similar to the 0.16% rate in the specimens collected in 1989–1990. However, the prevalence of HIV among childbearing women has changed over this time in different areas. From 1989 through 1993, the annual prevalence of HIV infection in the Northeast decreased from 4.1 per 1,000 population to 3.4 per 1,000, while the seroprevalence in the South increased from 1.6 per 1,000 in 1989 to 2.0 per 1,000 in 1991 and has remained at this rate through 1993. Based on the national HIV seroprevalence rate for 1993, an estimated 6,300 HIV-infected women gave birth and 1,600 children were born with HIV infection (assuming a 25% rate of maternal-child transmission) in that year.

Surveys in Health Care Settings

HIV seroprevalence rates among persons admitted to hospitals varies greatly. In 1991–1992, an anonymous serologic survey of 266,689 specimens collected from patients entering 39 acute care facilities revealed a median seroprevalence of 1.0% with a range of 0.1–5.8%. Hospitals with high rates of HIV infection tended to be in areas of the country with high rates of HIV infection and AIDS, mainly urban centers in the Northeast and along the Atlantic coast. Higher rates were found in men compared with women, blacks compared with whites, and patients aged 25 to 44 years compared with persons of other ages. A study of the admitting diagnosis for infected patients found that more than 70% were admitted for conditions other than HIV or AIDS. Extrapolating from this study, an estimated 163,000 HIV-infected persons were admitted to hospitals in 1990 for non–HIV-related conditions. The CDC has published guidelines that encourage routine HIV counseling and testing services in hospitals with an HIV seroprevalence of 1% or greater. A recent cost analysis has supported this recommendation.

Mycobacterium tuberculosis infection is frequently found among HIV-infected persons, and all persons with tuberculous infection or active tuberculosis need to be assessed for HIV infection. In 1993, pulmonary tuberculosis was added to the AIDS surveillance definition (extrapulmonary disease was already included). Of 81,254 persons reported to the CDC from January 1993 through March 1994 with AIDS-related opportunistic illnesses, 8,938 (11%) had tuberculosis. Among 20 tuberculosis clinics in 14 metropolitan areas surveyed in 1988–1989, the HIV seroprevalence ranged from 0% to 46% with a median rate of 3%. HIV-infected persons with tuberculosis tend to be located in the northeastern United States and along the Atlantic coast where rates were extremely high, approaching 50% in some clinics.

Population-Based Surveys

Large groups of persons who are tested on a routine basis provide unique opportunities for researchers and public health scientists. These include blood donors, civilian applicants for military service, and applicants to the Job Corps Residential Training Program conducted by the U.S. Department of Labor. These sources are valuable, but they are biased to the degree to which persons at high risk for HIV infection are restricted from these populations. Homosexual and bisexual men or those who have used intravenous drugs are actively discouraged from applying for military service and from donating blood. The HIV seroprevalence rate among voluntary blood donors in the United States is low and has decreased from 0.022% of donations in 1985 to 0.0067% of donations collected in late 1992. This decrease was accomplished by permanently deferring previously identified HIV seropositive donors.

Among civilian applicants for military service, the crude prevalence of HIV infection was 0.11% of 3.7 million applicants screened from October 1985 through December 1992. However, the seroprevalence rate has decreased over time for all applicants. In 1992, the HIV seroprevalence rate was 0.06% for men compared with

0.5% for women, and 0.22% for blacks compared with 0.10% for Hispanics, and 0.02% for whites, 0.02% for American Indians/Alaskan Natives, and 0.01% for Asians/Pacific Islanders. This decrease in HIV seroprevalence has not been readily interpretable due to the active discouragement of at-risk applicants.

Students who enter Job Corps training programs tend to be economically disadvantaged racial and ethnic minority youths drawn from both urban and rural areas. For students 16 to 21 years of age who entered the program from October 1987 through 1992, 3 per 1000 were infected with HIV. This rate was almost ten times the rate seen among applicants for military service. The rate of HIV infection increased over time among female students and was highest for older students and students from large urban areas in the Northeast and rural areas and smaller cities in the South.

HIV-Related Illnesses and Natural History

Patients may develop clinical illnesses soon after infection with HIV. This acute retroviral syndrome typically occurs within 2 to 6 weeks after HIV infection and may include fever, myalgia, arthralgia, photophobia, sore throat, lymphadenopathy, and maculopapular rash. Evidence from several studies has suggested that between 37% and 53% of adults may develop these symptoms following HIV infection. Using various methods, the interval between HIV infection and the development of detectable HIV antibody has been estimated to be an average of 45 days and almost all persons have detectable antibody well before 6 months postinfection.

Prospectively followed cohorts of HIV-infected persons have shed considerable light on the risk of developing AIDS or other clinical conditions in HIV-infected persons. In general, these studies have shown that the risk of AIDS increases over time. It is unusual for HIV-related illness to develop in the first few years after HIV infection. Only 1–2% of HIV-infected adults developed AIDS within 2 years of infection. The proportion who will develop AIDS rises steadily over time to at least 33–49% of adults within 7 years of infection and 50% within 10 years. A small proportion of HIV-infected persons may survive for 15 years or longer without developing AIDS-related illnesses and have become the subject of intense research interest.

Differences in the rate of progression to AIDS may be due to differences in viral strains including virulence, the inoculum size, and the immune function status of the host. For example, recipients of blood from donors who develop AIDS soon after donation are themselves more likely to develop AIDS more quickly than recipients of contaminated blood from other infected donors. These recipients with shorter incubation periods presumably received a transfusion containing a more virulent strain of HIV or a larger inoculum. Several studies have found that older age is associated with faster progression to AIDS. For example, older adults with hemophilia have been shown to develop AIDS faster than younger HIV-infected persons with hemophilia. This association suggests that underlying clinical conditions and the integrity of the immune system, and possibly other host factors, influence the natural history of HIV disease.

FUTURE DIRECTIONS

Surveillance systems for HIV infection and AIDS must evolve in accordance with clinical and public health needs for information. The reporting of AIDS cases will continue to be the best indicator of severe HIV-related immunosuppression and morbidity. However, the scope of information collected about AIDS cases and HIV infections will need to be expanded beyond demographic and risk factor characteristics to include access to health care and family planning services, drug use rehabilitation, and HIV and other sexually transmitted disease prevention programs. These data will help to identify gaps in these services and help to evaluate community prevention efforts.

Surveillance data will provide a basis for research, development, and application of many potentially controversial issues in the coming years. These include targeting of prevention efforts to specific populations and subpopulations or to broader audiences without regard to quantifiable differences in risk for HIV infection; community planning for clinical, social, and public health services; and assessment of the effectiveness of innovative prevention programs (such as needle exchange and condom availability in schools). Progress in the clinical management of HIV disease will influence surveillance data collection. As better clinical and laboratory markers than CD4$^+$ cell enumeration and improved treatments are developed, how and what we count as AIDS will have to evolve.

The collaborative surveillance system supported by the CDC and operated by all state and local health departments is clearly dependent on the work of thousands of dedicated clinicians, infection control practitioners, public health workers, laboratorians, and others. Keeping all participants in this system trained, informed, and motivated will require continued commitment and will be well worth the effort.

SUGGESTED READING

Buchbinder SB, Katz MH, Hessol NA, O'Malley PM, Holmberg SD. Long-term HIV-I infection without immunologic progression. *AIDS* 1994;8:1123–1128.

CDC. *HIV/AIDS Surveillance Report* 1994;6(2):1–39.

CDC. AIDS among racial/ethnic minorities—United States, 1993. *MMWR* 1994;43:644–647, 653–655.

CDC. *National HIV serosurveillance summary: update—1993*, vol 3. Atlanta, GA: U.S. Department of Health and Human Services, 1995.

Chamberland ME, Ward JW, Curran JW. Epidemiology and prevention of AIDS and HIV infection. In: Mandell GL, Douglas RG, Bennett JE, eds. *Principles and practice of infectious diseases*. New York: Churchill and Livingstone, 1994; 1174–1203.

Connor EM, Sperling RS, Gelber R, et al. Reduction of maternal-infant transmission of human immunodeficiency virus type 1 with zidovudine treatment. *N Engl J Med* 1994;331:1173–1180.

Diaz T, Chu SY, Byers RH, et al. The types of drugs used by HIV-infected injection drug users in a multistate surveillance project: implications for intervention. *Am J Public Health* 1994;84:1971–1975.

European Study Group on Heterosexual Transmission of HIV. Comparison of female to male and male to female transmission of HIV in 563 stable couples. *Br Med J* 1992;304:809–813.

Laga M, Manoka A, Kivivi M, et al. Non-ulcerative sexually transmitted diseases as risk factors for HIV-1 transmission in women: results from a cohort study. *AIDS* 1993;7:95–102.

McQuillan GM, Khare M, Ezzati-Rice TM, Karon JM, Schable CA, Murphy RS. The seroepidemiology of human immunodeficiency virus in the United States household population: NHANES III, 1988–1991. *J AIDS* 1994;7:1195–1201.

Osmond DH, Page K, Wiley J, et al. HIV infection in homosexual and bisexual men 18 to 29 years of age: the San Francisco young men's health study. *Am J Public Health* 1994;84:1933–1937.

Selik RM, Chu SY. HIV infection as leading cause of death among young adults in US cities and states: 1991. *JAMA* 1994;271:903.

USPHS/IDSA Prevention of Opportunistic Infections Working Group. USPHS/IDSA guidelines for the prevention of opportunistic infections in persons infected with human immunodeficiency virus: disease specific recommendations. *Clin Infect Dis* 1995:21 (suppl 1):S32–43.

Ward JW. Testing for retroviral infections: medical indications and ethical considerations. In: Schochetman G, George JR, eds. *AIDS testing*. New York: Springer-Verlag, 1994; 1–14.

Wortley PM, Chu SY, Diaz T, et al. HIV testing patterns: where, why, and when were persons with AIDS tested for HIV? *AIDS* 1995;9:487–492.

A Clinical Guide to AIDS and HIV,
edited by Gary P. Wormser.
Lippincott-Raven Publishers, Philadelphia © 1996.

2

Care of the Adult Patient with HIV Infection

Gary P. Wormser and *Harold W. Horowitz

*Division of Infectious Diseases, *Department of Internal Medicine, New York Medical
College, Westchester County Medical Center, Valhalla, New York 10595*

Skillful management of the HIV-infected patient involves blending common sense and compassion with up-to-date knowledge of the latest pertinent scientific discoveries. Care of HIV-infected patients is constantly changing and improving, which is reflected by objective increases in patient survival. These rapid changes impose additional challenges on the clinician for whom "routine" management often requires the use of investigational as well as approved therapies. A partial list of drugs already widely used in the care of HIV-infected patients, but that were not Food and Drug Administration (FDA) approved until well after the epidemic began, are zidovudine (AZT), didanosine (ddI), zalcitabine (ddC), stavudine (d4T), aerosol and parenteral pentamidine preparations, oral and parenteral ganciclovir preparations, fluconazole, itraconazole, atovaquone, clofazimine, foscarnet sodium, and interferon-α_2. Diagnostic procedures and methods are also in flux, continually being tailored to the specific needs of this patient population.

Recently acquired information on the natural history of HIV infection has indicated the importance of, and proper timing for, beginning prophylaxis for prevention of *Pneumocystis carinii* pneumonia and disseminated *Mycobacterium avium* complex (MAC) infection. These interventions will in turn have far-reaching consequences on the natural history of HIV infection and on management approaches in the years to come.

INITIAL ASSESSMENT

Table 1 outlines the initial assessment procedures. Although the diagnostic term AIDS is rigorously defined (albeit with several revisions) and has been immensely helpful for surveillance in following the epidemic (especially prior to the discovery of HIV), it is of limited value to clinicians in the care of individual patients. It is preferable to think in terms of HIV infection per se, and the clinical and immunologic consequences thereof. The definition of AIDS had been principally based on events that occur secondary to a state of advanced immunodeficiency. For exam-

TABLE 1. *Initial assessment of HIV-infected patients*

Strongly recommended for all patients
  History and complete physical examination
  Complete blood count with differential and platelet count
  Chemistry profile, including LDH, CPK, liver function tests
  $CD4^+$ cell count and percentage
  Treponemal antibody test
  Hepatitis B surface antigen, surface antibody, and core antibody
  PPD with control skin tests
  Papanicolaou smear for female patients
  Chest roentgenogram
Tests to be considered
  Antibody titers for toxoplasma and hepatitis C virus
  Stool for ova and parasites (for homosexual men and for persons who have traveled to at-risk
    geographic areas)
  Serum amylase level
  Triglyceride level
  Vitamin B_{12} and folate levels
  Glucose-6-phosphate dehydrogenase enzyme level (if initiating dapsone or primaquine)

CPK, creatine phosphokinase; LDH, lactate dehydrogenase; PPD, purified protein derivative (of tuberculin).

ple, the day after the diagnosis of *Pneumocystis carinii* pneumonia was made, the patient had AIDS; the day before the patient did not, despite the same degree of immunodeficiency. The latest revision of the case definition was the first to define a case based solely on laboratory criteria, in the absence of an opportunistic infection or neoplasm. Since 1993 all HIV-infected patients with a helper T-cell ($CD4^+$) count of <200 cells/mm^3 or a CD4 percentage of <14% are considered to have AIDS. The impact of this change on the number and demographic characteristics of reported AIDS cases is discussed in detail in Chapter 1.

Other diagnostic entities, such as "AIDS-related complex" (ARC) or "persistent generalized lymphadenopathy" (PGL), previously used to characterize certain HIV-infected individuals, are no longer helpful in patient management.

$CD4^+$ CELL COUNT

The most straightforward management approach for the HIV-infected patient is to focus attention on and monitor the course of HIV-induced immune deficiency. The most helpful, readily available laboratory tool to do this for adult patients is the number of helper T-cells ($CD4^+$) in peripheral blood.

$CD4^+$ cells are expressed either as a percentage of the total lymphocyte count, or as an absolute number, which is a calculated value derived from the percentage of $CD4^+$ cells multiplied times the total lymphocyte count. For healthy non–HIV-infected adults, the average $CD4^+$ cell count is approximately 1,000 cells/mm^3, but the values may range widely, from as low as approximately 500 to as high as 1,500 cells/mm^3.

A CD4$^+$ cell count of 200/mm^3 marks an especially important point in the course of HIV-infected patients, since serious opportunistic infections infrequently occur before this level of immune deficiency is reached. A CD4$^+$ cell count of 500/mm^3 is also an important juncture, since it has become customary to offer antiretroviral therapy to patients with counts at or below this level (see below).

As vital as the CD4$^+$ count has become in the general management of the HIV-infected patient, there are several noteworthy limitations. First, any single determination may be aberrant (Table 2). The reasons why a particular count may be inconsistent from other values for a specific patient are not always apparent. Since the CD4$^+$ count is dependent on the total lymphocyte count, the fluctuations and variability in the total white blood cell or differential count determinations will greatly impact test results. Inappropriate storage conditions and delayed transportation of blood samples to the laboratory may adversely affect CD4$^+$ lymphocyte determinations. In addition, factors such as test methodology, quality control, and type of laboratory equipment employed may influence the accuracy of the test.

Stress, exercise, season, use of exogenous glucocorticoids, serum cortisol level, and the presence of acute or chronic illness, have all been reported to affect CD4$^+$ cell counts. In addition, there is a normal diurnal variation of CD4$^+$ cells/mm^3 in HIV-infected patients, with the highest values present in the evening, implying that specimen collection times should be standardized. The effect of diurnal variation is greatest for persons who have relatively high CD4 cell counts.

Splenectomy is associated with a large and prolonged increase in peripheral blood CD4$^+$ lymphocyte count, often several hundred cells/mm^3 in magnitude. In these patients, the CD4$^+$ lymphocyte percentage reflects the level of immunodeficiency more accurately. Falsely low CD4$^+$ cell counts have been observed in up to 11% of blacks (and in lesser numbers of Asians and Caucasians) who lack or have a partial

TABLE 2. *Serial CD4$^+$ lymphocyte counts on peripheral blood samples of two HIV-infected patients*

Patient A[a]			Patient B[b]		
Date	Count	Percentage	Date	Count	Percentage
3/88	591	30	11/88	500	24
10/88	277	15	4/89	406	23
12/88	724	35	8/89	301	21
4/89	445	24	11/89	604	24
7/89	554	31	4/90	332	28
12/89	402	26	8/90	237	22
4/90	426	22	10/90	342	19
8/90	166	22	2/91	244	19
9/90	349	27			
12/90	408	24			
3/91	297	28			
8/91	353	22			

[a]AZT begun 7/88.
[b]AZT begun 12/88.

deficiency of the OKT4 epitope. Since the OKT4 monoclonal antibodies are widely used to identify T-helper cells, these individuals may appear to have no CD4$^+$ cells when in fact they have normal numbers of T-helper cells if identified by other monoclonal antibody markers (e.g., Leu3a).

Thus, the initial CD4$^+$ lymphocyte count for a patient, or counts significantly out of line with prior determinations, should be confirmed by repeat testing. During the first year of HIV infection the CD4 count falls approximately 400 cells/mm^3. Thereafter the average decline in CD4$^+$ cells is approximately 60 to 100 cells/mm^3 per year, except for those patients who, for unclear reasons, have entered into an accelerated phase, in which a decline of approximately 160 CD4$^+$ cells/mm^3 per year may be anticipated. Such patients are more likely to have detectable p24 antigen in serum and develop a serious opportunistic infection. In view of the usually observed rate of decline of the CD4$^+$ cell count, it is not surprising that the estimated mean duration of survival from time of onset of HIV infection to death in patients receiving standard preventive and therapeutic modalities (as described below), is more than 10 years (also see Chapter 1).

Caution should be exercised in overinterpreting small changes in CD4 test results. Patients often attach undue significance to minor rises or falls in these counts. They should be counseled that the overall trend of the CD4 count is more important than any single value (Fig. 1). In general, there is less test-to-test fluctuation in CD4 percentage compared with absolute number.

CD4 count enumerations are expensive tests ($100–200 per test in many commercial laboratories), and should not be done more frequently than is required for patient management. For patients with counts well above 600 cells/mm^3, once or at most twice yearly tests are sufficient. As counts approach 500 cells/mm^3, testing may be done every 3 to 4 months. When a level of 500 cells/mm^3 is reached, testing frequency should be reduced to once or twice annually until the counts fall to around 300 cells/mm^3, at which time they should be repeated every 3 to 4 months. At counts of 100 CD4$^+$ cells/mm^3 there is no need to do additional testing routinely, unless further management changes will depend on these values (see section on antiretroviral therapy below).

Since low CD4 cell counts are associated with the development of the most serious opportunistic infections, understanding why some patients have a more rapid reduction in count, or why a sudden acceleration in the rate of fall occurs in the course of some HIV-infected patients, is an extremely important concern.

OTHER LABORATORY MARKERS

Because of the variability (Table 2) and high cost of CD4 cell count determinations, other laboratory markers have been sought to assess prognosis and monitor the course of HIV-induced immunodeficiency. Two products of immune stimulation, neopterin and β_2-microglobulin, appear to be promising candidates. Neopterin is a metabolite of guanosine triphosphate produced by appropriately stimulated

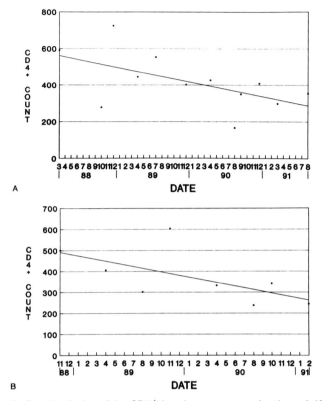

FIG. 1. A and **B**: Graphic display of the CD4$^+$ lymphocyte counts of patients A (**A**) and B (**B**) shown in Table 2. A downward trend over time can be seen.

macrophages. β_2-Microglobulin is a subunit protein of the class I histocompatibility antigens, present on the surface of all nucleated cells. High baseline serum levels of either molecule are associated with an increased risk of progression to AIDS. The mechanisms for the increased levels of these cellular products are not fully understood. Furthermore, the proper timing of standard therapeutic interventions (e.g., AZT and *Pneumocystis carinii* pneumonia prophylaxis) based on either an absolute level or a change in level of these substances is unclear. Therefore, the role of these tests in the care of an individual HIV-infected patient remains experimental.

History and Physical Examination

A thorough history and physical examination is necessary to uncover symptoms and physical findings that may at the outset require further evaluation. Particular attention should be given to systemic complaints, visual disturbances, neurologic abnormalities, and gastroenterologic or respiratory problems. Physical examination should carefully document the patient's weight, cutaneous or oral mucosal abnormalities, and presence of enlarged lymph nodes.

LABORATORY TESTING

A complete blood count with a platelet count is essential (Table 3). Mild leukopenia and anemia may be seen and are especially common in the setting of advanced immunodeficiency (CD4$^+$ cell count $<200/mm^3$). These hematologic abnormalities complicate the use of drugs that may further suppress the bone marrow, such as AZT or ganciclovir.

Depressed platelet counts may occur secondary to a variety of opportunistic processes including infections and lymphoma, or as an adverse effect of many of the drugs used to manage the HIV-infected patient. Equally or more common as a cause of thrombocytopenia, however, is the entity termed HIV-associated idiopathic thrombocytopenia purpura (ITP), which arises as a result of immune destruction of platelets that are coated with either immune complexes or antiplatelet antibody. Impaired marrow production of platelets may also be a contributing factor. Thrombocytopenia may occur at any level of CD4$^+$ cell count but is more common in advanced disease. In the absence of bleeding, no treatment is needed for patients with platelet counts above $20,000/mm^3$. At levels below this, AZT is probably the treatment of choice in the nonbleeding patient, with significant improvements in the platelet count occurring within 3 to 4 weeks of initiating therapy in at least 50% of patients (Table 4). (Paradoxically, although AZT regularly causes anemia and leukopenia, it does not typically cause thrombocytopenia and indeed can reverse it.) Intravenous gamma globulin, and possibly prednisone, may improve the count more quickly. Refractory cases usually respond to splenectomy, although irradiation of the spleen may also be effective.

Thrombotic thrombocytopenia purpura has also been reported in HIV infection. Although experience is much less than with HIV-associated ITP, therapy for this condition utilizing combinations of steroids, plasmapheresis, and antiplatelet agents has been successful.

Blood chemistry testing is useful to pinpoint abnormalities of liver function, which may be due to a variety of causes including chronic viral hepatitis. Interferon-α_2 may be considered for therapy of selected patients with hepatitis B or hepatitis C, although this usage should be regarded as investigational in the setting of HIV infection. Liver dysfunction may affect the pharmacokinetics of medications, which should be taken into account when any drug is prescribed. A baseline lactate dehydrogenase (LDH) is useful to serve as a basis for comparison during suspected bouts of *Pneumocystis carinii* pneumonia, since the LDH level is characteristically elevated in this form of pneumonia. A baseline creatine phosphokinase (CPK) may be helpful in detecting HIV-related myopathy or to serve as a basis for comparison should muscle pain or weakness develop during AZT therapy (AZT-induced myopathy).

TABLE 3. *Selected test results in HIV-infected patients*

Test	Expected result
Hemoglobin	Progressive reduction over time; 10–20% of asymptomatic HIV + persons are anemic vs. 70% of AIDS patients
Leukocyte count	Progressive reduction over time from 10% of asymptomatic HIV + persons to 65% of AIDS patients
Platelet count	Reduced in approximately 10% of asymptomatic HIV + persons and in up to 45% of AIDS patients
Neutrophil count	Reduced in 20–50% of AIDS patients
Lymphocyte count	Reduced in 70% of AIDS patients with opportunistic infections
CD4$^+$ lymphocyte count	Progressive reduction over time
CD8$^+$ lymphocyte count	Initially increased, falls later
CD4/CD8 ratio	Progressive reduction over time
Serum sodium	Hyponatremia present in ≥30% of AIDS patients, often attributed to renal salt wasting and (rarely) to hypoadrenalism
Serum potassium	Hyperkalemia may complicate therapy with trimethoprim-containing regimens or pentamidine because these drugs are sodium channel inhibitors and therefore function as potassium-sparing diuretics
Serum glucose	Pentamidine (especially by the IV/IM route) may cause hyper- or hypoglycemia and diabetes
Creatinine	Increased in a small proportion of cases, especially among black men who are intravenous drug users
Liver function tests	Abnormal in 90% but usually mildly, i.e., ≤twofold above upper limits of normal
Creatine phosphokinase	Usually normal; when elevated may indicate the presence of myopathy due to either HIV or AZT
Lactate dehydrogenase	Frequently mildly elevated; elevated in 90% of patients with *Pneumocystis carinii* pneumonia
Serum globulins	Hypergammaglobulinemia is usual
Amylase	Increased in 8%
Triglycerides	Elevated in 50% of HIV-infected patients
HBsAg	Present in approximately 10%
HBcAb	Present in 90%
Hepatitis C antibody	Positivity rates >50% among intravenous drug users and hemophiliacs
PPD	Positivity rates highest in Haitians, intravenous drug users, prisoners, and the homeless
Papanicolaou smear	Cervical dysplasia in one-third
Treponemal antibody test (e.g., MHA-TP)	Positive in 45% of HIV-infected homosexual men
Toxoplasma antibody	Present in 15–80%
Cytomegalovirus antibody	Present in 70–100%
Herpes simplex antibody	Present in 30–100%
Vitamin B$_{12}$ level	Abnormally low levels in 7–15% of HIV-infected patients
p24 antigen	Variably present; detectable immediately after HIV acquisition prior to seroconversion, and again in the later stages of immunodeficiency

PPD, purified protein derivative (of tuberculin).

Syphilis Serology

It has been observed that the prevalence of a positive serologic test for syphilis is five times higher among HIV-infected homosexual men compared with those without HIV infection. HIV-infected individuals with latent syphilis, based on the isolated finding of a positive serology, who have never been adequately treated or

TABLE 4. *HIV-associated thrombocytopenia—
treatment approaches*

With active bleeding
  Platelet transfusion
  Intravenous gamma globulin—1 g/kg/day × 2 days
Without active bleeding (platelet count <20,000/mm^3)
  First-line therapy
    Zidovudine (AZT)—500–1000 mg daily[a]
  Alternatives
    Prednisone—20–60 mg daily
    Intravenous gamma globulin[b]
    Splenectomy
    Irradiation of spleen

[a]Response is directly dependent on dosage.
[b]400mg/kg/day for up to 5 days as needed, with
maintenance doses of 400 mg/kg Q 3 weeks, depending on the response.

evaluated should undergo a lumbar puncture. Cerebrospinal fluid abnormalities, even if nonspecific, warrant strong consideration for the parenteral administration of penicillin in doses adequate for the treatment of neurosyphilis. In the absence of cerebrospinal fluid abnormalities, benzathine penicillin G at a dose of 2.4 million units should be given intramuscularly weekly for 3 consecutive weeks to those patients judged to have late latent syphilis. However, benzathine penicillin cannot be relied on in patients with neurosyphilis due to very low cerebrospinal fluid drug levels. HIV-infected patients with neurosyphilis should be treated with aqueous crystalline penicillin G at a dose of approximately 3 million units IV every 4 hours for 10 to 14 days. The serum Venereal Disease Research Laboratory (VDRL) or rapid plasma reagin (RPR) values should be closely followed after treatment in all patients, with particularly frequent testing done for patients with early syphilis (primary, secondary, or early latent, i.e., a year's duration or less).

Tests for Hepatitis B

Hepatitis B (HB) surface antigen is present in approximately 10% of HIV-infected patients. This infection may be associated with chronic liver disease and may pose an additional occupational hazard for health care workers with parenteral blood exposures to these patients. Patients without prior hepatitis B infection (i.e., with a negative test for HBcAb) should be considered for hepatitis B vaccination (see below).

PPD with an Anergy Panel

The purified protein derivative (PPD) skin test–positive HIV-infected patient has a 5–10% risk per year of developing active tuberculosis and consequently should receive chemoprophylaxis with isoniazid for 1 year (after active disease has been excluded). Induration at the PPD skin test site of 5 mm (versus the usual 10 mm) is regarded as indicative of tuberculous infection for HIV-infected patients. Patients who are anergic but who have had a positive tuberculin skin test in the past and did not receive prior antituberculous treatment should also be given chemoprophylaxis. Presently, it is impossible to judge the need for prophylactic therapy in an anergic person whose skin test history is unknown. Some authorities would give isoniazid prophylaxis to such individuals if they are deemed to be at high risk for past exposure to tuberculosis (i.e., members of a group in which the prevalence of tuberculous infection is $\geq 10\%$).

Papanicolaou Smear

Because of the high incidence of papillomavirus infection (31–67%) and cervical dysplasia (32%) among women with HIV infection, Papanicolaou smears should be performed at least annually. See Chapter 3 for a discussion of the management of HIV-infected women.

Chest Roentgenogram

In asymptomatic HIV-infected patients the chest roentgenogram is typically normal. A baseline film is very useful for comparison with later studies done for the evaluation of respiratory tract symptoms.

Toxoplasma Antibody

The seroprevalence of toxoplasma antibody in adults varies widely according to geographic location (from 15% to 80%). Since most cases of active toxoplasmosis among HIV-infected patients represent reactivation of latent infection, only those with a positive antibody test are, in general, at risk. This serologic result is helpful in the evaluation of neurologic abnormalities and may be a factor in guiding the choice of a chemoprophylactic regimen for prevention of *Pneumocystis carinii* pneumonia (see below). Seronegative persons should be counseled on how toxoplasmosis is acquired (i.e., through ingestion of undercooked meat containing tissue cysts of *Toxoplasma gondii* or any food contaminated with oocysts that originate in cat feces) and on ways to reduce this occurrence.

Hepatitis C Antibody

Coinfection with hepatitis C is very common among HIV-infected intravenous drug users and hemophiliacs (>50%). This form of hepatitis may explain abnormalities of liver function in these patients and, like hepatitis B, may pose an additional occuaptional risk for health care workers with needle-stick accidents. Commercially available α-interferon preparations will ameliorate chronic hepatitis C infection in approximately 50% of non–HIV-infected individuals. Comparable efficacy rates have been observed in a small group of HIV-infected patients without advanced immunodeficiency (see Chapter 7).

Stool Examination for Ova and Parasites

Homosexual men, or persons who have resided in areas endemic for *Strongyloides stercoralis* (most tropical and subtropical areas), should have stool examinations for ova and parasites. Patients who are infected with *Strongyloides* may be at risk for developing dissemination of this helminth as the immunodeficiency progresses. Consequently, all carriers should be treated, with thiabendazole being the treatment of choice. Homosexual men infected with *Giardia lamblia* or *Entamoeba histolytica* should also receive appropriate chemotherapy.

Serum Amylase

For unclear reasons, serum amylase levels are modestly elevated in approximately 8% of HIV-infected patients who have no clinical signs of pancreatic disease. In the few instances in which isoenzyme analysis has been done, approximately 75% of the serum amylase was of the salivary type, and in other cases the elevation was due to the presence of macroamylasemia. Results of a baseline amylase level may be helpful for use in comparison to subsequent testing in patients with abdominal pain, nausea, or vomiting, and in patients prior to treatment with ddI, which is associated with the development of pancreatitis in approximately 10% of patients receiving the drug.

Serum Triglyceride Level

The fasting serum triglyceride level is often elevated in HIV-infected patients and may be one factor contributing to the increased incidence of pancreatitis in this patient population. The elevated triglyceride level directly correlates with the serum α-interferon level, implying a possible etiologic role for the cytokine in the disordered lipid metabolism.

Vitamin B_{12} and Folate Levels

Vitamin B_{12} levels are modestly depressed in up to 15% of HIV-infected patients due to malabsorption, which may occur even in the absence of diarrhea or other clinical or laboratory abnormalities indicative of intestinal disease. Because low B_{12} or folate levels may be associated with increased hematologic toxicity from trimethoprim-sulfamethoxazole, pyrimethamine, trimetrexate, or AZT, replacement therapy should be given.

Glucose-6-Phosphate Dehydrogenase Levels

Regimens including the drugs dapsone or primaquine are being increasingly utilized in prevention and treatment of *Pneumocystis carinii* pneumonia for patients intolerant of trimethoprim-sulfamethoxazole (Chapter 5). Because of the risk of hemolysis in glucose-6-phosphate dehydrogenase (G-6-PD)–deficient patients, this enzyme should be assayed prior to administration of these agents (doses of dapsone of 50 mg or less per day, however, are not associated with G-6-PD–related hemolysis).

INTERVENTIONS FOR HIV-INFECTED ADULTS

The standard interventions are listed in Table 5.

Counseling

Various counseling activities are an integral part of the care of HIV-infected persons (Table 6). Counseling often first begins at the time that an individual requests or is advised to have HIV antibody testing. Because of the extraordinary psychosocial impact of a diagnosis of HIV infection, it is essential for the person being tested to have a clear understanding of the implications of the test results. The purpose and meaning of the test, the testing procedure itself, and the potential issues of discrimination should be explained to the patient. Informed consent is obtained prior to testing.

HIV test results should generally be communicated in person, at which time posttest counseling is done. This should include a discussion of coping strategies

TABLE 5. *Standard interventions for HIV-infected adults*

Counseling
Pneumococcal vaccine—once only
Influenza A and B vaccine yearly
Isoniazid for 1 year if PPD positive (now or in past)
Evaluation and treatment of syphilis (including asymptomatic seropositives)
Initiation of antiretroviral therapy: AZT for patients with CD4 counts $\leq$500 cells/mm^3
Initiation of *Pneumocystis carinii* pneumonia prophylaxis for patients with CD4 counts $\leq$200 cells/mm^3
Initiation of prophylaxis of *Mycobacterium avium* complex infections for patients with a CD4$^+$ count <100 cells/mm^3
Caloric dietary supplementation, as needed

PPD, purified protein derivative (of tuberculin).

TABLE 6. *Topics to be considered in counseling HIV-infected adults*

Methods of transmission of HIV
Partner notification (needle-sharing and/or sexual partners)
Food safety issues to prevent toxoplasmosis, cryptosporidiosis, and salmonellosis
Natural history of HIV infection, timing, nature and importance of interventions

---

after learning of a positive result, issues regarding potential discrimination, behavioral changes to reduce the risk of secondary transmission, available medical treatments, and the importance of notifying needle-sharing and/or sexual contacts. Food safety issues to reduce transmission of *Toxoplasma gondii* and enteric pathogens such as *Salmonella* sp. should also be discussed. These discussions should not be limited to the first or second patient visit but should continue throughout the long-term care of the individual.

Vaccinations

HIV-infected adults respond less well than their HIV-uninfected counterparts to many vaccines. Response to hepatitis B vaccine, influenza A and B vaccine, and pneumococcal vaccine depends upon the degree of immunodeficiency present at the time of vaccination. Asymptomatic HIV-infected patients with $CD4^+$ cell counts well in excess of $200/mm^3$ respond the best. The theoretical argument that antigenic stimulation of the immune system will lead to increased HIV replication and progression of disease has not been substantiated in vaccine trials to date.

Since the inactivated preparations appear safe and potentially beneficial, they should be routinely administered to HIV-infected individuals. The pneumococcal vaccine is given once, while the latest preparation of the influenza A and B vaccine is given annually during the fall. Patients who are susceptible to hepatitis B (HBcAb-negative) who remain at risk of exposure to this virus should be vaccinated. An exception would be the patient with a recent exposure to hepatitis B who may be incubating the virus. For unclear reasons, hepatitis B vaccination of such individuals has been associated with an increased rate of chronic HBsAg carriage.

Patients should be informed that the extent and duration of protective efficacy of these vaccines are still uncertain. Whether there may be a role for booster doses of the pneumococcal or hepatitis B vaccines in this patient population is unknown.

Haemophilus influenzae is also a potential cause of infection in HIV-infected adults, although the serotypes most frequently causing disease have only been elucidated in a few instances. If *H. influenzae* type b is confirmed as the cause of one-third of invasive infections, then use of the conjugate Hib vaccine may be considered. Data are limited, however, regarding the efficacy of this vaccine in HIV-infected adults.

Initiation of Antiretroviral Therapy

Antiretroviral therapy began in earnest in March 1987 when the FDA gave approval for the reverse transcriptase inhibitor, AZT. Since then additional antiretroviral drugs have been approved. Some, like didanosine (ddI), zalcitabine (ddC), stavudine (d4T) and lamivudine (3TC) are also nucleoside analogues and reverse transcriptase inhibitors, while others, such as saquinavir, ritonavir and indinavir are of entirely different chemical structure and target the viral protease enzyme (see Chapter 10). For several reasons clinicians newly involved in the care for HIV-infected patients may find the use of antiretroviral drugs especially challenging. First is an unfamiliarity with these recently and rapidly approved drugs; second is the tendency for clinical management of patients to be based in part on what seems biologically plausible, rather than on the results of rigorous scientific studies; and third, a sizable number of patients will request to be placed on a specific investigational therapy, usually based on very optimistic but typically highly preliminary observations that find their way into lay publications.

To summarize the status of antiretroviral therapy, it can be simply stated that while all of the approved drugs have biologic activity, this activity is suboptimal (Table 7). None of the drugs will eradicate HIV and none of the therapies is able to suppress the virus to a level where it can consistently no longer be cultured from plasma. Resistance has emerged during therapy, a factor that has contributed to the increasing use of combination therapies, with the expectation that this approach will follow the paradigm of antituberculosis treatment. However, there is as yet only limited evidence that combination antiretroviral therapy either substantively enhances efficacy or retards the emergence of drug resistance. Furthermore, all of the available drugs are associated with significant adverse effects, making even single agent therapy difficult for many patients to tolerate. Selected features of the first four antiretroviral drugs given FDA approval for use in adult HIV-infected patients are found in Table 8 (see Chapters 10 and 11).

TABLE 7. *Status of antiretroviral drug therapy*

Zidovudine (AZT) is the mainstay of therapy, used increasingly in combination with other drugs
No available agent yet able to eliminate HIV or to suppress HIV for prolonged periods; effect on duration of patient survival is modest
Emergence of resistance is common
When in the course of HIV infection to initiate antiretroviral therapy has not been established
Whether combination therapy will have greater efficacy or retard the emergence of resistance has not been established
All antiretroviral therapies carry risk for adverse effects; the impact of these agents on quality of life needs to be considered when recommending their use
The risks of antiretroviral treatment may outweigh the benefits for some HIV-infected patients
Knowledge of the use of antiretroviral therapy is rapidly expanding, making it likely that management approaches will continually change and improve

An approach to the use of antiretroviral drugs that we have found to be straight-forward and consistent with the available data is to offer AZT to patients who have a $CD4^+$ count of ≤ 500 cells/mm^3. We usually begin AZT at a dose of 500 to 600 mg/day (100 mg orally every 4 hours while awake or 200 mg three times per day). Starting AZT at this $CD4^+$ count has been associated with a delay in immunologic and clinical progression. Although the data are more limited, similar results have been observed for patients with $CD4^+$ counts above 500 cells/mm^3. The benefits of early AZT therapy, however, appear to be self-limited and apparently do not influence life expectancy. Consequently, particular attention should be paid to the tolerability of AZT therapy in these patients. If quality of life is appreciably reduced because of the drug's side effects, a better plan may be to defer AZT use until the $CD4^+$ count drops to 200 to 300 cells/mm^3. Conversely, if AZT is well tolerated, it is continued as monotherapy until a $CD4^+$ count of 200 to 300 cells/mm^3 is reached, at which point a second antiretroviral agent is added to, or substituted for, AZT. Alternative agents that may serve as monotherapy, or which may be combined with AZT, are listed in Table 9 (also, see Chapter 10).

The decision to alter therapy after this point is based on either drug intolerance or "deterioration." Deterioration is loosely defined and may be based on clinical parameters, such as the development of a new opportunistic infection or progressive weight loss, a fall in $CD4^+$ cell count, or an increase in "viral burden" (as measured by p24 antigen levels, viral culture, or quantitative polymerase chain reaction techniques, all of which are investigational).

Typically, patients with $CD4^+$ lymphocyte counts of 200 to 500/mm^3 are able to tolerate the 500 to 600 mg daily dose of AZT extremely well, although dose-limiting anemia and leukopenia may occur. Hematologic parameters should be carefully monitored in all AZT-treated patients. It is helpful to forewarn patients about headaches, insomnia, nausea, or vomiting that may complicate AZT usage during the first days of therapy, but that tend to abate spontaneously over time (Table 8). Long-term AZT administration may lead to darkening of the nails. We usually obtain a complete blood count and chemistry profile with CPK at 2-week intervals during the first 4 weeks of AZT treatment and then monthly or bimonthly thereafter, depending on individual tolerance.

Because AZT is generally less well tolerated in patients with lower $CD4^+$ cell counts, they should be especially closely monitored. AZT may be continued despite severe anemia if blood transfusion support is given. Alternatively, in an attempt to reduce the need for red blood cell transfusions, the dose of AZT can be lowered or another antiretroviral agent used (Table 9). Preliminary data from one study have suggested equivalent efficacy for a 300 mg daily dose of AZT. During AZT therapy the mean corpuscular volume of erythrocytes usually becomes elevated, and, curiously, when this does not occur, there is a much greater likelihood of developing severe anemia. Despite the macrocytosis, vitamin B_{12} or folate supplementation is not indicated, unless these vitamin levels are found to be deficient. Recombinant human erythropoietin at doses of 100 units/kg to 300 units/kg subcutaneously (or IV) three times per week has been shown to decrease erythrocyte transfusion re-

TABLE 8. Features of selected antiretroviral agents in HIV-infected adults

Generic name	Brand name	Common name	FDA-approved indications (1995)	Other uses	Recommended doses
Zidovudine	Retrovir	AZT	Monotherapy for persons with CD4+ ≤500 cells/mm³ Combination therapy with zalcitabine for persons with CD4+ ≤300 cells/mm³ (see ddC below) HIV-infected pregnant women	Idiopathic thrombocytopenia purpura (HIV associated) Combination therapy (See Table 9.) Health care workers with mucous membrane or percutaneous exposure to HIV-infected blood	100 mg po Q4H (600 mg/day)[a] for symptomatic patients 100 mg po 5x/day[a] for asymptomatic patients without AIDS
Didanosine	Videx	ddl	Monotherapy for persons with advanced HIV infection and prolonged prior AZT use, or intolerance to AZT, or clinical or immunologic deterioration during AZT therapy	In combination with AZT in patients with advanced immunodeficiency (i.e., CD4+ ≤200–300 cells/mm³)	≥60kg 200 mg BID of tablets 250 mg BID of powder <60 kg 125 mg BID of tablets 167 mg BID of powder Give on an empty stomach
Zalcitabine	Hivid	ddC	Monotherapy for persons with advanced HIV infection and intolerance to AZT or disease progression while on AZT Combination therapy with AZT for the following groups: 1) AZT naive and CD4 ≤300 cells/mm³ 2) Prior AZT and CD4 ≤300 cells/mm³ but ≥150 cells/mm³	See Table 9.	0.75mg TID
Stavudine	Zerit	d4T	Monotherapy for persons with advanced HIV infection who are intolerant of other approved therapies or who have had significant clinical or immunologic deterioration while receiving those therapies or for whom such therapies are contraindicated		≥60kg 40 mg BID <60 kg 30 mg BID

[a]Some authorities prefer a dosage of 200 mg TID based on the longer intracellular than serum $t^{1/2}$ and greater convenience for the patient. GFR, glomerular filtration rate.

TABLE 8 Continued. Additional features of antiretroviral agents

Drug	Selected adverse effects	Preparations	Dosage in renal insufficiency	Dosage in hepatic disease	Selected drug interactions
AZT	Anemia, granulocytopenia, myalgia and myopathy, cardiomyopathy, nausea, headache, insomnia, darkening of fingernails, lactic acidosis	Capsules: 100 mg Syrup: 50 mg/5 ml; IV formulation	For severe renal dysfunction: reduce dose to 300–400 mg/day; the drug is not cleared by hemo or peritoneal dialysis	Insufficient data but prudent to reduce dose or avoid drug	Avoid if possible drugs that also cause bone marrow depression (e.g., ganciclovir, interferon-α_2) Probenecid increases blood levels
ddI	Pancreatitis, peripheral neuropathy, liver dysfunction, hyperuricemia, diarrhea	Chewable tablets: 25 mg, 50 mg, 100 mg, 150 mg Powder: 100 mg, 167 mg, 250 mg, 375 mg	Limited information: GFR 10–50 ml/min; give dose Q24H GFR <10 ml/min; give dose Q48H Dose after hemo or peritoneal dialysis (GFR <10 ml/min) Note magnesium and aluminum content[a]	Reduce dose or avoid drug	Avoid drugs that cause peripheral neuropathy or pancreatitis; drugs whose absorption can be affected by reduced gastric acidity (e.g., ketoconazole) should be administered at least 2 hours prior to dosing with ddI; the magnesium and aluminum cations in ddI preparation may affect absorption of certain drugs (e.g., tetracyclines, quinolones)
ddC	Peripheral neuropathy, pancreatitis,	0.375 mg tables 0.75 mg tablets	GFR—10–50 ml/min, 0.75 mg Q12H GFR—<10 ml/min, 0.75 mg Q24H	No dosage reduction anticipated but use	Avoid drugs that cause peripheral

Drug	Adverse effects	Dosage form / Renal dosing	Hepatic	Drug interactions
ddC	liver dysfunction, hepatic failure, lactic acidosis, cardiomyopathy, oral ulcers	Insufficient data on clearance by hemo or peritoneal dialysis	cautiously due to potential hepatotoxicity	neuropathy; treatment with ddC should be interrupted when the use of a drug that has the potential to cause pancreatitis is needed (e.g., IV pentamidine); Probenecid and cimetidine reduce elimination of ddC; bioavailability reduced when coadministered with magnesium/aluminum containing antacid products (25% reduction)
d4T	Peripheral neuropathy, pancreatitis, hepatic dysfunction	15 mg, 20 mg, 30 mg, and 40 mg capsules. GFR dosage: (see below)	Insufficient data	Avoid drugs that cause peripheral neuropathy; do not give with AZT as there may be antagonism

GFR dosage:

GFR	≥60 kg	<60 kg
>50 ml/min	No change	No change
26–50 ml/min	20 mg Q12H	15 mg Q12H
10–25 ml/min	20 mg Q24H	15 mg Q24H
<10 ml/min	Insufficient data	
Hemo or peritoneal dialysis	Insufficient data	

[a] All oral formulations contain buffering agents because didanosine is rapidly degraded at acidic pH; to achieve adequate acid neutralizing for the tablet preparation, each dose must consist of 2 tablets; a 2-tablet dose of buffered didanosine contains 529 mg sodium; the magnesium and aluminum content should be considered when the drug is prescribed for long periods to patients with renal insufficiency

TABLE 9. *Antiretroviral drugs and drug combinations*

Monotherapy	Combination therapy[a]
Zidovudine is standard	Zidovudine plus Didanosine
Alternatives	Zidovudine plus Zalcitabine
Didanosine	Zidovudine plus Lamivudine[b]
Zalcitabine	Zidovudine plus Saquinavir
Stavudine	Zidovudine[b] plus Ritonavir
Ritonavir	Zidovudine[b] plus Indinavir
Indinavir	Zalcitabine plus Saquinavir

[a]Zidovudine plus stavudine is not recommended as combination therapy since these drugs appear to share the same phosphorylation pathway, and therefore combined therapy might decrease the intracellular concentrations of both agents. Combinations of any two of the agents didanosine, zalcitabine, and stavudine are not recommended until more information is available concerning the risk of peripheral neuropathy, since this is a well-recognized adverse effect of each of the drugs individually. Triple therapy with two nucleoside analogues plus a protease inhibitor may be the most potent antiretroviral combination therapy available, and is being increasingly used.
[b]Other nucleoside analogues besides Zidovudine may also be considered for combination therapy.

quirements significantly in anemic patients with endogenous erythropoietin levels of less than 500 mU/ml. Erythropoietin may be considered an alternative approach to blood transfusion support, AZT dosage reduction, or antiretroviral drug substitution, although the high cost and the inconvenience of chronic subcutaneous injections are drawbacks to this modality.

AZT dosage should be decreased to approximately half the full dose if the neutrophil count falls below 1,000 to 1,250 cells/mm^3 and should be stopped in patients who develop severe granulocytopenia (<500–750 cells/mm^3). This effect of AZT on the bone marrow may be offset by the use of granulocyte colony-stimulating factor (GCSF), but this is an expensive and impractical form of therapy for long-term use.

Other medications such as ganciclovir, cytotoxic chemotherapeutic agents, and high-dose trimethoprim-sulfamethoxazole, which are all myelosuppressive, are difficult to use in conjunction with AZT. As a general approach, we temporarily discontinue AZT (and other antiretroviral agents) during the acute therapy of intercurrent serious opportunistic infections. When discontinuing AZT, the physician must watch for the rapid progression of myelopathy or meningoencephalitis, but this appears to be extremely rare. Whenever possible, AZT is resumed following the completion of acute therapy of these infections.

Although there is a theoretical reason to believe that drugs such as acetaminophen or aspirin would increase AZT toxicity through competition for hepatic glucuronidization, when studied, enhanced rather than impaired clearance of AZT has actually been observed. Concomitant administration of probenecid, however, will increase AZT blood levels because of a reduction in AZT metabolism; probenecid also causes impaired renal excretion of the 5' glucuronide metabolite of AZT. Drug interactions should always be watched for in HIV-infected patients due to the large number and variety of simultaneously administered medications (Table 8). For example, ritonavir is a potent inhibitor of certain cytochrome P450 enzymes, and may cause large, undesired increases in the blood level of several highly metabolized drugs. This kind of drug interaction should be considered when prescribing the other available protease inhibitors.

The combination of AZT with acyclovir has been evaluated in several studies based on three considerations. First, although acyclovir has little or no antiretroviral activity as a single agent, potentiation of the anti-HIV activity of AZT has been observed *in vitro*, although not consistently. Second, if herpes viruses act as cofactors for disease progression, then an inhibitor might slow the course of HIV infection. Third, high-dose acyclovir might serve to reduce the frequency of cytomegalovirus infections, in a manner similar to what has been observed in renal transplant recipients.

AZT in combination with acyclovir does not alter the pharmacokinetics of either drug and is well tolerated even with daily doses of acyclovir of over 2,000 mg. Controlled studies, however, have failed to demonstrate a reduction in the frequency of cytomegalovirus infection in acyclovir recipients, possibly because acyclovir blood levels are not as high in these patients as in renal transplant recipients who may have impaired renal function. There is also no evidence that acyclovir enhances the antiretroviral activity of AZT *in vivo*. Notwithstanding these negative results, a survival advantage has been observed in several studies among acyclovir recipients. Doses of acyclovir as low as 600 mg per day appear to be associated with this effect. In two studies that provided information on the cause of death, it is of interest that Kaposi's sarcoma occurred less frequently in the acyclovir recipients (6 vs. 15 cases in the two studies combined), which might have a bearing on the recent discovery of a new herpes virus–like agent in Kaposi's sarcoma tissue. Unfortunately, none of the studies was done utilizing *Mycobacterium avium* complex prophylaxis, making it somewhat unclear if the results are still applicable. In our practice chronic acyclovir therapy is reserved for patients with recurrent herpes simplex virus infections. Further clarification of this issue is needed.

The role of antiretroviral therapy combined with one or more of a variety of drugs with immunomodulating activity is also under active investigation. These therapies, however, cannot be recommended at present (see Chapter 13). None of the antiretroviral agents is curative in HIV infection. Opportunistic infections and further reduction in CD4$^+$ lymphocyte counts still occur, even as early as within 6 months after drug initiation. Because of this it is likely that many changes in the approach to antiretroviral therapy will occur over the next few years, representing perhaps the most dynamic area in clinical management.

CHEMOPROPHYLAXIS OF OPPORTUNISTIC INFECTIONS

Pneumocystis carinii Pneumonia Prophylaxis

HIV-infected patients are at risk for such serious opportunistic infections as *Pneumocystis carinii* pneumonia (PCP), cytomegalovirus retinitis, cryptococcosis, toxoplasmosis, or disseminated *M. avium* complex infection, principally when the $CD4^+$ lymphocyte count falls below 200 cells/mm^3. Without specific chemoprophylaxis, it has been estimated that up to 75% of HIV-infected individuals with such low $CD4^+$ lymphocyte counts will develop PCP, an infection that has a mortality rate of up to 30% per episode.

The discovery that this form of pneumonia can be largely prevented by chemoprophylaxis was a major achievement in the care of HIV-infected patients. The preferred agent is trimethoprim-sulfamethoxazole (160 mg trimethoprim, 800 mg sulfamethoxazole) given orally once daily, on alternate days, or three times weekly (Table 10). Daily therapy is less well tolerated than the intermittent regimens. Advantages of trimethoprim-sulfamethoxazole over other prophylactic therapies in-

TABLE 10. *Primary chemoprophylaxis of selected opportunistic infections in adults with HIV infection*

Infection	Indication	Preferred regimen	Alternative regimen
Pneumocystis carinii pneumonia	$CD4^+$ <200/mm^3	Trimethoprim (160 mg)–sulfamethoxazole (800 mg); TIW[a]	Dapsone 100 mg daily;[a] aerosol pentamidine 300 mg monthly
Mycobacterium avium complex— disseminated	$CD4^+$ <100/mm^{3b}	Rifabutin 300 mg daily	Clarithromycin 500 mg BID
Tuberculosis	Positive tuberculin skin test	Isoniazid 300 mg daily plus pyridoxine 50 mg/d × 12 months[c]	Rifampin 600 mg daily × 12 months
Toxoplasmosis	Toxoplasma antibody positive and $CD4^+$ <100/mm^3	Trimethoprim-sulfamethoxazole (any regimen used for *Pneumocystis carinii* pneumonia prophylaxis)	Dapsone 50 mg daily plus pyrimethamine 50 mg Q week plus folinic acid 5 mg daily; or dapsone 200 mg Q week plus pyrimethamine 75 mg and folinic acid 25 mg Q week
Cytomegalovirus retinitis	$CD4^+$ <100/mm^3	None established[d]	None

[a]For other regimens see Chapter 5.
[b]Disseminated *Mycobacterium avium* complex infections usually occur at $CD4^+$ cell counts <60/mm^3; therefore, some authorities would begin prophylaxis at $CD4^+$ cell counts <75/mm^3.
[c]Rifabutin when used for prevention of disseminated *Mycobacterium avium* complex infection is believed to be adequate to provide prophylaxis for tuberculosis as well.
[d]Acyclovir is not effective; oral ganciclovir under investigation.

clude greater efficacy, low cost, convenience of oral administration, and potential effectiveness in preventing extrapulmonary pneumocystosis and in preventing infections other than pneumocystosis, such as salmonellosis, shigellosis, pneumococcal infection, *H. influenzae* infection, isospora infection, cyclospora infection, nocardiosis, and listeriosis. A particularly desirable feature of trimethoprim-sulfamethoxazole chemoprophylaxis is its effectiveness in preventing cerebral toxoplasmosis. The principal disadvantage of trimethoprim-sulfamethoxazole is that it is not well tolerated by approximately 50% of patients. The most frequent cause of intolerance is hypersensitivity reactions, particularly rashes and fever.

For patients with CD4$^+$ lymphocyte counts <200/mm^3 who are not already receiving AZT, we prefer to begin trimethoprim-sulfamethoxazole before AZT, and if the hematologic parameters, liver chemistries, and renal function are stable at 2 weeks, then introduce AZT in standard doses.

Alternative therapies for the trimethoprim-sulfamethoxazole–intolerant patient include dapsone (100 mg daily) and once monthly aerosol pentamidine, at a dose of 300 mg delivered by the Respirgard II jet nebulizer (Marquest, Englewood, CO) (Table 10) (see Chapter 5). The dose of pentamidine is diluted in 6 ml of sterile water and delivered at 6 L/min from a 50-pound/square inch (PSI) compressed air source until the reservoir is dry. Since dapsone provides systemic therapy, is relatively inexpensive, is at least as effective as aerosol pentamidine, and may provide protection from reactivation of toxoplasma infection (when combined with pyrimethamine, see below), it has become for many physicians the first alternative to trimethoprim-sulfamethoxazole. Although dapsone is a sulfone antibiotic with some structural similarity to sulfonamides, approximately 60% of patients who react to trimethoprim-sulfamethoxazole will tolerate dapsone.

Several caveats should be kept in mind when using dapsone. Any patient with a prior life-threatening reaction to a sulfonamide, such as anaphylaxis or Stevens-Johnson syndrome, should not be challenged with dapsone. In addition, before using dapsone, G-6-PD levels should be measured to avoid the problem of hemolytic anemia that can occur in G-6-PD–deficient patients. Dapsone should be used with caution in patients who are concomitantly receiving rifampin, since this drug causes a seven- to tenfold reduction in the serum level of dapsone due to hepatic microsomal enzyme induction. Although it had been conjectured that the bioavailability of dapsone would be impaired by reduced gastric acidity, a recent study found that raising the gastric pH does not affect the drug's absorption.

When combined with pyrimethamine (Table 10), dapsone is effective in preventing toxoplasmosis; there is insufficient information to recommend dapsone alone for this purpose. Consequently, a dapsone plus pyrimethamine regimen should be employed for toxoplasma seropositive patients with CD4$^+$ lymphocyte counts of <100 cells/mm^3.

Pentamidine should probably be reserved for patients who are intolerant of both trimethoprim-sulfamethoxazole and dapsone, due to its high cost, requirement for special equipment, relatively lower efficacy (especially at CD4 counts of <100 cells/mm^3), and ineffectiveness against extrapulmonary *P. carinii* infection. In addition, use of aerosol pentamidine requires cooperative patients, may be associated with aerosolization and transmission of respiratory tract pathogens such as *Mycobacterium tuberculosis* to health care workers and other patients, has an unknown effect on lung tissue from long-term exposure and unknown risks for health care personnel, and will not prevent toxoplasmosis. The most frequent toxicities of aerosolized pentamidine are bronchospasm and coughing, which occur in approximately one-third of patients during the inhalation period. These relatively minor problems can be largely prevented by pretreatment with an inhaled β-adrenergic agonist. Hypoglycemia and pancreatitis are much less common with aerosol pentamidine compared with intravenous administration, but may still rarely occur.

Some authorities prefer to desensitize the trimethoprim-sulfamethoxazole intolerant patient by using an escalating dosage regimen administered over a time period ranging from as long as several weeks to as short as 5 hours. Success rates of approximately 50% have been reported, but none of the studies evaluated a large enough number of patients to provide a definitive assessment of safety or efficacy. Patients who have previously experienced only cytopenias or liver function abnormalities during high-dose trimethoprim-sulfamethoxazole therapy of PCP, without other manifestations to suggest hypersensitivity, will usually tolerate the lower drug doses used for prophylaxis; desensitization is rarely necessary.

It should be noted that patients may need to have their PCP prophylaxis therapy changed several times before arriving at a regimen that is well tolerated. However, given the frequency and seriousness of PCP in the nonprophylaxed patient, devising an adequate regimen deserves the highest priority.

It is important to emphasize that when patients who are compliant with trimethoprim-sulfamethoxazole prophylaxis develop respiratory tract symptoms and an abnormal chest roentgenogram, PCP is unlikely to be the cause. In contrast, in our experience PCP remains the most common cause of this clinical picture in patients receiving aerosol pentamidine, although the roentgenographic findings may be atypical for this form of pneumonia (e.g., upper lobe infiltrates).

Although most HIV-infected patients with PCP have a CD4$^+$ lymphocyte count of 200 cells/mm^3, approximately 5% have higher counts. Identification of those HIV-infected patients with higher CD4$^+$ lymphocyte counts who are at risk for pneumocystosis may be problematic. Patients with thrush, or those who have had a prior bout of PCP, should receive pneumocystis prophylaxis regardless of the CD4$^+$ lymphocyte count. Some authorities begin prophylaxis for all HIV-infected patients with a CD4 lymphocyte percentage ≤20%, regardless of the absolute CD4 count.

Prevention of *Mycobacterium avium* Complex Infections

Disseminated *Mycobacterium avium* complex (MAC) infections are almost uniquely associated with AIDS patients compared with other immunocompromised populations. In the United States, MAC infections occur in up to 40% of HIV-infected patients with CD4$^+$ lymphocyte counts below 100 cells/mm^3. Since treatment of active infection requires a multidrug regimen that provides only modest success, prevention is greatly preferred.

In two randomized, placebo-controlled, multicenter studies, the drug rifabutin (a semisynthetic derivative of rifamycin S with structural similarities to rifampin), was successful in reducing the frequency of MAC bacteremia by approximately 50%. As a result the United States Public Health Service recommended that chemo-prophylaxis for MAC infections be initiated for all eligible HIV-infected patients who have CD4$^+$ cell counts of <100 cells/mm^3. Before prophylaxis is prescribed, patients should be evaluated to ensure that they do not have active mycobacterial disease, especially *M. tuberculosis* infection. This is to avoid giving rifabutin inadvertently as a single agent for active tuberculosis, which would pose a substantial risk for the emergence of drug resistance to both rifampin and rifabutin. In an asymptomatic patient, a normal chest radiograph and a nonreactive tuberculin skin test are usually sufficient to begin rifabutin therapy. The recommended dose of rifabutin is 300 mg orally per day. The drug is well tolerated but may cause rash, nausea, elevated liver function tests, neutropenia, and rarely uveitis.

Like rifampin, rifabutin may cause an orange-brown discoloration to the urine (which should be mentioned to the patient prior to starting the drug) and may induce hepatic microsomal enzymes and thereby affect the metabolism of a wide array of drugs. Vigilance is necessary for drug-drug interactions, although rifabutin appears to be a less potent enzyme inducer than rifampin. Clarithromycin and azithromycin are also being evaluated for their prophylactic potential against disseminated MAC infection. Preliminary analysis of a placebo-controlled multicenter study evaluating the prophylactic efficacy of clarithromycin at a dose of 500 mg twice daily demonstrated a 68% reduction in MAC bacteremia. A survival advantage was also shown in the clarithromycin-treated group.

In current practice either rifabutin or clarithromycin is acceptable to use for MAC prophylaxis. In a patient for whom there is the need to give both tuberculosis and MAC prophylaxis (for example, a patient at high epidemiologic risk for tuberculosis but who is anergic), rifabutin is a convenient choice since it should be effective for both infections, and would avoid having to add isoniazid.

MANAGEMENT OF SPECIFIC COMPLICATIONS

Fever

The majority of HIV-infected patients will develop fever at some point in the course of their illness. Aside from primary HIV infection, sustained fevers are rarely, if ever, attributable to HIV infection itself and are usually due to serious but treatable superimposed infections (Table 11). Management of the febrile HIV-infected patient is integrally related to establishing a specific etiology for the fever. Finding the source of fever, however, can at times be very challenging. Fever may be related to nonopportunistic infections presenting typically or atypically, oppor-

TABLE 11. *General principles in the approach to the HIV-infected patient with fever*

Except for primary HIV infection, sustained fevers are due to causes other than HIV infection itself
Serious opportunistic infections usually first occur in patients with CD4$^+$ lymphocyte counts of less than 200 cells/mm^3
Multiple opportunistic infections and/or neoplasia may occur simultaneously, even in the same organ or tissue
Serodiagnostic studies and tuberculin skin testing may be ambiguous
Growth of some opportunistic organisms, e.g., cytomegalovirus of *Mycobacterium avium* complex, from urine or sputum samples may not indicate active infection

tunistic infections (sometimes multiple), hypersensitivity reactions to medications, and malignancies, particularly lymphomas. Furthermore, nosocomial infections from intravascular catheters, decubiti, and urinary tract infections must not be overlooked in the hospitalized febrile HIV-infected patient.

It is important at the outset to know whether the patient is highly immuno-compromised (i.e., has a CD4$^+$ lymphocyte count <200 cells/mm^3) and is thus predisposed to serious opportunistic infections. If not, evaluation may be directed toward the discovery of less unusual microbial pathogens and conditions, for example sinusitis, herpes zoster infection, or tuberculosis.

It is also important to note epidemiologic clues that may help in identifying specific infectious risks. For example, Haitians, as well as intravenous drug users from major metropolitan areas, have an increased risk of tuberculosis. Patients from the southwestern United States (and occasionally those who have previously resided there) are at risk for disseminated *Coccidioides immitis* infection. Histoplasmosis may be a consideration in individuals who have resided in areas endemic for this fungus in the United States or elsewhere, including certain areas of the Caribbean such as Puerto Rico.

An approach to the evaluation of fever in the HIV-infected patient with advanced immunodeficiency is found in Table 12. If the source of fever has not been identified on routine diagnostic studies such as blood and urine cultures or chest roentgenogram, then further testing is necessary. Blood cultures for fungi and mycobacteria should be obtained (two are sufficient). Mycobacterial blood cultures should include lysis of the cellular fraction of the specimen, followed by plating on a standard solid mycobacterial culture medium or by liquid culture with radiometric detection. Multiple cultures of stool, urine, and sputum for mycobacteria should also be considered. Stool acid-fast smears and cultures are helpful in the diagnosis of disseminated *M. avium* complex infection, since the intestinal tract is often involved in the disease process. However, single positive cultures from stool and sputum for nontuberculous mycobacteria may represent contamination or colonization and not indicate true infection. Stool acid-fast cultures may also be useful in the diagnosis of *M. tuberculosis* infection, although usually the sputum is culture positive in these instances.

Although cytomegalovirus infection may be a cause of fever in these patients,

TABLE 12. *A diagnostic approach for evaluation of fever in HIV-infected patients*

Evaluate if patient falls into a group at high risk for serious opportunistic infections, i.e., CD4$^+$ cell count less than 200 cells/mm^3

Direct history to determine possible geographic, ethnic, or lifestyle risk factors for specific infections; pay particular attention to neurologic, respiratory, dermatologic, visual, and gastrointestinal complaints

Note medication list

Physical examination

Laboratory tests: CBC; chemistry profile, including liver function tests; urine analysis; cultures of blood, urine, and sputum for bacteria; chest roentgenogram; stool culture if diarrhea present

If initial cultures are negative, culture blood, urine, sputum, and stool for mycobacteria and blood, urine, and sputum for fungi; do serum cryptococcal antigen, toxoplasma titer, and VDRL; do PPD with controls unless known to be anergic; sputum for IFA test for *Pneumocystis carinii*

If no source yet identified, consider:
   Gallium scan of lung
   Computed tomography of abdomen
   Examination by ophthalmologist for CMV retinitis
   Lymph node biopsy if enlarged node is accessible
   Bone marrow biopsy and aspiration (especially if anemic)
   Skin lesion biopsy (if present)
   Lumbar puncture if clinical signs warrant
   Bronchoscopy with bronchial alveolar lavage and/or biopsy (if respiratory tract signs or abnormalities are present)
   Liver biopsy (if liver function studies are abnormal)

CMV, cytomegalovirus; IFA, immunofluorescent antibody; PPD, purified protein derivative (of tuberculin).

positive cultures for this virus from urine, pharynx, bronchial lavage fluid, or even blood are so frequent that they cannot be relied on to pinpoint the cause of fever. For the same reasons, serology for cytomegalovirus is also nondiagnostic. It is of utmost importance to attempt to establish the pathogenicity of an organism that has been cultured, since specific treatment for microorganisms such as cytomegalovirus or *M. avium* complex may be at best partially effective, potentially toxic, inconvenient (require multiple drugs or intravenous administration), or prolonged. Further, administration of ganciclovir for cytomegalovirus infection may preclude the use of AZT, due to potential additive bone marrow suppression.

Additional diagnostic studies should include a test for serum cryptococcal antigen, since it is positive in 75–95% of HIV-infected patients with cryptococcosis. Sputum should be obtained (induced if necessary) for detection of *P. carinii* using an immunofluorescent monoclonal antibody assay. This is especially important for patients with respiratory complaints, an abnormal chest roentgenogram, or gallium-67 uptake by the lung on scintigraphy. If an induced sputum sample is nondiagnostic or unavailable, bronchoscopy for bronchial alveolar lavage and/or biopsy should be considered for patients with objective pulmonary signs or test abnormalities.

Serodiagnosis of *Histoplasma capsulatum* and *Coccidioides immitis* is helpful for selected patients. Also, Giemsa-stained preparations of the buffy coat of peripheral blood may be useful in the diagnosis of disseminated histoplasmosis. An experimental test for a histoplasma polysaccharide antigen was positive on urine and/or serum samples in more than 95% of AIDS patients with histoplasmosis, according to the test's originator.

A careful funduscopic examination by an ophthalmologist may help establish the diagnosis of disseminated cytomegalovirus infection (Fig. 2). Although the patient with cytomegalovirus retinitis usually reports visual disturbances, this is not uniformly true, particularly in patients with an altered mental status.

Biopsies for culture, special stains, and histologic examination of sites such as bone marrow, lymph nodes, gastrointestinal tract, or skin lesions may be very helpful in the diagnosis of disseminated fungal, mycobacterial, or cytomegalovirus infection, bacillary epithelioid angiomatosis, lymphoma, and Kaposi's sarcoma, when other modalities of diagnosis are either nondiagnostic or negative. It is particularly helpful to perform a lymph node biopsy in patients who have a single group of lymph nodes that are disproportionately enlarged or that have rapidly increased in size.

Computed tomography may be used to locate intraabdominal masses or enlarged lymph nodes for biopsy. In patients with an elevated alkaline phosphatase level and

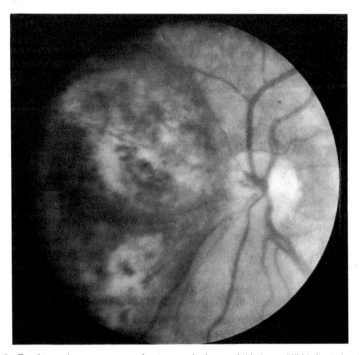

FIG. 2. Funduscopic appearance of cytomegalovirus retinitis in an HIV-infected patient.

fever, a liver biopsy for histologic examination and culture may be useful. This procedure is not often necessary, however, since other sources of culture material are usually diagnostic.

Before embarking on any biopsy procedure it is important to determine if the patient has a potential bleeding diathesis, such as thrombocytopenia. Platelet transfusions, intravenous infusions of immunoglobulin G preparations, or other measures to elevate the platelet count at least transiently may be required for patients with platelet counts below 50,000 to 100,000/mm^3, depending on the bleeding time and the type and urgency of the invasive procedure to be done (Table 4). Partial thromboplastin times and (less often) prothrombin times may be prolonged in HIV-infected patients. Usually this is due to the presence of a lupus-like anticoagulant, found in up to 70% of HIV-infected patients, particularly those with opportunistic infections. The "anticoagulants" are immunoglobulins that interfere with several *in vitro* coagulation assays. The presence of these anticoagulants can be confirmed by several diagnostic tests, such as the ½ + ½ correction or the Russell's viper venom time. The majority of patients who have these factors are not predisposed to bleeding unless the level of coagulation factors is abnormal, or qualitative/quantitative platelet abnormalities coexist.

Empiric Treatment for Infection in the HIV-Infected Patient

The empiric use of broad-spectrum antibiotics is not routinely indicated for the febrile HIV-infected patient, since these drugs may be toxic, lead to increasingly resistant organisms, or confound the diagnostic evaluation. However, if the patient is clinically unstable or profoundly neutropenic (fewer than 500 neutrophils/mm^3), broad-spectrum antibiotics should be administered promptly. Certain other indications for empiric therapy are found in Table 13.

When an opportunistic infection (or infections) is diagnosed, specific therapy should be initiated (Table 14). It is important to note that treatment of opportunistic infections in HIV-infected patients is rarely curative. More often, chronic maintenance therapy for an indefinite period is necessary after completion of the acute treatment.

Diarrhea

Diarrhea is a frequent complaint in HIV-infected patients, occurring in at least 20–30% of patients at some point during their course. There is a large differential diagnosis ranging from common bacterial pathogens, such as *Campylobacter jejuni* and *Salmonella* sp., to previously rare protozoans, such as cryptosporidia and microsporidia (see Table 15 for a partial listing). An infectious etiology has been found in up to 85% of cases. If diarrhea persists despite negative initial cultures and smears, colonoscopy and possibly gastroduodenoscopy are warranted for biopsy and cultures (Table 16).

TABLE 13. *Clinical situations in which empiric therapy may be useful in HIV-infected adults prior to confirmation of diagnosis*

Condition	Microorganism to which therapy is directed	Recommended therapy
Clinically unstable (septic appearing) or profoundly neutropenic (<500 PMNs/ mm³)	*Staphylococcus aureus* *Streptococcus pneumoniae* *Haemophilus influenzae* *Salmonella* sp. Aerobic gram-negative rods	Third-generation cephalosporin with or without an aminoglycoside
Lobar pneumonia	*Streptococcus pneumoniae* *Haemophilus influenzae* *Moraxella catarrhalis* *Staphylococcus aureus* *Legionella* sp. *Klebsiella* sp. *Escherichia coli*	Third-generation cephalosporin plus erythromycin
Ring-enchancing mass lesion(s) on cranial MRI or CT, especially if serum toxoplasma titer is positive	*Toxoplasma gondii*	Pyrimethamine plus sulfadiazine plus folinic acid
Diffuse pulmonary infiltrates and hypoxia, especially if not on trimethoprim-sulfamethoxazole chemoprophylaxis	*Pneumocystis carinii*	Trimethoprim-sulfamethoxazole
Dysphagia or odynophagia	*Candida albicans*	Fluconazole
PPD+ and ill-appearing, especially with abnormal chest roentgenogram (or if PPD− and anergic, but at high epidemiologic risk for tuberculosis)	*Mycobacterium tuberculosis*	Isoniazid, rifampin, pyrazinamide, ethambutol

CT, computed tomography; MRI, magnetic resonance imaging; PPD, purified protein derivative (of tuberculin); PMN, polymorphonuclear (leukocytes).

If an infectious agent is either not diagnosed or not effectively treated with available antimicrobials, as for example with cryptosporidia or microsporidia, antiperistaltic agents such as loperamide may be tried. Somatostatin analogue in doses of 100 to 300 µg three times daily subcutaneously or intramuscularly has been used successfully in a small number of patients to reduce the diarrhea associated with cryptosporidia infection or when no pathogen could be identified.

AIDS Cachexia

AIDS wasting syndrome (or AIDS-related cachexia as it is frequently called) is increasingly common as HIV-infected patients survive longer due to improved prophylaxis and treatment of opportunistic infections. It is a major cause of morbidity in this population. For surveillance purposes, the Centers for Disease Control and

TABLE 14. *Guide to therapy of opportunistic infections in HIV-infected patients*

Infection	Specific treatment	Alternative treatment	Maintenance therapy
Fungal infections			
Oral candidiasis (thrush)	Clotrimazole troches (10 mg) 5×/day	Nystatin oral suspension 100,000 units/cc; 5 cc QID swish/swallow; or ketoconazole 200–400 mg/day; or fluconazole 100 mg/day	Same as initial therapy but may reduce frequency of administration
Candida esophagitis	Fluconazole 100 mg/day PO or IV	Ketoconazole 200–400 mg/day PO; or amphotericin B 15–25 mg IV/day	Same as initial therapy
Histoplasmosis	Amphotericin B ≥0.5 mg/kg/day; 2 g total dose	Itraconazole 200 mg PO BID	Itraconazole 200–400 mg/day PO, or amphotericin B 50–80 mg biweekly
Cryptococcosis	Amphotericin B, ≥0.5 mg/kg/day; 1–2 g total dose	Amphotericin B, 0.3 mg/kg/day plus flucytosine 100–150 mg/kg/PO daily, or fluconazole 400 mg PO or IV/day	Fluconazole 200–400 mg PO/day
Coccidioidomycosis (without CNS involvement)	Amphotericin B, ≥0.5 mg/kg/day; ≥1 g total dose	Fluconazole 400 mg/day, or itraconazole 200 mg PO BID	Fluconazole 400 mg/day, or itraconazole 200 mg PO BID
Aspergillosis	Amphotericin B, 0.5–1.5 mg/kg/day; ≥2 g total dose	Itraconazole 200 mg PO BID	? Itraconazole 200 mg PO BID
Viral infections			
Localized herpes zoster	Acyclovir 800 mg PO 5×/day × 7–10 days	Famciclovir 500 mg PO Q8H × 7–10 days	None
Disseminated varicella zoster	Acyclovir 10 mg/kg IV Q8H × 10 days	Foscarnet 40–60 mg/kg IV Q8H × 10 days	Consider high-dose oral acyclovir if recurrences are seen
Localized, nonhealing herpes simplex virus infection, nasolabial, genital, or perianal areas	Acyclovir 200 mg PO 5×/day ≥10 days	Foscarnet 40–60 mg/kg IV Q8H ≥10 days	Acyclovir 200 mg PO TID or 400 mg PO BID
Cytomegalovirus retinitis	Ganciclovir 5 mg/kg IV Q12H × 14–21 days	Foscarnet 60 mg/kg IV Q8H × 14–21 days	Ganciclovir 5 mg/kg IV Q24H, or foscarnet 90 mg/kg IV Q24H, or oral ganciclovir 1 gm PO Q8H, or ganciclovir ocular implant (experimental)
Progressive multifocal leukoencephalopathy (JC virus infection)	None	None	None

Continued on next page

TABLE 14. *Continued*

Infection	Specific treatment	Alternative treatment	Maintenance therapy
Parvovirus B19	Immunoglobulin G IV 0.4 g/kg × 5 days	None	If relapse occurs within 6 months after initial treatment, give single-day infusions of 0.4 g/kg IgG every 4 weeks
Protozoal infections			
Pneumocystis carinii pneumonia[a]	Trimethoprim (15–20 mg/kg/day with Sulfamethoxazole (75–100 mg/kg/day) in 3–4 divided doses IV or PO × 21 days plus a tapering dose of corticosteroids if PaO$_2$ <70 or A-a gradient >35 mm Hg One possible regimen is prednisone 40 mg PO BID × days 1–5, prednisone 40 mg PO daily × days 6–10, prednisone 20 mg daily × days 11–21	Pentamidine 3–4 mg/kg IV daily × 21 days, or trimethoprim 20 mg/kg/day PO in 4 divided doses plus dapsone 100 mg PO daily × 21 days, or atovaquone elixir 750 mg PO BID with meals × 21 days, or trimetrexate 45 mg/m^2 IV daily × 21 days plus folinic acid 20 mg/m^2 IV Q6H × 24 days, or clindamycin 600 mg IV Q6H plus primaquine 15 base PO daily × 21 days, plus steroids when indicated, for all of the above regimens	Trimethoprim (160 mg)–sulfamethoxazole (800 mg) PO TIW, or dapsone 100 mg PO daily (dapsone plus pyrimethamine regimens are preferred for toxoplasma antibody + patients, see Table 10), or aerosol pentamidine 300 mg once/month by the Respirgard II nebulizer
Cerebral toxoplasmosis	Pyrimethamine 50–100 mg/day PO with sulfadiazine 1 g PO QID plus folinic acid 5 mg/day PO, until resolution or stabilization, with improvement of clinical signs and CT abnormalities	Clindamycin up to 1,200 mg IV Q8H with pyrimethamine 50–100 mg/day PO with folinic acid 5 mg PO/day	Pyrimethamine 25 mg/day Sulfadiazine 1 g/day Folinic acid 5 mg/day
Microsporidial enteric infection	Albendazole 400 mg PO BID (experimental)	None	? Same as initial therapy
Cryptosporidiosis	Paromomycin 500–750 mg PO QID 160 mg trimethoprim–800 mg sulfamethoxazole PO QID × 10 days	Azithromycin 500–1,250 mg/day Pyrimethamine 75 gm PO, folinic acid 5 mg PO daily × 10 days	Same as initial therapy if response 160 mg trimethoprim–800 mg sulfamethoxazole TIW, or pyrimethamine 25 mg/day plus folinic acid 5 mg/day
Isospora belli enteric infection			
Cyclospora	Trimethoprim (160 mg)–sulfamethoxazole (800 mg) PO QID × 10 days	None	Trimethoprim (160 mg)–sulfamethoxazole (800 mg) PO TIW

Helminthic infection			
Strongyloides stercoralis	Thiabendazole 25 mg/kg Q12H × ≥5 days	Ivermectin 200 μg/kg × ≥1 dose (experimental)	None
Bacterial infections			
Nocardiosis	Sulfisoxazole 1–2 g PO QID × ≥6 weeks	Minocycline 100–200 mg PO BID, or others based on susceptibility testing	Continue therapy at 1 g sulfisoxazole PO QID
Salmonella bacteremia	Ciprofloxacin 750 mg PO BID × 6 weeks	Amoxicillin 500 mg PO TID; trimethoprim 160 mg–sulfamethoxazole 800 mg PO TID	? None, if ciprofloxacin is used as primary therapy; otherwise, continue primary therapy
Mycobacterium tuberculosis	Isoniazid 300 mg PO daily with pyridoxine 50 mg PO daily, with rifampin 600 mg PO daily, with pyrazinamide 15–30 mg/kg per day PO (once daily or in 3–4 divided doses, up to a daily maximum of 2 g), with ethambutol 15–25 mg/kg daily; all × 2 months (if multiply resistant strain suspected, use ≥5 drugs)	Same except may substitute streptomycin 20–40 mg/kg (maximum 1 g) IM daily for ethambutol	Isoniazid 300 mg PO daily with pyridoxine 50 mg PO daily, with rifampin 600 mg PO daily; both × ≥6 months total course (including initial 2 months)
Mycobacterium avium complex	Clarithromycin 500 mg PO BID with ethambutol 15–25 mg/kg PO daily	Add or substitute rifabutin 300–600 mg PO daily, ciprofloxacin 500–750 mg PO daily, clofazimine 100 mg PO daily, amikacin 7.5 mg/kg IV Q 12–24H	Continue initial therapy
Bacillary epithelioid angiomatosis	Erythromycin 500 mg PO QID × ≥2–4 weeks	Doxycycline 100 mg PO BID	None, unless relapses occur
Helicobacter cinaedi cellulitis and/or bacteremia	Doxycycline 100 mg PO or IV Q12H × 2–6 weeks	Gentamicin 3–5 mg/kg/day IV	None
Rhodococcus equi	Vancomycin 15 mg/kg IV Q12H plus rifampin 600 mg PO or IV/ day × 4–8 weeks	Macrolide plus rifampin 600 mg IV or PO daily	Macrolide plus rifampin 600 mg PO daily

[a]Recent evidence suggests that *Pneumocystis carinii* is a fungus.

TABLE 15. *Microorganisms and/or conditions that have been associated with diarrhea in HIV-infected patients[a]*

Microorganisms
  Bacteria
    Campylobacter jejuni
    Shigella sp.
    Salmonella sp.
    Mycobacterium avium complex
    Enterocyte adherent bacteria
  Protozoans
    Cryptosporidia
    Giardia lamblia
    Isospora belli
    Microsporidia
    Cyclospora
  Helminths
    Strongyloides stercoralis
  Viruses
    Cytomegalovirus
    Adenovirus
    Rotavirus
    Astrovirus
    Calicivirus
    HIV itself (? cause of AIDS enteropathy)
Turmors
  Lymphoma
  Kaposi's sarcoma (uncommon cause of diarrhea)
Miscellaneous
  Side effects of medications
  Clostridium difficile colitis

[a]Listing not meant to be exhaustive.

TABLE 16. *Approach to the evaluation of the HIV-infected patient with diarrhea*

Standard evaluation
  Stool sample for
    Culture and sensitivity for routine enteric pathogens
    Ova and parasite examination[a]
    Cryptosporidia smear[a]
    Mycobacterial culture and smear
    Clostridium difficile (antigen, toxin, or culture assay)
Further evaluation if above negative or nondiagnostic
  Colonoscopy with biopsy
  Gastroduodenoscopy with biopsy[b]

[a]Examination of several stool samples will enhance yield.
[b]Electron microscopic examination necessary to detect microsporidia.

Prevention has defined the HIV wasting syndrome as involuntary weight loss of more than 10% of baseline body weight plus either chronic diarrhea (at least two loose stools per day for at least 30 days) or chronic weakness and documented fever (at least 30 days, intermittent or constant), in the absence of a concurrent illness or condition other than HIV infection to explain the symptoms. Metabolic disorders, alterations in cytokines, anorexia, endocrine dysfunction, and malabsorption are among multiple described factors working independently or in concert to cause AIDS wasting.

In the patient who has had an opportunistic infection or neoplasm or has an extremely low CD4$^+$ lymphocyte count, meeting the strict definition of AIDS wasting is dependent upon the extent to which an evaluation is performed to exclude more specific etiologies for wasting. Often the cause of weight loss is multifactorial and changes over time. In fact, unintentional weight loss of more than 10% of body weight has been reported in 50% of patients with AIDS in some studies. Physicians are frequently faced with the problem of continued weight loss in a patient who is already being treated for another problem that may be contributing to weight loss, such as *M. avium* complex infection.

Successful treatment of an underlying infection or condition causing weight loss remains the cornerstone of management. Medications should be reviewed to determine if any are causing diarrhea, anorexia, or vomiting, symptoms that often contribute to weight loss. In the face of no other identified or easily treated cause for wasting, several therapeutic strategies have emerged. Unfortunately, few agents have been tested in a randomized, placebo-controlled fashion, and most studies have involved few patients.

Perhaps the best studied and most widely used agents for AIDS wasting are those that are employed with the intent of stimulating appetite. In two large randomized placebo-controlled studies, megestrol acetate (800 mg of the liquid preparation daily) was demonstrated to increase food intake leading to a mean weight gain of approximately 8 pounds during a 12 week period, which was associated with improvement of well-being. Dronabinol in doses of 2.5 mg twice daily to 5 mg four times daily has also been associated with significant weight gain in a small number of patients, including a few who had failed megestrol acetate, but is associated with frequent intolerance. It is still not certain that either of these agents increases body mass. At present megestrol acetate (800 mg daily of the liquid preparation) is our first line therapy for treatment of AIDS wasting.

Anabolic agents such as recombinant human growth hormone, stanozolol (an anabolic steroid), and testosterone are all under study with some encouraging preliminary findings. The place of these agents in the treatment of AIDS wasting is dependent upon the outcome of larger studies.

Since cytokine dysregulation may play a prominent role in weight loss, agents capable of modulating these factors have been tested in small numbers of patients with AIDS wasting. Oral corticosteroids (dexamethasone or prenisolone), which may act to both enhance appetite and alter cytokine release, and thalidomide have been shown anecdotally to increase weight, sometimes remarkably in extremely ill individuals. Pentoxifylline, however, a tumor necrosis factor inhibitor, did not lead to increased weight gain in a small study of AIDS patients with wasting. Larger randomized trials with these types of agents are needed before they can be recommended.

For patients with mechanical or neurologic problems that reduce oral intake, use of parenteral or enteral nutrition should be entertained (see Chapter 7). Both types of feeding can lead to stabilization of weight loss or to weight gain in the HIV-infected patient with wasting. However, both have attendant risks including high rates of infection, and parenteral nutrition is extremely expensive.

Cutaneous Manifestations

Patients with HIV infection are at risk for a variety of cutaneous lesions. One of the most important to recognize is Kaposi's sarcoma. This lesion is typically nodular and violaceous (Fig. 3), and can occur at any skin or mucous membrane site. The number of lesions will vary from a few to innumerable, at which point they may coalesce. Lymphatic involvement is suggested by the development of edema, which can be severe and places the patient at risk for bacterial cellulitis. Kaposi's sarcoma is discussed in more detail in Chapter 8.

The earliest cutaneous process to occur in HIV infection is a nonspecific and mild morbilliform eruption that often occurs during the mononucleosis-like illness associated with primary HIV infection. This self-limited exanthem occurs within 2 months of onset of HIV infection and is accompanied by fever and often lymphadenopathy, pharyngitis, and aseptic meningitis (Fig. 4). Many additional infections may involve the skin or mucous membranes during the course of HIV infection (Table 17). One of the most common is herpes simplex virus infection. In HIV-infected patients, herpes simplex infections are not restricted to nasolabial or genital areas. These infections can be disfiguring and on occasion can cause severe destruction of soft tissue, cartilage, and even bone (Fig. 5). Because of the severity and atypical locations of this infection, the diagnosis may be initially overlooked. Viral culture by swab (of moist lesions) or of biopsy tissue is helpful in establishing the diagnosis. Despite the advanced nature of certain of these lesions, a highly satisfactory response is usually seen with acyclovir therapy (Table 14).

Herpes zoster infections commonly occur in HIV-infected patients and may antedate other opportunistic infections by several years. Although zoster may disseminate with both an acute and chronic course, and may recur after acyclovir therapy, in the large majority of patients infection remains localized to a single dermatome, heals uneventfully, and does not recur. Other commonly encountered viral infections of the skin or mucous membranes in HIV-infected patients include molluscum contagiosum, human papilloma virus infection, and hairy leukoplakia.

Bacterial infections of the skin include impetigo, folliculitis, ecthyma, and bacillary epithelioid angiomatosis. Bacillary epithelioid angiomatosis is a newly recognized cutaneous infection caused by the rickettsia-like organisms *Bartonella henselae* and *Bartonella quintana*. Infection with these agents is not confined to the

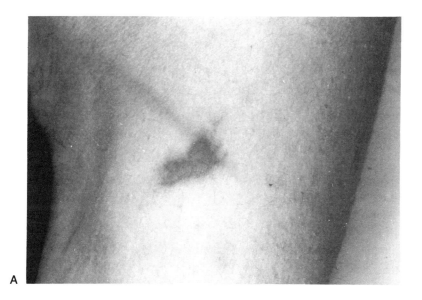

A

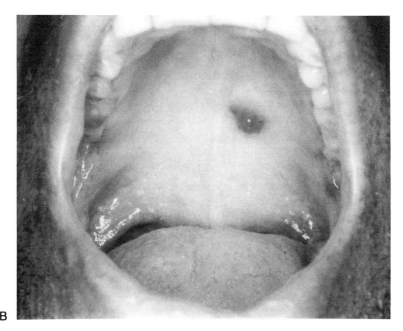

B

FIG. 3. Kaposi's sarcoma lesion on upper arm (**A**) and palate (**B**) of HIV-infected patients.

FIG. 4. A widely distributed eruption of pinkish macules and papules is characteristic of the acute exanthem of primary HIV infection. (Figure courtesy of C. J. Cockerell.)

TABLE 17. *Infections of the skin or mucous membranes of HIV-infected patients[a]*

Infection	Approach to Management
Abscesses	Incision and drainage
Angular cheilitis	Topical antifungal and corticosteroid preparation (hydrocortisone cream)
Bacillary epithelioid angiomatosis (Bartonella infection)	Erythromycin (Table 14)
Botryomycosis	Systemic antibiotics
Candida infection	Topical or systemic antifungal preparation
Condylomata acuminata	Podofilox (or equivalent) or various ablative therapies
Cryptococcosis	Systemic antifungal preparation (Table 14)
Cytomegalovirus infection	Ganciclovir or foscarnet (Table 14)
Dermatophyte infection	Topical or oral antifungal preparation
Ecthyma	Systemic antibiotics
Exanthem of primary HIV infection	None
Folliculitis	Topical or systemic antibiotics (if bacterial)
Furuncles	Systemic antibiotics
Gingivitis[b]	Plaque removal; chlorhexidine mouth rinse
Hairy leukoplakia	None needed but acyclovir is effective
Herpes simplex virus infection	Acyclovir (Table 14)
Histoplasmosis	Systemic antifungal preparation (Table 14)
Impetigo	Systemic antibiotics
Molluscum contagiosum	Curettage or cryosurgery
Mycobacterial infections	See Table 14 and Chapter 5
Necrotizing gingivitis	Debridement; povidone-iodine irrigation; systemic antibiotics; chlorhexidine mouth rinse
Necrotizing stomatitis	Debridement including bone sequestra; povidone-iodine irrigation; systemic antibiotics; chlorhexidine mouth rinse
Periodontitis	Plaque removal; root planing and curettage; irrigation with povidone-iodine; systemic antibiotics; chlorhexidine mouth rinse
Pneumocystosis	Trimethoprim-sulfamethoxazole (Table 14)
Pyomyositis	Systemic antibiotics
Scabies	5% permethrin or 1% lindane
Syphilis	Penicillin
Varicella zoster infection	Acyclovir (Table 14)

[a]Management often optimized by consultation with specialist, the choice of which (e.g., dermatologist, dentist, gynecologist) is dependent on the specific condition and site of involvement.
[b]See also necrotizing gingivitis and necrotizing stomatitis.

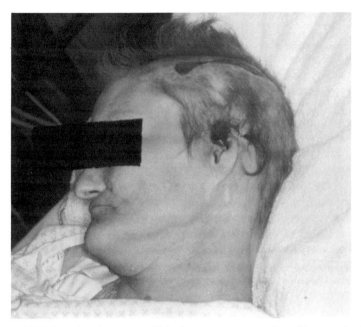

FIG. 5. This HIV-infected patient had multiple discrete cutaneous sites of herpes simplex virus infection. A destructive lesion of the pinna is shown; a separate scalp lesion is also present.

skin; there may be involvement of the liver, heart valves, and other sites. Bacillary epithelioid angiomatosis is characterized by small, red to purple papules with a clinical appearance similar to cherry angiomata or pyogenic granulomata; these lesions are occasionally mistaken for Kaposi's sarcoma (Fig. 6). Lesions may be few in number or numerous and can involve mucosal surfaces. Some lesions may involve subcutaneous tissue, underlying muscle, and even bone. Histologic examination of a skin biopsy specimen is the most commonly used method of confirming the diagnosis. Erythromycin is effective therapy (Table 14).

Fungal infections of the skin and mucous membranes are very common, ranging from superficial dermatophyte infections to highly unusual opportunistic fungal diseases. Candida infections of the oral pharynx or vagina are very frequent, particularly at $CD4^+$ cell counts below $200/mm^3$, at which point continuous antifungal therapy may be necessary to suppress these infections (Table 14). Although topical antifungal agents such as clotrimazole troches are highly effective in prevention of recurrences, our preference is to use an oral systemic agent, such as fluconazole, for patients with $CD4^+$ counts below 100 cells/mm^3, because of the additional benefit of preventing certain invasive fungal diseases, like cryptococcosis.

Cutaneous lesions in HIV-infected patients with advanced immunodeficiency (<200 $CD4^+$ cells/mm^3) are often an important diagnostic clue to the presence of a

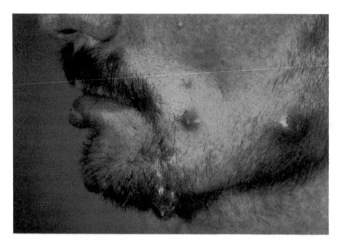

FIG. 6. Reddish nodules of bacillary epithelioid angiomatosis on the skin surface of the face of an HIV-infected patient. Some of the nodules have a somewhat acuminant shape and are crusted. (Figure courtesy of C. J. Cockerell.)

systemic opportunistic infection. There should be a low threshold for dermatologic consultation and biopsy of unexplained skin lesions with samples obtained for histology, special stains, and viral, bacterial, mycobacterial, and fungal cultures.

In addition to Kaposi's sarcoma and a wide variety of cutaneous infections, there are also many other conditions and diseases that involve the skin of HIV-infected patients (Table 18). It is not clear that all of these are manifestations or complications of HIV infection per se; some may represent coincidental findings. Included among these conditions is a nonspecific pruritus that can be highly symptomatic for the patient and potentially complicated by secondary bacterial infections due to excoriation. This unexplained pruritus may be confused with drug reactions. Emollients, topical corticosteroids, antihistamines, topical or systemic antifungal preparations, and topical or systemic antibiotics rarely provide significant relief of the itching. Symptomatic improvement sometimes results from ultraviolet light A or B phototherapy. Patients should be given instructions on how to optimize skin care, including use of mild soaps, correct application of emollients (for example, applying moisturizing creams immediately after bathing), and avoidance of factors that dry out the skin.

One of the most commonly observed skin conditions associated with advanced HIV infection is seborrheic dermatitis, occurring in up to 80% of patients (Fig. 7). Why this lesion develops is unclear but overgrowth of certain cutaneous fungi, such as *Pityrosporum*, may contribute to its development. Compared with seborrheic dermatitis in non–HIV-infected patients, the lesions in AIDS patients tend to be more florid and may be characterized by intense erythema and thick scaly plaques

TABLE 18. *Noninfectious conditions of the skin or mucous membranes of HIV-infected patients*

Alopecia
Aphthous ulcers
Calciphylaxis
Eosinophilic folliculitis/eosinophilic pustular folliculitis[a]
Erythema elevatum diutinum
Granuloma annulare
Hives
Hyperpigmentation
Ichthyosis
Kaposi's sarcoma
Leukocytoclastic vasculitis
Lymphoma
Morbilliform drug eruption
Papular urticaria
Pityriasis rubra pilaris
Photodermatitis
Porphyria cutanea tarda
Pruritic papular eruption[a]
Pruritus nodularis
Psoriasis
Reiter's syndrome
Salivary gland enlargement
Seborrheic dermatitis-like eruption
Transient acantholytic dermatosis
Xerosis
Xerostomia

[a]As reported in HIV-infected patients, these conditions have overlapping clinical features.

involving many cutaneous sites outside of the expected distribution, including the upper anterior chest, back, groin, and extremities. The scalp may be severely involved. In some patients, widespread involvement may mimic erythroderma or psoriasis. Treatment of seborrheic dermatitis includes application of topical corticosteroid creams (hydrocortisone cream is the most appropriate preparation for use on the face), as well as topical antifungal preparations (e.g., ketoconazole). Scalp disease often requires keratolytic agents and medicated shampoos (e.g., selenium or tar shampoos or ketoconazole shampoo) with accompanying corticosteroid gels or solutions. In selected cases, ultraviolet phototherapy or treatment with grenz rays may be beneficial.

Eosinophilic pustular folliculitis is a widespread acneiform papular and pustular eruption that characteristically involves the face, trunk, neck, and extremities. This entity accounts for at least some of the cases referred to by the term "pruritic papular eruption." The severe pruritus associated with this lesion helps to distinguish it from bacterial folliculitis. Because of the intensive itching, it is not uncommon for patients to present primarily with prurigo nodularis and lichen simplex chronicus as a consequence of rubbing and scratching. Ultraviolet B phototherapy analogous to that used for psoriasis is an effective treatment. Itraconazole in doses of 200 to 400

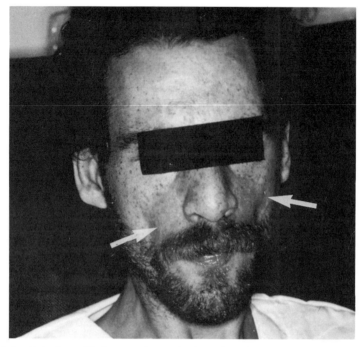

FIG. 7. Seborrheic dermatitis-like eruption on the face of an HIV-infected patient; note butterfly appearance (*arrow*).

mg per day led to complete or partial response of itching and lesions in 21 of 28 (75%) patients with eosinophilic folliculitis in a recent open trial. These promising results need to be confirmed by other studies.

Aphthous ulcers of the oral mucosa occur somewhat more frequently in HIV-infected patients than in the general population, and are very much more severe. These ulcers may enlarge to 1 to 2 cm, may be multiple, and may persist for weeks. They may be a major impediment to swallowing and mastication. The etiology is unknown, but they usually respond to topical corticosteroids. Systemic corticosteroid therapy is rarely needed. Outside of the United States, thalidomide has been used successfully. Very large necrotizing oral ulcers are occasionally also seen in HIV-infected patients. They may represent aphthous ulcers superinfected with bacteria, or they may be a form of necrotizing stomatitis. They respond to a combination of topical steroids plus systemic antibiotics directed at anaerobic and gram-negative aerobic bacteria.

Stenotic Biliary Tract Disease

Stenotic biliary tract disease is being increasingly recognized in HIV-infected individuals. These patients typically have fever and epigastric or right upper quadrant pain. Blood chemistries reveal a markedly elevated alkaline phosphatase level, with relatively lower bilirubin and hepatocellular enzyme elevations. Dilated intra- or extrahepatobiliary ducts are frequently found on ultrasound examination or by computed tomography. Papillary stenosis and sclerosing cholangitis may be present together or individually on endoscopic evaluation. Cytomegalovirus and/or cryptosporidia are often present in bile or observed on histologic preparations of ampulla of Vater tissue, or papillary or peripapillary duodenal tissue. *Mycobacterium avium* complex infection, microsporidia, Kaposi's sarcoma, and lymphoma have also been demonstrated in periampullary or biliary ductal tissue. However, in 45% of cases, no opportunistic infection or neoplasm has been discovered. The role of HIV itself in the entity is unknown. Endoscopic sphincterotomy may be useful in relieving pain and reducing fever. However, the alkaline phosphatase level may continue to rise, suggesting progression of intrahepatic sclerosing cholangitis or the presence of diffuse hepatic parenchymal disease (see Chapter 7).

Renal Manifestations

Clinically apparent renal disease occurs in 10–30% of AIDS patients in certain geographic areas. In HIV-infected populations in which many patients are young black men who use intravenous drugs, proteinuria of greater than 0.5 g/24 h has been reported to occur in more than 40% of AIDS patients, with nephrotic-range proteinuria in up to 10%. In other HIV-infected populations, the incidence of clinically apparent renal disease appears to be much lower.

AIDS patients with renal disease have been divided into three groups based upon the presentation of renal disease. Group 1 consists of patients who suddenly develop renal failure because of an acute insult to the kidneys, such as dehydration, sepsis, hypotension, hypoxia, or nephotoxic agents, including nonsteroidal antiinflammatory agents, pentamidine, foscarnet sodium, trimethoprim-sulfamethoxazole, or radiocontrast dye. In general, the clinical course of acute renal failure and response to treatment in AIDS patients is similar to that of nonimmunocompromised patients, and these patients benefit from dialysis when it is required. Both hemodialysis and peritoneal dialysis have been used successfully.

Group 2 consists of HIV-infected patients with renal disease due to HIV-associated nephropathy. For unclear reasons the majority of these patients (approximately 90%) are young black men, about half of whom have used intravenous drugs. (It is of interest that blacks also appear to develop idiopathic and heroin-associated variants of focal and segmental glomerulosclerosis much more commonly than other races). These patients have nephrotic syndrome and even in the absence of ischemic or nephrotoxic injury, a rapidly progressive course to uremia over 6 to 12 months. An interesting clinical finding is the notable absence of hypertension during both early and late stages of disease, despite severe renal failure. Changes in the kidney consist of focal or global glomerulosclerosis and prominent tubulointerstitial disease. Immunofluorescence studies have revealed deposits of complement (C3,C1q), IgM, and sometimes IgG, but not IgA, localized predominantly to segments of glomerular sclerosis and less frequently to the mesangium. The focal and segmental glomerulosclerosis is reminiscent of the glomerular lesions seen in patients using illicit drugs intravenously before the AIDS epidemic. The etiology of these lesions is unknown. CD4 receptors have been demonstrated on glomerular cell membranes, suggesting that direct infection of these cells by HIV may be involved. Proviral HIV DNA has been demonstrated in kidney tissue of HIV-infected patients both with and without clinical evidence of renal disease. Those patients with advanced HIV-induced immunodeficiency fare poorly on dialysis with complications of severe cachexia, malnutrition, and opportunistic infections, frequently leading to death within months. The therapeutic role of steroids or other immunosuppressive agents in this group is unclear. In anecdotal cases there have been beneficial effects both from corticosteroids and AZT.

Although HIV-associated glomerulosclerosis is the most distinctive and common type of chronic nephropathy in HIV-infected patients, other types of glomerular lesions may occur. Included among these are diffuse mesangial hyperplasia and a variety of immune complex–mediated glomerulopathies, such as IgA nephropathy. Exactly how these relate to HIV infection is unclear.

Group 3 consists of patients who have end-stage renal disease of diverse causes unrelated to HIV infection (e.g., heroin-induced nephropathy or diabetic glomerulosclerosis). HIV infection may precede or follow the development of chronic renal failure. Seroprevalence surveys in chronic hemodialysis units have shown HIV seropositivity rates ranging from 0.77% in broad-based geographic studies to 12–40% in inner-city hemodialysis units. These patients usually have a progressive downhill course once the diagnosis of frank AIDS is made. The majority have died within 1 year with marked cachexia unresponsive to nutritional support by hyperalimentation. However, patients with asymptomatic HIV infection on chronic dialysis can live for years, although the risk of peritonitis in those receiving chronic ambulatory peritoneal dialysis is approximately twice as high as for patients without HIV infection. The effect of chronic dialysis on the natural history of HIV infection per se remains to be defined.

Cardiac Manifestations

Cardiac abnormalities are common in AIDS patients, judging from an up to 77% prevalence at postmortem examination. However, they are much less often recognized antemortem, unless sensitive testing procedures are done specifically to identify them. Aside from electrocardiographic abnormalities, the cardiac conditions most likely to be appreciated clinically are cardiomyopathy (including myocarditis) and pericardial effusion (Table 19). Cardiac disease is most common in HIV-infected individuals with advanced immunodeficiency and reportedly directly contributes to the death of 1.1–6.3% of patients.

Electrocardiographic abnormalities occur in up to 44% of HIV-infected patients and may be due to myocarditis or pericarditis, or may reflect the presence of fever,

TABLE 19. *Cardiac manifestations in HIV-infected patients*

Myocarditis
    Idiopathic
    Infectious—toxoplasmosis, cytomegalovirus infection, coxsac-
       kievirus infection, cryptococcosis, aspergillosis, candidiasis,
       mycobacterial infection, nocardiosis
    HIV-related (?)
Pericarditis
    Idiopathic
    Infectious—tuberculosis, *Mycobacterium avium* complex in-
       fection, cytomegalovirus infection, nocardiosis, toxoplas-
       mosis, salmonellosis, cryptococcosis, herpes simplex infec-
       tion
    Neoplastic—Kaposi's sarcoma, lymphoma
Endocarditis
    Infectious—*Staphylococcus aureus* and others
    Nonbacterial thrombotic endocarditis (marantic)
Cardiomyopathy
    Myocarditis
    Postinfectious (presumed)
    Nutritional deficiencies—selenium, vitamin B_1
    Toxins—alcohol, cocaine
    Drug-induced—Adriamycin, interferon, AZT
Primary pulmonary hypertension
Arrhythmias
    Underlying cardiac disease
    Fever/sepsis
    Electrolyte abnormalities
    Medications—IV pentamidine, interferon

sepsis, electrolyte disturbances, or drug toxicities. The findings are generally minor and consist of low-voltage, ST-T wave changes, bundle branch block, and intraventricular conduction delays. However, ventricular tachycardia has been reported that may result in congestive heart failure or sudden death. Intravenous pentamidine (but not aerosol pentamidine) may cause QT interval prolongation and lead to *torsades de pointes*, a polymorphic ventricular tachycardia.

Symptoms and signs of congestive heart failure and/or embolic phenomena are the usual presenting manifestations of HIV-associated cardiomyopathy. Although most commonly felt to be due to active myocarditis, or to be postinfectious in origin, nutritional deficiencies of selenium or vitamin B_1, and abuse of ethanol or cocaine may play a role. Congestive heart failure has also been attributed to the use of AZT and to high-dose α-interferon for the treatment of Kaposi's sarcoma. Doxorubicin hydrochloride, which is included in some combination chemotherapy protocols for Kaposi's sarcoma, is a well-known cause of cardiomyopathy.

Myocarditis is a relatively common cardiac finding at postmortem examination in HIV-infected patients. Although infections such as toxoplasmosis (the most commonly recognized infectious cause), cytomegalovirus infection, coxsackievirus infection, cryptococcosis, aspergillosis, candidiasis, mycobacterial infection, and nocardiosis are potential etiologies, most often the cause is not identified.

The pathogenesis of myocarditis in the absence of an infectious agent is unclear. HIV can be demonstrated by a variety of techniques in the myocardium of certain cases implying a possible direct or indirect etiologic role for HIV itself. However, CD4 antigen has not been detected in normal human myocardium, and there has been no histologic evidence of HIV infection of the myocyte specifically. One group has hypothesized that an autoimmune process, as evidenced by the presence of serum antibodies to cardiac antigens, may play a role in pathogenesis.

Specific treatment for myocarditis is rarely possible except when caused by opportunistic infections, which are usually diagnosed based on cultures obtained from sites outside of the myocardium. In the absence of an alternative diagnosis, we empirically treat patients with a positive toxoplasma serology for toxoplasmosis. "Idiopathic" cases sometimes resolve spontaneously or in one case coincident with the introduction of antiretroviral therapy.

Pericardial effusions occur in up to 38% of AIDS patients and are the most common cause of clinical cardiovascular symptoms and signs. Although these effusions are often small, remain asymptomatic, and spontaneously resolve in 50% of cases, rarely cardiac tamponade may develop. Pericardial effusion may be "idiopathic" in origin or be caused by infection or neoplasms. In some instances, idiopathic effusions have been associated with chronic pulmonary disease and isolated right ventricular dilation. *M. tuberculosis* is the most commonly identified infectious cause, responsible for 22–50% of cases. Other infectious agents that have caused pericarditis in HIV-infected patients include *M. avium* complex, cytomegalovirus, nocardia, *T. gondii*, *Salmonella typhimurium*, and cryptococcus. Malignant effusions may be due to lymphoma or Kaposi's sarcoma. Successful treatment of cases due to tuberculosis, toxoplasmosis, salmonellosis, and cryptococcosis has been possible. However, pericardial effusions due to *M. avium* complex infection, lymphoma, or Kaposi's sarcoma are usually refractory to treatment. Drainage procedures such as pericardiotomy or pericardiocentesis have proved beneficial in selected patients with symptomatic disease.

Endocarditis in HIV-infected persons may be due to infection, but is more commonly due to nonbacterial thrombotic endocarditis (marantic endocarditis), which accompanies many wasting illnesses. Intravenous drug users who continue to inject drugs are at risk for infective endocarditis due principally to *Staphylococcus aureus*, but also to gram-negative organisms and fungi.

Primary pulmonary hypertension, with or without cor pulmonale, has been reported in a small number of HIV-infected patients. Echocardiograms have shown right atrial enlargement, right ventricular enlargement, or paradoxical septal motion. In several patients, underlying lung infections were also present. The etiology is unknown. However, a role for HIV has been speculated either as the primary cause, or as an inciting agent for an immune response that leads to pulmonary vascular damage. Primary pulmonary hypertension should be suspected in an HIV-infected patient who presents with dyspnea on exertion in the presence of a normal chest roentgenogram.

Rheumatologic Manifestations

Arthralgia, arthritis, myopathies (which are mentioned elsewhere in this chapter and in Chapter 6), various forms of vasculitis, a sicca syndrome, and numerous autoimmune phenomena are the principal rheumatologic complications of HIV infection. Intermittent arthralgias without synovitis may occur during primary HIV infection and in up to one-third of patients at a later time. Although sometimes intensely painful, the cause is unknown and treatment is symptomatic.

Joint infections are surprisingly uncommon among HIV-infected adults. Anecdotally, we have seen a case due to *S. aureus*, and other reported pathogens include *Sporothrix schenckii*, *Cryptococcus neoformans*, *Histoplasma capsulatum*, *Pseudomonas* sp., *Neisseria gonorrhoeae*, *Nocardia asteroides*, *Mycobacterium haemophilum*, *Salmonella* sp., and *Campylobacter fetus*. Microbiologic studies are an essential component in the evaluation of joint fluid in the HIV-infected patient with arthritis.

Reactive arthritides and Reiter's syndrome are the most frequently recognized forms of arthritis in HIV infection, occurring in 2–10% of adults depending on geographic area. The majority of North American patients with Reiter's syndrome have the human leukocyte antigen (HLA)-B27 allele. Organisms known to trigger reactive arthritis are, however, rarely discovered. It should be noted that reactive arthritis or Reiter's syndrome may be the first clinical manifestation of HIV infection. Psoriasis is also common in HIV infection occurring in 5–20% of patients and is complicated by psoriatic-like arthritis in up to one-half of cases.

A less etiologically well-defined type of oligoarthritis termed "HIV-related arthritis" has been described, which is characterized by subacute painful involvement of the knees and ankles with fewer than 10,000 leukocytes/mm^3 on synovial fluid analysis. Proposed pathophysiologic mechanisms include direct HIV infection of joints; immune complex deposition; and an atypical form of reactive arthritis occurring in the absence of HLA-B27, antecedent genitourinary or enteric infections, and inflammatory synovial fluid.

For patients with these forms of arthritis or with Reiter's syndrome, nonsteroidal antiinflammatory agents are the mainstay of treatment. A trial of sulfasalazine may be warranted in instances of sustained inflammation, but steroids and other immunosuppressive medications are potentially harmful and may increase the risk of developing opportunistic infections and Kaposi's sarcoma.

Several types of vasculitis have been reported in HIV-infected patients, including those of the polyarteritis nodosa type. The latter patients present primarily with a peripheral sensory or sensorimotor neuropathy. The etiology for the vasculitis is unknown in most cases, although cytomegalovirus infection is one recognized cause.

A syndrome characterized by massive parotid enlargement and xerostomia that superficially resembles Sjögren's syndrome is a well-reported but relatively infrequent complication. In adults the syndrome appears to have an immunogenetic basis and is found principally in blacks who have the DR5 allele. It is characterized by markedly elevated numbers of $CD8^+$, $CD29^+$ lymphocytes in blood that infiltrate various glandular and extraglandular tissues. Consequently, it has been designated as the "diffuse infiltrative lymphocytosis syndrome." Unlike classic Sjögren's syndrome, autoantibodies are usually absent. Extraglandular involvement may include the liver, lung, gastrointestinal tract, kidney, thymus, and nervous system. The possibility of HIV infection should always be considered in an individual with unexplained bilateral parotid enlargement. Anecdotally, we have observed striking resolution of parotid enlargement following irradiation of the gland.

Various autoimmune phenomena have been associated with HIV infection including the production of autoantibodies. Aside from antiplatelet antibodies that may be responsible for thrombocytopenia, antibodies directed at other targets, including red blood cells, leukocytes, and nuclear and cardiolipin antigens, are usually clinically silent. The same can probably be said for the presence of circulating immune complexes and cryoglobulins.

Neurologic Manifestations

Nearly 50% of HIV-infected adults at some point will manifest a clinically apparent neurologic disorder (Table 20). Direct HIV infection seems to play an important role in certain CNS manifestations. Complicating the primary neurologic disease process caused by HIV are various potential opportunistic infections, as well as lymphomas, conditions which may cause diffuse or focal neurologic abnormalities.

The neurologic history and examination should attempt to ascertain the duration, course, and focality of the disease process. Frequently cerebrospinal fluid (CSF) analysis is required. CSF studies should include cell counts and cytology; protein and glucose determination; VDRL; cultures for bacteria, mycobacteria, and fungi; gram and acid-fast stains; India ink examination; and cryptococcal antigen determination. If there are no focal findings on physical examination, lumbar puncture can be performed prior to radiologic imaging. Computed tomography or magnetic resonance imaging frequently provides useful information. Neurologic consultation is helpful and should be a standard aspect of the care of these patients.

Diagnostic considerations (Table 20) and therapies are discussed in detail in Chapter 6.

FUTURE PROSPECTS

Studies of novel chemo- and immunotherapeutic approaches to control HIV infection are likely to increase at an ever-expanding pace during the remainder of the 1990s and into the 21st century. Particular emphasis will be given to the use of combination therapies. Such therapeutic strategies will be designed to take advantage of potential additive or synergistic antiviral effects, and to prevent or retard the emergence of resistant strains. Putative benefits of any new therapy will continue to be judged against the efficacy and safety profile of AZT.

TABLE 20. *Common neurologic presentations in HIV-infected adults and usual etiologies*

Meningitis
  HIV
  Syphilis
  Cryptococcosis
  Tuberculosis
  Lymphoma (primary outside of CNS)
  Listeria (rare)
  Bacterial (e.g., pneumococcus, salmonella) (rare)
Encephalitis
  HIV
  Herpes simplex infection
  Cytomegalovirus infection
  Toxoplasmosis
Dementia
  HIV
  Progressive multifocal leukoencephalopathy
  Cytomegalovirus infection
  Toxoplasmosis
  Alcohol abuse
Focal CNS disease
  Toxoplasmosis
  Primary CNS lymphoma
  Progressive multifocal leukoencephalopathy
  Cryptococcosis (rare)
  Tuberculosis (rare)
  Aspergillosis (rare)
  Nocardiosis (rare)
Transient ischemic attacks/strokes
  Toxoplasmosis
  Syphilis
  Cryptococcosis
  Herpes zoster vasculitis
  Tuberculosis
  Aspergillosis
  Marantic endocarditis
  Embolus from mural thrombus (2° to cardiomyopathy)
  Vasculitis
  Idiopathic
  Coagulopathy and thrombocytopenia
  Anticardiolipin antibody
Myelopathy/myelitis
  Vacuolar myelopathy
  Human T-cell lymphotropic virus type I
  Varicella-zoster infection
  Lymphoma/plasmacytoma
  Syphilis
  Cytomegalovirus infection
  Tuberculosis
  Epidural or intramedullary abscess
Peripheral neuropathy
  Autoimmunity
  HIV
  Drug toxicity
  Cytomegalovirus infection (polyradiculopathy)
Myopathy
  HIV
  AZT

Because of the effectiveness of *Pneumocystis carinii* pneumonia and *Mycobacterium avium* complex prophylaxis, a reduction in the frequency of these infections will occur, and other complications, particularly cytomegalovirus infections and lymphoma, will become relatively more prominent. These conditions in turn will engender intensive efforts directed at improved diagnostic, therapeutic, and preventive measures. Advances that may come from these efforts will in turn further alter the natural history of HIV infection and lead to different research priorities.

ACKNOWLEDGMENTS

The authors thank Drs. R. Lerner and N. Goldberg for their helpful advice and Mrs. Eleanor Bromesco for typing the manuscript.

SUGGESTED READING

Calabrese LD. Human immunodeficiency virus (HIV) infection and arthritis. *Rheum Dis Clin North Am* 1993;19:477–488.

CDC. USPHS/IDSA guidelines for the prevention of opportunistic infections in persons infected with human immunodeficiency virus: a summary. *MMMR* 1995;44(RR-8):1–34.

Coodley GO, Loveless MO, Merrill TM. The HIV wasting syndrome: a review. *J Acquir Immune Defic Syndr* 1994;7:681–694.

Francis CK. Cardiac Involvement in AIDS. *Curr Probl Cardiol* 1990;15:569–639.

Hoover DR, Saah AJ, Bacellar H, et al. Clinical manifestations of AIDS in the era of *Pneumocystis* prophylaxis. *N Engl J Med* 1993;329:1922–1926.

Kaplan JE, Masur H, Holmes KK. Prevention of opportunistic infections in persons infected with human immunodeficiency virus. *Clin Infect Dis* 1995;21(suppl1):S1–S141.

Lederman MM. Host-directed and immune-based therapies for human immunodeficiency virus infections. *Ann Intern Med* 1995;122:218–227.

Lenderking WR, Gelber RD, Cotton DJ, et al. Evaluation of the quality of life associated with zidovudine treatment in asymptomatic human immunodeficiency virus infection. *N Engl J Med* 1994;330:738–743.

Loes SK, de Saussure P, Sourat J-H, Stalder H, Hirschel B, Perrin LH. Symptomatic primary infection due to human immunodeficiency virus type 1: review of 31 cases. *Clin Infect Dis* 1993;17:59–65.

Miralles P, Moreno S, Perez-Tascon M, Cosin J, Diaz MD, Bouza E. Fever of uncertain origin in patients infected with the human immunodeficiency virus. *Clin Infect Dis* 1995;20:872–875.

Prego V, Glatt AE, Roy V, Thelmo W, Dincsoy H, Raufman JP. Comparative yield of blood culture for fungi and mycobacteria, liver biopsy, and bone marrow biopsy in the diagnosis of fever of undetermined origin in human immunodeficiency virus-infected patients. *Arch Intern Med* 1990;150: 333–336.

Ray MC, Gately LE III. Dermatologic manifestations of HIV infection and AIDS. *Infect Dis Clin North Am* 1994;8:583–605.

Sande MA, Carpenter CCJ, Cobbs CG, Holmes KK, Sanford JP, for the National Institute of Allergy and Infectious Diseases. State of the art panel on anti-retroviral therapy for adult HIV-infected patients. *JAMA* 1993;270:2583–2589.

Stone HD, Appel RG. Human immunodeficiency virus-associated nephropathy: current concepts. *Am J Med Sci* 1994;307:212–217.

A Clinical Guide to AIDS and HIV,
edited by Gary P. Wormser.
Lippincott-Raven Publishers, Philadelphia © 1996.

3

Clinical Management of HIV-Infected Women

Kathryn Anastos, *Risa Denenberg, and †Laurie Solomon

*Montefiore Medical Center, and Department of Medicine, Albert Einstein College of Medicine, Bronx, New York 10467; *Family Nurse Practitioner; †Department of Obstetrics and Gynecology, Albert Einstein College of Medicine; and Ambulatory Obstetric and Gynecology Services, Bronx Lebanon Hospital Center, Bronx, New York 10461*

EPIDEMIOLOGY

Although HIV infection/AIDS is now a leading cause of death for women of ages 25 to 44 years in the United States, North American women with HIV infection constitute less than 2% of the worldwide burden of HIV in women. Early 1995 estimates of cumulative HIV infection worldwide include 17 to 23 million infected adults, of whom approximately 10 million are women. Although 7.8 million (over 75%) of these women reside in sub-Saharan Africa, which has an annual incidence rate of new HIV infections in women of 368/100,000, incidence rates are also high in the Caribbean (199/100,000), and Southeast Asia (141/100,000). In sub-Saharan Africa, both the incidence and the prevalence of HIV infection are higher in women than in men.

HIV infection, unheard of as a cause of death in U.S. women in 1981, is now the leading cause of death for women 25 to 44 years old in 17 United States cities and in many states. AIDS has been the leading cause of death for African-American women in that age group since 1989. The highest prevalence and incidence rates of AIDS in women occur in New York City, which accounts for 25% of the total AIDS cases in U.S. women. Although early in the HIV epidemic (1982 to 1987) AIDS in women was concentrated in urban areas, recent epidemiologic trends demonstrate rising incidence rates in smaller cities and rural areas, especially in the southeastern United States. Through December 1994, 58,428 women with AIDS in the United States have been reported to the Centers for Disease Control and Prevention (CDC), representing 13% of the cumulative U.S. AIDS caseload. The 14,081 women reported with AIDS in 1994 represent 18% of the total number of cases reported that year.

Worldwide, 90% of HIV-infected women have acquired their infection heterosexually. In the United States most women are infected through their own injection drug use (IDU) or through heterosexual exposure. Currently, heterosexual transmission continues to rise more rapidly than other types of exposure for women. From 1981 through 1986, approximately 1800 women with AIDS were reported to the CDC; 21% had acquired infection heterosexually and 52% through injection drug use. In 1994, 14,081 women with AIDS were reported to the CDC; 41% had acquired infection through injection drug use and 38% through heterosexual exposure. Nineteen percent had no specific HIV exposure. There is considerable evidence in developed countries that HIV is more efficiently transmitted sexually from men to women compared with the reverse. Studies have demonstrated a 3- to 18-fold increased rate of transmission from males to females. This difference in efficiency of transmission by gender of the index case has not been demonstrated in Africa. It has been suggested that the presence of genital ulcers results in greater enhancement of female-to-male transmission than the reverse. Thus, the high prevalence of genital ulcer disease in Africa could result in the observed equal rates of transmission by gender of the index case.

NATURAL HISTORY OF HIV DISEASE IN WOMEN AND ITS IMPLICATIONS FOR MANAGEMENT

Although the natural history of HIV infection in women remains poorly defined through mid-1995, preliminary information provides no cogent evidence that the disease course in women differs substantially from that in men. Conflicting data exist concerning the relative prevalence by gender of AIDS-defining conditions and possible differences in survival after a diagnosis of AIDS is made; however, most large studies have demonstrated minimal or no gender differences in disease progression by any measure. Indeed, data are conflicting concerning whether a survival advantage, if it occurs, accrues to women or to men. Gynecologic disease, however, may differ in multiple ways from that in HIV-uninfected women.

AIDS-Defining Conditions

Although a few small studies have found *Pneumocystis carinii* pneumonia (PCP) to occur in less than 20% of women with AIDS, with concomitant higher rates of *Candida* esophagitis and cryptococcal meningitis, nearly all large data sets indicate that PCP is the most common AIDS-defining diagnosis in women, as it is in men, in the United States. PCP is nearly unknown in much of Africa in either gender.

The CDC has reported that among all United States cases of AIDS through 1990, the only significant gender differences in AIDS-defining illnesses, excluding Kaposi's sarcoma, were *Candida* esophagitis (occurring 50% more frequently in women) and opportunistic herpesvirus infections (occurring 32% more frequently in women). Investigators in New York City found very similar results in a clinical study of 800 women and men in the Bronx, New York. In all studies, Kaposi's sarcoma is severalfold more common in men because of its high prevalence in homosexual men.

Survival with AIDS

Through mid-1991 all reports suggested a moderate to marked gender difference in survival with AIDS, with the survival advantage always accruing to men. Recent data from the Community Program for Clinical Research on AIDS also found a moderate survival disadvantage in women. However, from 1991 through 1994, there have been several reports suggesting little or no male survival advantage. In one European study male gender conferred a 2.5-fold increased risk of death. Three studies have suggested that shorter survival after a diagnosis of AIDS in women is highly associated with not receiving PCP prophylaxis and antiretroviral therapy.

CLINICAL MANAGEMENT OF HIV-INFECTED WOMEN

Thus, there is no cogent evidence suggesting that clinical management of HIV-infected women, with the exception of gynecologic screening and treatment, should differ significantly from that of HIV-infected men. Prophylactic therapy for PCP and *Mycobacterium avium* complex (MAC) disease should be provided to HIV-infected patients with impaired immune function without regard to gender. Similarly, the scant available evidence suggests that the efficacy of antiretroviral therapy is similar in women and men.

However, some authorities suggest that antifungal prophylaxis be provided to women differently from men. Specifically, providers who have demonstrated that there is a high rate of *Candida* esophagitis in their population of women patients with HIV infection have suggested that antifungal prophylaxis with fluconazole 100 mg daily by mouth be initiated when the CD4 cell count falls below $100/mm^3$. Other clinicians, in the absence of cogent evidence to guide therapy and in light of recent evidence demonstrating no survival benefit from fungal prophylaxis in men, feel that fungal prophylaxis specifically for women is not warranted. In our clinical practice systemic antifungal therapy is used to suppress frequently recurring *Candida* in any mucosal site (vagina, esophagus, oral), but is not used prophylactically.

GYNECOLOGIC DISEASE AND MANAGEMENT

While the majority of gynecologic manifestations occurring in women with HIV infection also occur in uninfected women, some general observations regarding their frequency and morbidity are summarized in Table 1.

Gynecologic screening can be incorporated into primary HIV clinical care by various routes. Guidelines for routine care are provided in Table 2. Consideration must be given to the extra time that is often required to take an ob/gyn history and

TABLE 1. *Gynecologic manifestations in HIV-infected women compared with non−HIV-infected women*

Condition	Increased frequency	Increased morbidity
Vaginitis	+	+
Urinary tract infection	−	?
Cervical dysplasia	+	+
Menstrual problems	?	−
Pelvic inflammatory disease	?	+
Genital herpes virus	+	+
Genital warts	+	+

perform the breast and pelvic examinations. Women often state a preference for a female gynecologic provider, but are also generally pleased when their usual primary care provider provides this type of care. Fragmentation of care is probably the largest factor contributing to poor gynecologic services for HIV-infected women. If gynecologic care is to be provided outside of the site where primary care services are provided, a mechanism for communication of results to the primary care provider must be established.

Cervical Cytologic Abnormalities

Multiple sources of data available since 1990 have indicated that women infected with HIV have a higher prevalence of cervical intraepithelial neoplasia (CIN) than do uninfected women. Recent data have indicated that HIV infection itself (odds

TABLE 2. *Routine gynecologic screening in HIV infection*

Annually
  Breast examination
  Mammography starting at age 50
  Papanicolaou smear if CD4>400
Every six months
  Pelvic examination
  Pap smear, if CD4<400
  STD screen: gonorrhea, chlamydia, VDRL
  Wet mount
Abnormal Pap smear
  Infection or inflammation: treat and repeat
  Atypia of undetermined significance: colposcopy
  Dysplasia: colposcopy
Patient education
  Rationale for frequent gynecologic visits and care
  Strategies for implementing safer sex with male and
    female partners
  Contraceptive counseling
  Information regarding pregnancy, perinatal transmission of
    HIV, and HIV testing of children at risk

ratio = 3.5) and HIV-related immune dysfunction as measured by CD4 cell counts (O.R. = 2.7), are both independently associated with CIN.

The accuracy of Papanicolaou (Pap) smears as a screening method for detecting cervical cancer in HIV-infected women has been questioned. However, recent data suggest that Pap smears in HIV-infected women have a sensitivity and specificity that fall well within the previously published ranges of sensitivity and specificity of Pap smears in a general population of women.

Our clinical guidelines for screening for cervical cytologic abnormalities include performing Pap smears annually for women with CD4 cell counts of more than 400/mm^3, but every 6 months if the CD4 cell count is less than 400/mm^3. In spite of the importance of such screening, these clinical guidelines should be altered as indicated for individual patients. For example, we may decide not to perform Pap smears at the recommended frequency for a woman who has had prior negative Pap smears, and whose HIV disease is in a very advanced stage with ongoing opportunistic processes that confer a poor prognosis.

Gynecologic Infections

Sexually Transmitted Diseases and HIV Transmission

There is clearly a need for female-controlled methods for reducing transmission of sexually transmitted diseases (STDs). Unfortunately, barrier methods, with or without spermicide, may cause local allergic or inflammatory reactions, which increase vaginal discomfort and may even cause abrasions or ulcerations. Intrauterine devices (IUDs) increase the risk of STD transmission and pelvic inflammatory disease to an unacceptable degree for women who are immunocompromised. In addition, IUDs often lead to heavy blood loss during menstruation.

HIV-infected women whose partners are also HIV-infected often ask whether they need to use barriers. Clinicians can point out that barriers offer some protection from the burden of other sexually transmitted infections such as chlamydia and herpes, which their sexual partner may harbor. Barriers may also prevent the back-and-forth transmission of silent human papillomavirus (HPV) infection, which may lead to cervical dysplasia. Providers should acknowledge the lack of specific information about the effect of repeated exposure to HIV through semen or vaginal secretions for an individual already HIV-infected. However, while reinfection may not technically occur, such exposure may cause local immune activation in the reproductive tract, which has been theorized to result in more rapid disease progression.

Clinical Management of Gynecologic Infections

Although there are no currently published data to provide definitive information concerning the association of HIV infection and gynecologic infections, preliminary results from multiple clinical studies indicate that the prevalence of treatable gynecologic infections among HIV-infected women receiving screening examinations is 50% to 70%. In some clinical settings this has included a 2% prevalence of both asymptomatic gonorrhea and asymptomatic *Chlamydia trachomatis* infections. These findings mandate that screening gynecologic care be provided for all HIV-infected women receiving primary care services for HIV infection.

Gynecologic infections may be an early sign of progression of HIV-related illness. These infections—genital ulcers (sometimes of unknown etiology), vaginitis, urinary tract infections, postpartum endometritis (which also may occur postabortion or postcryotherapy), and pelvic inflammatory disease (PID)—may be recurrent and difficult to treat. In general this may be a clue to underlying progression of immunodefiency. Thus, infections that have unusual presentations, are recurrent, or are refractory to treatment warrant close attention and follow-up.

In general, screening for and managing gynecologic infections includes taking an appropriate sexual history, asking about symptoms, performing speculum and bimanual examinations, and obtaining relevant laboratory specimens. It is also important to consider the woman's overall state of health, and the status of immune competence. Patients with low CD4 cell counts are often neutropenic, increasing their susceptibility to infection, and complicating response to treatment. Further, these women may not mount an elevated white blood cell count in response to systemic infection, rendering an important diagnostic test less useful. Erythrocyte sedimentation rates (ESR) are often elevated in chronic illness, and thus become a less useful clue in the diagnostic evaluation of acute infection, for example in PID. Some clinicians have observed that immunocompromised women with acute PID may present with fewer symptoms than their immunocompetent counterparts, even with more severe PID. Yet, other clinicians have noted that PID in HIV-infected women appears to have a more severe presentation and disease course. Consideration of the stage of HIV illness is a useful tool in planning treatment and follow-up, and must be clearly communicated when a gynecologic referral is made.

STDs should be treated following CDC guidelines, and tests of cure should be obtained. Treatment of sexual partners, where appropriate, should be arranged. Counseling regarding safer sex must be reinforced frequently, as a way to preserve overall health and freedom from the burden of new infections.

Based on anecdotal reports, full-course therapy is recommended for vaginitis and urinary tract infection, rather than any abbreviated course. For example, it is preferred to use a full 7-day course of topical metronidazole to treat *Trichomonas* vaginitis, or a full 7 days of antifungal topical treatment to treat vaginal candidiasis. Single-dose treatment of vaginal candidiasis with fluconazole (150 mg po) has not been evaluated in immunocompromised women, although we have found it to be effective in our clinical practice. It also seems prudent, whenever possible, to have the HIV-infected woman return to ascertain if the treatment has been successful, even in the case of a "minor" vaginitis or urinary tract infection. Strong consideration should be given to hospitalization of the immunocompromised woman with PID.

Particularly troublesome are the recurrent and hard to treat infections. Immune deficiency predisposes many women to recurrent outbreaks of genital herpes, which may eventually become resistant to acyclovir. Genital warts may rapidly turn into a florid infection that fails to respond to ordinary local treatments such as application of trichloroacetic acid. Vaginal candidiasis may recur, or fail to clear with local treatment. Each case merits an individual evaluation; however, it is important to be prepared to resort to aggressive therapy and supportive comfort measures. Patients may require lifelong treatment with acyclovir for persistent herpes lesions. Referral for cryotherapy, liquid nitrogen, or laser therapy may be required for treating difficult genital warts. Systemic antifungal agents often need to be used for treating and then preventing recurrent vaginal candidiasis. Further, the patient's comfort may depend on the clinician's familiarity with the safe use of "home remedies" such as sitz baths, soothing lotions and creams, nutritional considerations, and judicious use of pain medications. Persistence, sensitivity, and consideration on the part of the clinician is likely to be rewarded with improvement, or at least enhanced comfort, for these individuals.

Menstruation, Menopause, and Use of Exogenous Hormones

HIV-infected women frequently report changes in their menstrual cycles, and such problems can adversely affect a woman's health during HIV-related illness. Blood loss from heavy menses can predispose to or exacerbate anemia. Irregular or absent periods may signal significant systemic illness. Decreased estrogen levels may predispose a woman to vaginitis and urethritis, as well as cause discomforting "hot flushes," which may be mistaken for the "night sweats" common in HIV infection.

It is currently unclear if amenorrhea is more common in HIV-infected women. When present in a premenopausal female, amenorrhea may be due to various conditions such as pregnancy, ovarian cyst, thyroid disorder, pituitary tumor, premature ovarian failure, or autoimmune disease. It may be compounded by multiple other factors common in a cohort of HIV-infected women including stress, prescription medications, use of street drugs (particularly heroin), chronic illness, malnutrition, and weight loss. It remains to be clarified what, if any, effect antiviral agents such as zidovudine have on the menstrual cycle. Amenorrhea may be evaluated as described in Table 3.

The role of exogenous hormones as therapy or replacement in HIV infection has yet to be adequately addressed. In providing gynecologic care, it is common to prescribe estrogens, progestin, and combinations of both for various conditions. In HIV infection, attention must be given to potential interactions between exogenous hormones and the many drug therapies currently in use or being developed for use by these patients. Of particular concern are interactions with medications that are metabolized in the liver, including certain antibiotics, diphenylhydantoin, barbiturates, bronchodilating agents, and corticosteroids. It is unknown whether or not

TABLE 3. *Amenorrhea: decision tree*

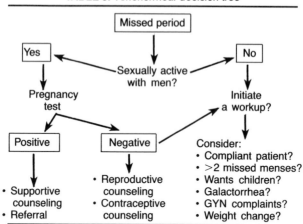

there are significant interactions with antiretrovirals. Another general concern is the effect of exogenous hormones on immune function. It is known that differences in male and female immune response are, at least in part, mediated by sex hormones (in particular, estrogens, progesterones, and testosterone). Physiologic replacement doses do not give rise to the same concerns as would the use of higher doses, such as the amount of progestin present in certain contraceptive preparations (injected or implanted progesterone). Megestrol acetate (Megace), a progestin used for HIV-associated wasting, may cause irregular vaginal bleeding.

Physiologic hormone replacement in natural, surgical, or premature menopause is indicated for symptoms of estrogen depletion such as hot flushes, atrophic vaginitis, urethritis, vaginal dryness and itching, and discomfort during urination. A combination of estrogen and progestin is always used when the uterus is present, in order to offset the risk for development of endometrial cancer from unopposed estrogens. Replacement hormones may also prevent osteoporosis and ischemic heart disease, and their use should be considered for HIV-infected women, as for all women, especially those whose HIV disease is in its early stages.

Reproductive and Sexual Health

HIV-infected women merit the same rights and access as other women to reproductive choices. Clinicians often admit to feelings of discomfort when HIV-infected patients express an interest in pregnancy, or admit to engaging in unprotected sexual activity. Providers deserve opportunities to discuss these complicated and difficult issues. It is helpful to recognize that HIV infection does not erase normal desires. It is also useful for clinicians to understand that setting aside value judgments in order to engage and help patients is not the same as abandoning one's own values.

Taking an appropriate and comprehensive sexual and reproductive history allows the medical provider many opportunities to educate, support, and intervene. It may also bring up difficult and unpredictable topics. For example, if asked, a history of childhood sexual abuse may be reported by many women. In fact, children who are sexually abused are at increased risk as adults of both substance abuse and acquiring HIV infection. A disclosure of this type provides the opportunity for offering support and assistance (Table 4).

Discussion of safer sexual practices and use of condoms should not be confused with the need to discuss reproductive control and choice. The clinician should describe the spectrum of contraceptive choices with women (Table 5) and provide the gynecologic care needed for appropriate use of the method selected.

It is important to keep in mind that intimate and sexual relationships for women may take place with women. Lesbian patients need to have their partners and families included in care planning, and clinicians need to know safer sex guidelines for women who have sex with women. A common response to discovery of HIV infection is for individuals (both male and female) to shun sexual relations for some period of time. This often is a symptom of depression and altered self-esteem and may be accompanied by poor appetite and sleep disturbance. HIV-infected individuals need support and encouragement to continue expression of healthy and safe relationships where affection and sexual intimacy are experienced.

The clinician may be the first person to whom an HIV-infected woman can talk frankly about these concerns. It is important to recognize sexual dysfunction as a normal initial response to learning one's HIV status. Patients may need to go through the established stages of grieving—both in anticipation of their own death and for the loss of their previous self-image as healthy and whole. The message that sexual dysfunction (like poor sleep and appetite) is most likely temporary and that sexual interest will resume is most hopeful, and sets the stage for teaching about safer sex practices.

TABLE 4. *Disclosure of sexual abuse*

Prior sexual abuse plays a role in current drug abuse, eating disorders, psychiatric disorders, adolescent pregnancy, and HIV transmission. In obtaining a history of sexual abuse, the provider is able to intervene in positive ways:
Provide assurance to the patient that any abuse that occurred was not her fault
Validate the experience of sexual abuse and reassure the individual that she is not alone
Assure the patient that she will be in control during the gynecologic examination
Assess if she is in a safe living situation at the present time
Assess if there are any children living with her who are currently at risk of sexual abuse
Incorporate the knowledge of the prior sexual abuse into current and future education regarding safer sexual practices
Make appropriate referrals for counseling, crisis intervention, safe housing, or other services

TABLE 5. *Contraceptive choices for HIV-infected women*

Oral contraceptives
    Pros   High contraceptive efficacy, menstrual regulation; decreased incidence of premen-
                  strual symptoms; decreased incidence of dysmenorrhea; scanty menstrual blood
                  losses; decreased menstrual-related anemia; theoretical decreased risk of PID,
                  arthritic syndromes, and acne; good treatment for dysfunctional bleeding
    Cons   Bothersome side effects in some women; contraindicated in smokers and in pa-
                  tients with undiagnosed vaginal bleeding, hypertension, blood clotting disorders
                  or liver disease; potential increased incidence of gingivitis, vaginitis, and respira-
                  tory infections; known and unknown interactions with other medications; possible
                  reduced immune function in immune compromised women; does not reduce
                  transmission of STDs
Condoms with spermicides
    Pros   Excellent choice when acceptable to both partners
    Cons   Allergic reaction to latex or spermicides by either partner; failure rate; product vari-
                  ability and requires more education in correct usage than generally
                  acknowledged
Diaphragm with spermicide or cervical cap
    Pros   Good contraceptive choice with most failures related to inexact usage
    Cons   Does not prevent (though may limit) transmission of STDs
Other barriers (creams, gels, suppositories, foams, sponges)
    Pros   Augments effectiveness of condoms
    Cons   Inadequate for contraception or STD prevention unless used with condoms; allergic
                  reactions of sensitivity
IUD (intrauterine device: loop, coil, Progestisert, Cooper-7)
    Pros   Easy to use, once inserted
    Cons   Risk of infections is high: *not* a good choice for immune compromised women
Surgical sterilization (bilateral tubal ligation)
    Pros   Excellent method of contraception for women who are certain that they will never
                  desire more children
    Cons   A decision for permanent sterilization should not be made in the early months (per-
                  haps the first year) after diagnosis of HIV infection; tubal ligation does not prevent
                  transmission of STDs; it should never be considered reversible
Norplant (progesterone implants)
    Pros   Contraceptive efficacy with long duration (5 years)
    Cons   Irregular bleeding; uncertain hormonal interactions in HIV infection; slight risk of in-
                  fection at site of insertion that may be increased in immune compromise;
                  uncertain interaction with medications commonly used in HIV infection
Depo-provera (intramuscular progesterone)
    Pros   Contraceptive efficacy with short duration (3 months)
    Cons   Inconvenience and discomfort of injections every 3 months; irregular bleeding; un-
                  certain hormonal interaction in HIV illness; uncertain interaction with medications
                  commonly used in HIV infection

HIV AND PREGNANCY

As discussed above, HIV infection per se does not erase the normal desires and hopes for a future with children among women and their families. Where possible, the medical provider should initiate a discussion about future plans for childbearing with all HIV-infected women. Given the epidemiology of HIV infection, women of childbearing age are disproportionately affected and face considerable obstacles in their reproductive decision making. When discussions of childbearing goals are conducted, interventions can be planned for couples that may in fact enhance the family's health. For example, in the HIV discordant couple in which the woman is HIV infected and her partner is not, strategies can be employed to reduce risk. The couple could inseminate the man's semen and reduce his risk of contracting HIV from unprotected intercourse. This can be done at home with simple instructions and without medical intervention. Reducing the male partner's risk of contracting HIV infection will increase the likelihood that the child will have at least one healthy parent. If the couple finds this unacceptable and is willing to risk transmission to the male, the partners can learn fertility awareness and limit his exposure.

The HIV discordant couple in which the male partner is infected can consider options such as adoption or insemination with sperm from a sperm bank or a male donor. Such couples should be advised that HIV transmission that occurs during a pregnancy (or perhaps in the attempt to achieve pregnancy) may greatly increase the risk of HIV transmission to the fetus. There are currently no available techniques to free sperm of HIV to make it safe for insemination, but such techniques may be developed in the future. Thus, for many reasons, it is imperative that health care providers who care for HIV-infected women and their families be well informed about all aspects of HIV infection and pregnancy and all factors that may affect perinatal transmission.

Currently, there are 15,000 to 20,000 HIV-infected children in the United States, with 7,000 infants born annually to HIV-infected women. Of these 7,000 HIV-exposed children, approximately 1,100 to 1,800 (15–25%) will be HIV-infected. It has been estimated that there will be 10 million HIV-infected children globally by the year 2000. The vast majority of these children are infected perinatally: during pregnancy, labor, delivery, or postpartum via breastfeeding. The risk of perinatal transmission has been associated with advanced disease stage, low CD4 cell count, and high viral burden.

Effect of Pregnancy on HIV

Although data are conflicting, there is a consensus that normal pregnancy is associated with a decrease in cell-mediated immunity, causing some concern that pregnancy may accelerate HIV disease progression. However, preliminary data suggest that pregnancy may have little effect on HIV disease progression. Some reports state that 45% to 75% of asymptomatic pregnant women develop symptoms 28 to 30 months postpartum. These studies are based on relatively short periods of follow-up. In the few studies in which infected pregnant women have been compared with infected nonpregnant women, little or no difference has been observed in the rates of clinical or immunologic deterioration. HIV-infected pregnant women need careful monitoring of CD4 cell counts and symptoms of systemic infection. Low CD4 cell counts have been shown to be predictive of the development of serious infections during pregnancy.

Effect of HIV-infection on Pregnancy

The majority of obstetrical problems that adversely affect perinatal outcome (preterm labor, intrauterine growth retardation, fetal distress, etc.) have not been demonstrated to be influenced by HIV infection. Some reports from Zaire, however, indicate that there is an increased risk of prematurity in women who are HIV-infected. Larger studies are needed to assess the impact of HIV on pregnancy.

Perinatal Transmission

Rates of transmission of HIV from a pregnant woman to her baby range from 15% to 30% and vary geographically, with the highest rates in Africa (30%), and the lowest in Europe (15%). Perinatal transmission rates in United States studies range from 18% to 26%. Multiple factors have been found to be associated with the rate of maternal-infant HIV transmission. In one study of 30 HIV-infected women, those with a high viral burden (>190,000 copies of HIV RNA/ml blood) were more likely to transmit HIV to their infants than women with lower viral burden (80% vs. 0%). Maternal seroconversion with its associated high titer viremia has been found to be associated with elevated rates of vertical transmission. Advanced HIV immune suppression in the mother, as evidenced by decreased CD4 cell counts or by symptomatic clinical disease, has been associated with increased rates of vertical transmission. Intriguing recent reports from Africa have demonstrated a strong association between maternal vitamin A deficiency and higher rates of mother-to-infant transmission of HIV.

A multicenter, randomized, placebo-controlled trial has demonstrated a substantial reduction in the risk of perinatal HIV-1 transmission when zidovudine (ZDV) was administered to HIV-infected pregnant women during late pregnancy and intrapartum, and to their infants in the early neonatal period (first 6 weeks after birth). This study demonstrated a 67.5% reduction in mother-to-child transmission in the treated compared with the placebo group (8.3% vs. 25.5%). The study included women who had not previously received long-term ZDV therapy, were in early stages of HIV disease, and had access to prenatal care. It is thus unclear whether a comparable protective effect occurs for women with CD4 cell counts less than $200/mm^3$ or for those who may harbor ZDV-resistant HIV strains because of prior long-term therapy with ZDV.

Communicating the hopeful news that ZDV may reduce transmission may be interpreted by patients that they are now able to have a baby "safely." It is important to emphasize to HIV-infected women contemplating childbearing that although use of ZDV may reduce the risk of perinatal transmission, it does not eliminate this risk. The medical and support staff must keep abreast of information regarding transmission as it develops, reminding women that at this time there are no guarantees. Reproductive counseling should be conducted as with inheritable illnesses, that is, in a nonjudgmental manner.

Other pharmacologic strategies to influence vertical transmission of HIV are currently under active investigation, utilizing both active and passive immune mechanisms. These include use of HIVIG (an immunoglobulin obtained from asymptomatic HIV-infected individuals), vaccines, and monoclonal antibodies.

OBSTETRICAL MANAGEMENT

It is of primary importance to provide the HIV-infected pregnant woman with the appropriate background for an informed reproductive choice. If she chooses to continue her pregnancy, the antepartum care should be tailored to her specific needs with ample psychosocial supportive services made available. All routine antepartum tests need to be done including tests for hepatitis B antigen and screening for tuberculosis and cutaneous anergy. Baseline antibody titers for *Toxoplasma gondii* should be obtained as with all pregnant women. Hepatitis B, pneumococcal, and influenza vaccines may be safely administered during pregnancy to susceptible individuals. CD4 cell counts should be closely monitored during pregnancy and PCP prophylaxis started for counts below $200/mm^3$, utilizing trimethoprim/sulfamethoxazole (TMP/SMX) in standard dose or inhaled pentamidine. Neonatal kernicterus has not been observed in newborns whose mothers received TMP/SMX.

Guidelines for the use of ZDV in pregnancy have been published by the U.S. Public Health Service (Table 6) and should be discussed with HIV-infected pregnant women. Clinicians should offer oral ZDV therapy after 14 but before 34 weeks of gestation. ZDV therapy should continue during the entire antepartum period, should be administered intravenously in appropriate doses intrapartum, and should be

TABLE 6. *Recommended use of zidovudine to reduce the risk of mother-to-child HIV transmission*

Maternal therapy
    Second and third trimester 100 mg PO 5 doses/day; therapy should start as early in the second trimester as possible; monitor CBC at 2 weeks, 4 weeks, then monthly, creatinine and liver function tests (LFTs) monthly
Intrapartum
    Intravenous ZDV during labor and delivery in a 2 mg/kg loading dose over ½ to 1 hour followed by continuous infusion of 1 mg/kg per hour until the cord is clamped
    For patients undergoing induction of labor, intravenous therapy should begin at the time induction of labor begins; for an elective cesarean section, intravenous therapy should begin 4 hours before the time of surgery
Newborn
    ZDV syrup, 2 mg/kg PO 4 doses/day for 6 weeks; therapy should start within 8 to 12 hours of birth
    If the infant remains NPO and cannot begin oral ZDV within 8 to 12 hours of life, intravenous ZDV (1.5 mg/kg over ½ hour every 6 hours) can be given
    At present, there is insufficient pharmacokinetic information to recommend dose modifications for premature infants

ZDV, zidovudine (AZT).

given by oral suspension to the neonate for the first 6 weeks of life. Mothers should be monitored with a complete blood count at 2 weeks and 4 weeks, and then monthly, and with monthly liver function tests and creatinine determinations. ZDV appears to be well tolerated by mothers and their infants; the only observed short-term infant toxicity was a decrease in mean hemoglobin of approximately 1g/dl. Because many investigators believe that as many as 50% of HIV-infected infants acquire HIV intrapartum, intravenous ZDV during labor and oral ZDV for the new-born may be considered even when maternal therapy has not been implemented before the onset of labor.

While these results represent hope for HIV-infected pregnant women and their families, the decision to initiate this protocol must rest with the pregnant woman. Overzealous pressure to use ZDV during pregnancy may be interpreted by patients as coercive, in disregard for their autonomy to decide what is the best course of action. It also should be explained to all pregnant women that this protocol may or may not benefit women who do not fit the profile of women who enrolled in the original trial, particularly women who are not ZDV naive or who have CD4 cell counts below 200/mm^3. Further, the long-term safety of this regimen for children remains unknown.

Clinicians should as much as possible avoid invasive procedures (e.g., amniocentesis, fetal scalp sampling, internal scalp electrodes, periumbilical cord blood sampling, etc.) during labor because of the risk posed to the fetus by direct contact with maternal blood or secretions. In general, amniotomy should be reserved for situations in which the information obtained would markedly benefit the laboring patient. Finally, women in labor should be carefully assessed initially and periodically for any signs of chorioamnionitis, and antibiotics initiated as needed.

It is well documented that HIV infection of the fetus can occur early in pregnancy. However, it is felt with HIV, as with hepatitis B, that a substantial proportion of mother-to-infant transmission occurs intrapartum, and thus could perhaps be prevented by cesarean delivery. No single study of mother-to-child transmission of HIV (none of which was designed to address mode of transmission) has demonstrated a statistically significant association of cesarean delivery with a lower rate of vertical transmission. However, a metanalysis of the association of cesarean delivery and rates of vertical transmission was performed by Villari et al. of seven studies (six prospective, one retrospective). In all of the reports the odds ratio was less than 1.0 and overall the odds ratio was 0.69 with a 95% confidence interval of 0.51 to 0.94, thus supporting a hypothesis of a protective effect. HIV infection alone, however, is not currently considered to be an indication for cesarean delivery.

Postpartum care should be tailored to the individual woman's needs. Although there is little information regarding the postpartum course in HIV-infected women, no differences between HIV-infected and -uninfected women have been noted. Data suggest that breast-feeding confers a risk of mother-to-infant transmission equal to that of pregnancy, labor, and delivery. Women in developed countries should be made aware of this risk, and should be advised not to breast-feed their babies. The mother and child should be referred for ongoing care to physicians with expertise in HIV primary care.

SUGGESTED READING

Anastos K, Greenblatt R. Epidemiology and natural history of HIV infection among women. *HIV Adv Res Ther* 1994;4(3):11–20.

Anastos K, Vermond S. Epidemiology and natural history of HIV infection among women. In: Kurth A, ed. *Until the cure: caregiving for women with HIV*. New Haven: Yale University Press, 1992.

Carpenter CCJ, Mayer KH, Stein M, Leibman BD, Fisher A, Fiore TC. Human immunodeficiency virus infection in North American women: experience with 200 cases and a review of the literature. *Medicine* 1991;70:307–325.

Centers for Disease Control and Prevention. Update: acquired immunodeficiency syndrome—United States, 1992. *MMWR* 1993;2:547–557.

Centers for Disease Control and Prevention. Heterosexually acquired AIDS—United States, 1993. *MMWR* 1994;43:155–159.

Centers for Disease Control and Prevention. Update: AIDS among women—United States, 1994. *MMWR* 1995;44:81–84.

Conference Abstracts. HIV infection in women: setting a new agenda. February 1995. Washington D.C., available from Philadelphia Sciences Group, Publishing Division 11232 Midlothian Turnpike, Suite 325, Richmond, Virginia 23235-9620.

Connor EM, Sperling RS, Gelber R, et al., for the Pediatric AIDS Clinical Trial Group protocol 076 study group. Reduction of maternal-infant transmission of human immunodeficiency virus type 1 with zidovudine treatment. *N Engl J Med* 1994;331:1173–1180.

Denenberg R. *Gynecologic care manual for HIV positive women*. Durant, OK: Essential Medical Information System, 1993.

Mann J, Tarantola D, eds. *AIDS in the world*, vol. 2, Global AIDS Policy Coalition. London, New York: Oxford University Press, in press.

Minkoff H, DeHovitz JA. Care of women infected with the human immunodeficiency virus. *JAMA* 1991;266:2253–2258.

Minkoff H, DeHovitz JA, Duerr A, eds. *HIV infection in women*. New York: Raven Press, 1995.

Padian NS, Shiboski G, Jewell N. Female-to-male transmission of human immunodeficiency virus. *JAMA* 1991;266:1664–1667.

Schoenbaum E, Webber MP. The underrecognition of HIV infection in women in an inner city emergency room. *Am J Public Health* 1993;83:363–368.

Wright TC, Ellerbrock TV, Chiasson MA, Van Devanter N, Sun X, and the New York Cervical Disease Study. Cervical intraepithelial neoplasia in women infected with human immunodeficiency virus: prevalence, risk factors, and validity of papanicolaou smears. *Obstet Gynecol* 1994;84:591–597.

A Clinical Guide to AIDS and HIV,
edited by Gary P. Wormser.
Lippincott-Raven Publishers, Philadelphia © 1996.

4

HIV Infection in Infants, Children, and Adolescents

Samuel Grubman and *James Oleske

*Departments of Pediatrics and Pediatric Allergy and Immunology, Saint Vincent's Hospital and Medical Center, New York, New York 10011; and *Division of Allergy Immunology and Infectious Diseases, University of Medicine and Dentistry of New Jersey/New Jersey Medical School, Newark, New Jersey 07103*

In a discussion of HIV infection in infants, children, and adolescents, it is inevitable that comparisons should be made with HIV infection in adults. In the various age groups, there are differences in the disease's epidemiology and transmission, diagnosis, clinical manifestations, prognosis, and treatment. This chapter gives an overview of pediatric HIV infection, with an emphasis on those aspects of disease that differ between adults and younger people. It also addresses the question of developing standards of care for children with HIV infection and social issues complicating the delivery of care.

EPIDEMIOLOGY AND TRANSMISSION

In the United States, 6611 cases of pediatric AIDS (birth to 13 years of age) had been reported through the end of June 1995 to the Centers for Disease Control and Prevention (CDC). Perinatal transmission accounts for 89% of all cases of AIDS in this age group. Virtually all new cases of HIV infection in infants occur as a result of perinatal transmission. Using an estimated average perinatal transmission rate of 24.5%, over 5,000 HIV-infected infants have been born in the United States over the past three years. The estimated total number of HIV-infected children in the United States is currently between 10,000 and 20,000.

The rate of increase in new AIDS cases in the pediatric age group is increasing at an alarming rate. A 23.6% increase in pediatric AIDS cases occurred in 1993 compared with 1992.

Adolescence is a developmental stage of life normally characterized by experimentation, risk taking, and sexual exploration within the context of feelings of invulnerability. This makes it a uniquely high-risk period for acquisition of HIV. Although fewer than 1% of the reported cases of AIDS in the United States have been among adolescents, the impact of HIV disease in this age group is more serious than this figure might suggest. Of all reported AIDS cases in the United States through June 1995, 18% were among those aged 20 to 29, with 4% of the total among those aged 20 to 24. The latency period from the acquisition of HIV infection to the development of AIDS in adults suggests that a significant proportion of HIV-infected young adults under 29 acquired their infection as teenagers. In sub-Saharan Africa, it is estimated that 75% of all new cases of HIV infection occur in individuals less than 20 years of age. In the United States, an analysis of the age of acquisition of HIV using a "back-calculation" model revealed that the median age of acquisition of HIV fell from over 30 years in 1980, to 25 years during the period from 1987 to 1991 and that during this same time 25% of newly infected people were under the age of 22 years. Seroprevalence data from the Job Corps in the United States indicate that disadvantaged and out-of-school youth are at highest risk for HIV infection.

The rising rates of other sexually transmitted diseases and unplanned pregnancies among adolescents are suggestive of a substantial risk for sexually transmitted HIV infection in this age group. Of the 12 million people nationally who contracted a sexually transmitted disease in 1991, two-thirds were under the age of 25. Sexual exposure, including heterosexual, homosexual, bisexual, and sexual abuse, has been a prominent mode of HIV transmission among adolescents with AIDS, with heterosexual transmission the identified risk factor in 33% of adolescent females with AIDS and homosexual transmission in 42% of adolescent males diagnosed with AIDS in 1993. While intravenous drug use is relatively uncommon among adolescents, the disinhibiting effects of drug use—particularly alcohol, cocaine, and crack—as well as the cost of dependence result in increased sexual risk taking, including prostitution, and contribute to the further spread of HIV. In the United States, the cumulative male-to-female ratio of reported AIDS cases among adolescents is approximately 2.2:1, reflecting the influence of cases of AIDS among patients with hemophilia.

Transmission from mother to infant (vertical transmission) can occur both prenatally and at the time of delivery. Studies done with fetal tissue suggest that prenatal transmission of HIV can occur as early as the eighth week of gestation. HIV has been cultured as early as the 12th week of gestation from fetal brain, thymus, liver, spleen, and lung and has been identified using other techniques in fetal brain tissue as early as 14 weeks gestation. Although the actual mixing of maternal and fetal circulation is prevented by the placenta, cellular elements and soluble factors can cross the placenta. CD4 positive cells have been demonstrated in the lining of the stroma of the chorionic villi, which is in close contact with maternal blood. HIV-specific immunoglobulin (Ig)A-containing immune complexes have been documented in amniotic fluid. The fact that up to a third of infants present with AIDS-defining symptoms in the first 2 years of life is consistent with early prenatal infection in these infants.

There is now ample evidence that HIV transmission also occurs, perhaps in the majority of perinatally infected infants, during the peripartum period. Serial serologic evaluations of infants has documented the appearance of HIV-specific IgM, IgG3, and IgG1 antibodies in some who lacked HIV-specific IgM antibodies at birth, thereby providing evidence for HIV transmission around the time of delivery. Only 35% to 50% of infected infants test positive for HIV by culture or polymerase chain reaction (PCR) of peripheral blood within the first week of life, and fewer than one in four have a positive p24 antigen capture assay. In a small study on eight HIV-infected neonates, immune complex dissociated p24 antigen was detected in cord blood in 63%. By 3 months of age, however, over 90% of infected infants have a positive HIV culture and PCR, suggesting an increased viral load consistent with peripartum infection and ensuing viremia. HIV transmission at the time of delivery is most likely associated with exposure to maternal body fluids, including blood and vaginal secretions. This is supported by recent studies evaluating the impact of the mode of delivery on transmission rates. Data from the European Collaborative Study of 1,254 maternal-infant pairs indicated that the odds of transmission of HIV via C-section relative to vaginal delivery are about 0.5. An earlier study, however, did not support a lower rate of transmission with C-sections. A UCLA-based study of 68 maternal-infant pairs found increased risk of transmission with increased peripartum exposure to maternal blood such as with fetal scalp monitoring, episiotomy, or severe lacerations. A study of HIV transmission to twins reported an increased transmission rate to the first-born of twins, implying significant peripartum transmission with the first-born having increased exposure to maternal secretions at the time of delivery. This mode of transmission is consistent with the documented peripartum transmission of other blood-borne viruses, such as hepatitis B virus. Studies evaluating the rate of transmission of HIV from mother to infant have yielded estimates ranging between 13% and 58%, with transmission rates varying by geographic location with lower transmission rates reported from industrialized countries compared with developing countries. A meta-analysis of 21 independent transmission studies revealed an estimated perinatal transmission rate of 24.5%.

Why some infants become infected and others do not is not yet known; ongoing research is investigating whether there are maternal factors that can predict the likelihood of perinatal transmission. Studies evaluating the impact of maternal antibody against gp120 on transmission rates have been inconsistent with several studies indicating an inverse correlation and others showing no correlation. A study looking at the ability of maternal antibodies to neutralize autologous virus showed that neutralizing antibodies are more frequently found in mothers who do not transmit HIV perinatally compared with transmitting mothers. Women who are more immunocompromised (lower CD4 count and increased p24 antigenemia) or symptomatic with HIV-related disease at the time of delivery seem to be more likely to transmit infection to their newborns. This is consistent with the belief that the main determinant of transmission is the level of maternal viral burden at the time of pregnancy and delivery. The risk of perinatal transmission appears to be greatest at the time of initial maternal infection prior to the development of HIV-specific immunity and coincident with high levels of viremia, and at the later stages of disease when viremia increases and HIV-specific immunity wanes.

The impact of the use of antiretroviral therapy on perinatal transmission has recently been investigated in the AIDS Clinical Trial Group (ACTG) study 076—a randomized, double blind, and placebo-controlled trial of zidovudine to prevent HIV transmission from mothers to their infants. HIV-infected pregnant women with $CD4^+$ lymphocyte counts over 200 cells/µl and not on antiretroviral therapy were randomized to receive either zidovudine or placebo. The zidovudine regimen consisted of 100 mg orally five times daily initiated at 14 to 34 weeks' gestation, 2 mg/kg intravenously over 1 hour at the beginning of labor followed by 1 mg/kg/hour intravenous drip until delivery, and 2 mg/kg/dose orally every 6 hours to the newborn for the first 6 weeks of life. An interim analysis of the first 364 births revealed a transmission rate of 8.3% in the zidovudine group versus 25.5% in the placebo group, or a 67.5% reduction in the risk for HIV transmission with zidovudine ($p = .00006$). The study was terminated after this review and all of the enrolled women were offered antiretroviral therapy.

In a smaller study of 68 infants born to HIV-infected mothers, 26 were given zidovudine during pregnancy and/or labor. Only three of these 26 women had been on antiretroviral therapy prior to conception. One of 26 (4%) women who received zidovudine transmitted HIV to her infant compared with 12 of 42 (28.6%) women who did not receive zidovudine. None of the infants in this study had received postpartum zidovudine.

The results of these studies are consistent with our current understanding of the impact of maternal viral load on perinatal transmission given the documented reduction in p24 antigenemia and increase in $CD4^+$ lymphocyte counts during initial therapy with zidovudine. Whether or not this documented reduction in transmission will hold true for women who are chronically on antiretroviral therapy or have more profound immunodeficiency ($CD4^+$ lymphocyte count <200 cells/µl) needs to be further evaluated. The role of vaginal topical treatments as well as local (mucosal) and systemic HIV vaccines is another urgent area for research. Likewise, HIV-infected pregnant women should be considered as an appropriate group to be offered participation in clinical trials.

Postpartum transmission of HIV infection from mother to newborn via breast-feeding has been reported and documented in women who acquired HIV infection after delivery through sexual relations and blood transfusion. In an Australian cohort of 11 women with documented postpartum acquisition of HIV who were breast-feeding their newborns, three transmitted HIV to their infants yielding an estimated risk of 27% for breast-feeding during primary maternal HIV infection. These cases may be accounted for by the significant HIV viremia and presumed increased infectivity in the first 3 to 6 months after acquisition of HIV infection. Whether breast-feeding is a significant mode of transmission in women who are already HIV infected during pregnancy and clinically stable has recently been elucidated. A meta-analysis of studies with varying perinatal transmission rates from different parts of the world suggests that breast-feeding increases the rate of perinatal transmission of HIV by 14% (95% CI 7–22%). The risk-benefit ratio for breast-feeding in HIV-infected women is affected by the infant mortality rate associated with infectious disease or malnutrition in conjunction with the relative risk for bottle-fed infants. Where sterile formula is readily available, this ratio is clearly in favor of bottle-feeding, and infected women should bottle-feed rather than breast-feed their infants. However, for parts of Africa and many other Third-World areas, the situation is much less clear and favors breast-feeding in areas where the infant mortality attributable to bottle-feeding is greater than 1 in 7.

Iatrogenic acquisition of HIV through transfusions and the use of unsterile needles is an ongoing problem in many countries in which blood products are not screened and disposable needles are not used. Recent reports of hospital-acquired HIV infection in Romania and the former Soviet Union are examples of this continuing problem. Over 200,000 children are sexually abused in the United States each year, and sexual abuse of infants, children, and adolescents is a documented mode of transmission of HIV infection. Despite this, sexual transmission of HIV is not a reportable category of HIV exposure for children and many barriers exist to identifying children infected with HIV through sexual abuse. None of 63 U.S. sexual abuse evaluation centers recently surveyed had a protocol for HIV testing. A study from Duke University reported that 14.6% of the HIV-infected children followed had been sexually abused. In this study sexual abuse was found to be prevalent in HIV-infected children irrespective of whether it was the documented mode of transmission, a fact that has important implications for siblings of children who are known to be HIV infected. Among 15 sexually abused children and adolescents with a known HIV-infected attacker seen at Children's Hospital AIDS Program (CHAP) in Newark, New Jersey, three became infected.

DIAGNOSIS

In adolescents and children older than 18 months, definitive diagnosis of HIV infection is made in the same way as it is in adults, by using the enzyme-linked immunoadsorbent assay (ELISA) and confirmatory Western blot assays. These provide serologic evidence of a humoral immune response to HIV by detecting HIV-specific IgG antibodies. However, since maternal IgG antibody is transferred to infants across the placenta, all infants born to HIV-infected women have a positive ELISA at birth. An IgG antibody response cannot be used to diagnose HIV infection definitively in infants until they are 18 months of age, when maternal antibody is no longer present and the infants' own humoral immune response should have been mounted. To determine infection status prior to 18 months, several direct viral detection assays are currently being used, including HIV viral culture, PCR, the standard p24 antigen capture assay, and the immune complex dissociated p24 antigen capture assay.

Viral culture is performed on peripheral blood mononuclear cells cocultured with uninfected mononuclear cells that can support HIV growth and detect latent HIV-infected cells by stimulating viral replication. Evidence of p24 antigen or reverse transcriptase activity indicates the presence of HIV in such samples. The sensitivity of this test is age dependent, exceeding 90% in infants by 3 months of age and nearly 100% by 6 months of age. The PCR assay facilitates the detection of minute amounts of HIV proviral DNA that has become incorporated into the DNA of infected cells. The sensitivity and specificity of PCR as a diagnostic tool is similar to HIV culture, and like HIV culture has a sensitivity of over 90% by 3 months and close to 100% by 6 months of age. The use of these assays for diagnostic purposes has been recommended for infants born to HIV-infected women, after 1 month of age. A presumptive diagnosis of HIV infection can be made with one positive HIV culture or PCR assay on non-cord blood and a definitive diagnosis made with a confirmatory test on a different blood sample. HIV infection can be reasonably excluded with two negative HIV cultures or PCR results, both of which are performed at ≥ one month of age, and one of which is performed at 24 months of age. The current standard of care requires a negative HIV ELISA and Western blot at 18 months of age to rule out HIV infection definitively.

While the ELISA assay tests for anti-HIV antibody, the antigen capture assay tests directly for the HIV p24 antigen levels in serum. There have been isolated false-positive antigen capture assay results reported in infancy and the question remains whether it is possible that viral particles can be transferred from mother to infant without actual infection ensuing. After the first few weeks of life, though, this test is very specific and can be used to help establish the diagnosis if it is positive. Antigen capture is not at all sensitive, with less than 50% of infected infants positive in the first year of life. Thus, it cannot be used to rule out HIV infection, and although it is available and relatively easy to run, it is not the assay of choice in diagnosing infants. The reason for the low sensitivity of the standard p24 antigen capture assay is that maternal HIV-specific IgG antibody can result in antibody excess immune complexes that cause a negative result. Through a modification in the assay that involves immune complex dissociation (ICD), the sensitivity of this assay has been greatly enhanced while maintaining its specificity. Although the ICD p24 antigen capture assay can be used as an alternative to HIV culture and PCR to help establish a diagnosis in infancy, because of the lack of published data it should not be used to rule out HIV infection at this time.

Non-IgG serologic assays are being investigated as less-expensive alternatives to HIV culture and PCR. These assays would be potentially more useful in developing countries since they require less sophisticated laboratory technology. Anti-HIV IgM and IgA assays are capable of detecting infant antibody responses because these classes of antibody do not cross the placenta. IgM antibody testing has certain inherent problems that have limited its usefulness, including the relatively short duration of the IgM response resulting in a limited window of positivity and the possibility that maternal passively transferred IgG directed against infant IgM (reagin antibody) may cause false-positive reactions. In contrast, there has been more success using the HIV-specific IgA assay. The sensitivity of this assay is low at birth but increases with age to about 50% at 3 months and 70–95% by 6 months of age. *In vitro* antibody production is a functional assay that looks for anti-HIV antibody production by an infant's lymphocytes. Research on its development is ongoing and has met with some success.

Unfortunately, viral-specific diagnostic assays are not universally available to practitioners, especially those outside of major medical centers in the United States and in developing countries, and a presumptive diagnosis frequently requires correlating clinical symptomatology with surrogate laboratory parameters in HIV-exposed infants. The 1987 CDC classification system for HIV infection for infants defined an HIV-infected infant using HIV-specific clinical symptomatology in conjunction with laboratory evidence of both cellular and humoral immune dysfunction. The most frequently used laboratory parameter of immune function is the CD4$^+$ lymphocyte count. In infants and children as in adults, a depressed CD4$^+$ lymphocyte count or reversed CD4/CD8 ratio is indicative of immunocompromise. However, healthy infants and children normally have much higher counts than healthy adults (Table 1). The median CD4$^+$ lymphocyte count for adults in a sample of uninfected subjects was 1027, while the median CD4$^+$ lymphocyte count for infants 1 to 6 months of age in the same study was 3211 and for those 7 to 12 months of age 3128. Whereas the absolute number of CD4$^+$ lymphocytes is higher in infants and children, the percentage of CD4$^+$ lymphocytes is relatively stable from infancy to adulthood with a normal median value of approximately 50%. It is important to be familiar with the normal age-specific lymphocyte counts when evaluating the immune status of infants and children. The revised 1994 CDC Pediatric HIV Classification System includes three immunologic categories of HIV-infected children based on age-adjusted CD4$^+$ cell values (Table 2).

Most infants and children with HIV infection have hypergammaglobulinemia, which is indicative of polyclonal B-cell activation. Hypergammaglobulinemia has been described as the most common laboratory abnormality in HIV-infected children, followed by a reversal of CD4/CD8 ratio. Normal immunoglobulin levels in

TABLE 1. *Normal CD4 lymphocyte counts for children*

	Age (months)				
	1–6	7–12	13–24	25–74	Adults
Absolute CD4 count					
Meidan	3211	3128	2601	1668	1027
Range	1153–5285	967–5289	739–4463	505–2831	237–1817
Percent CD4					
Median	51.6	47.9	45.8	42.1	50.9
Range	36.3–67.1	32.8–63.0	31.2–60.4	32.2–52.0	34.7–67.1
CD4/CD8 ratio					
Median	2.2	2.1	2.0	1.4	1.7
Range	0.9–3.5	0.8–3.4	0.6–3.4	0.7–2.1	0.4–3.0

TABLE 2. *1994 revised classification system for human immunodeficiency virus infection in children under 13 years of age: immune categories*

	0–11 months	1–5 years	6–12 years
No evidence of suppression	CD4≥1500 ≥25%	CD4≥1000 ≥25%	CD4≥500 ≥25%
Evidence of moderate suppression	CD4 750–1499 15–24%	CD4 500–999 15–24%	CD4 200–499 15–24%
Severe suppression	CD4<750 <15%	CD4<500 <15%	CD4<200 <15%

infants and children are also age specific and need to be considered when evaluating a child for hypergammaglobulinemia. Elevated β_2-microglobulin and neopterin levels have been reported in HIV-infected children. Other laboratory abnormalities seen in pediatric HIV infection (some of them nonspecific) include (a) hypogammaglobulinemia, seen in 3–5% of cases; (b) anemia, which is usually secondary to chronic disease and has been associated with disease progression (other causes such as iron deficiency, sickle cell, and lead toxicity must be ruled out); (c) thrombocytopenia, seen in about 10–20% of HIV-infected children and documented to be associated with antiplatelet antibody in 80% of these; and (d) leukopenia. Other clinical manifestations possibly indicative of pediatric HIV infection are discussed below. The laboratory abnormalities seen in adolescent HIV infection are similar to those seen in adults and discussed elsewhere in this volume.

CLINICAL MANIFESTATIONS

HIV in infants and children is a chronic disease with multiorgan system involvement; indeed, there is probably not an organ system that is not affected by HIV. As in adults, HIV disease presents in infants and children with a broad spectrum of manifestations, some of them specific to young people. The newly revised CDC classification system of HIV disease in children divides children into four clinical categories: (a) N—no signs/symptoms, (b) A—mild signs/symptoms, (c) B—moderate signs/symptoms, and (d) C—severe signs/symptoms (Table 3). Most of the symptomatic clinical manifestations of pediatric HIV disease are related to either direct HIV infection or the immunosuppression secondary to it. There is a wide range of clinical symptomatology from common nonspecific findings to severe manifestations of common childhood illnesses, AIDS-defining conditions, and end-organ dysfunction.

Common signs and symptoms seen in children with HIV infection that are not AIDS defining include lymphadenopathy, hepatomegaly, splenomegaly, parotitis, recurrent diarrhea, failure to thrive, and recurrent fevers. It is important to evaluate children for specific infectious etiologies for these conditions, although HIV or the ensuing immunodeficiency may be the sole cause. Common oropharyngeal signs

TABLE 3. *1994 revised classification system for human immunodeficiency virus infection in children under 13 years of age*

	Clinical categories			
	(N) No signs/ symptoms[a]	(A) Mild signs/ symptoms[b]	(B) Moderate signs/ symptoms[c]	(C) Severe signs/ symptoms[d]
No evidence of suppression	N1	A1	B1	C1
Evidence of moderate suppression	N2	A2	B2	C2
Severe suppression	N3	A3	B3	C3

Children whose HIV infection is not confirmed are classified using the above system with a letter E (perinatally Exposed) before the classification (e.g., "E/N2").

[a]No signs or symptoms or only one of those in category A.

[b]Two or more of the following: lymphadenopathy, hepatomegaly, splenomegaly, dermatitis, parotitis, recurrent or persistent upper respiratory infection or sinusitis, recurrent or persistent otitis media.

[c]Symptomatic conditions not listed in category A or C (including LIP).

[d]Any of the conditions in the 1987 surveillance case definition of AIDS with the exception of LIP, which is in category B.

include persistent thrush, severe painful gingivitis, HIV-specific periodontal disease, recurrent aphthous stomatitis, and recurrent herpetic gingivostomatitis. Some of these conditions are extremely common, and as with adults, lymphoproliferation manifesting as lymphadenopathy may be the first objective sign of disease.

As is true in other immunosuppressed conditions, children with HIV infection may have severe manifestations of relatively self-limited and usually non–life-threatening conditions common in childhood. There are several common childhood illnesses that manifest themselves more seriously in children with HIV infection, including severe recurrent fungal skin and nail infections (tinea, *Candida*), recalcitrant molluscum contagiosum, severe condylomata, recurrent and chronic otitis media and sinusitis, recurrent upper respiratory tract infections, as well as reactive airways disease.

Also included in this group are severe and life-threatening manifestations of varicella and measles. Prolonged disease with varicella is common in the immunocompromised child and includes progression to pneumonitis, hepatitis, pancreatitis, and encephalitis. In one study of HIV-infected children with varicella, 7 of 8 children had evidence suggestive of varicella pneumonitis. In another study, 7 of 17 HIV-infected children with varicella developed chronic, recurrent, or persistent disease. HIV-infected children with varicella should be treated aggressively with acyclovir as soon as there is evidence of disease. Varicella-exposed children should be given varicella zoster immune globulin (VZIG) in an attempt to prevent or modify the course of the disease. The incidence of zoster in HIV-infected children is close to that of children with leukemia. Measles can also be life-threatening in the HIV-infected child. Three of six HIV-infected children with measles followed at

Children's Hospital AIDS Program in Newark, New Jersey, from 1990 to 1991 died of this infection. Even with appropriate immunization, many HIV-infected children, especially those with low CD4$^+$ lymphocyte counts, do not mount protective antibody responses against measles and continue to be susceptible because of their impaired humoral immune response. Any HIV-infected child who is exposed to measles should receive intramuscular serum immune globulin as prophylaxis. Children already on intravenous immune globulin (IVIG) therapy may be protected, but should receive an additional dose of IVIG if the exposure occurs more than 2 weeks after their last infusion. Some children with life-threatening manifestations of measles such as pneumonitis are being treated with IV ribavirin on compassionate use basis.

Opportunistic Infections

In both adults and children, the opportunistic infections related to the immunodeficiency caused by HIV infection are varied and frequently difficult to treat. AIDS-defining opportunistic infections in children often represent primary infection with the organism rather than the recrudescence that is typically the case in adults. This may be why *Pneumocystis carinii* pneumonia (PCP) is a more severe illness in infants than in adults. Adult opportunistic infections that are rarely seen in children under 8 years of age include toxoplasmosis, cryptococcal disease, and other disseminated fungal infections such as coccidioidomycosis and histoplasmosis. Their relative infrequency in children probably relates to lack of exposure to the etiologic agents. These infections, however, are seen in adolescents. On the other hand, tuberculosis has become a problem in children born into households in which adults may be infected with both HIV and tuberculosis. HIV-infected children, like adults, are more susceptible to the rapid progression of *Mycobacterium tuberculosis* from infection to disease (tuberculosis). While space limitations preclude a comprehensive review of opportunistic infections in children, we will discuss some points that are particularly salient for pediatric HIV infection. Specific antimicrobial therapy for these infections is found in Table 4 using weight-specific doses of drugs.

The most common opportunistic infection in infants and children is PCP, accounting for 29% of reported AIDS indicator diseases in children in 1993. Prior to the widespread use of PCP prophylaxis beginning in 1991–92, PCP accounted for a higher percentage of reported AIDS indicator diseases and up to 65% of opportunistic infections in the pediatric population. Over half of all cases of PCP in infants and children occur in the first 3 to 6 months of life. Mortality is high even with therapy, and the median survival following an episode is 1 to 4 months. The clinical presentation of PCP varies; acute disease with rapid onset of respiratory failure is common in the first year of life. Diagnosis can be made using induced sputum, bronchoalveolar lavage, or lung biopsy. The use of gallium scans as a diagnostic modality is not standardized in children. Lymphoid interstitial pneumonitis (LIP) is an

TABLE 4. *Pharmacologic treatment of HIV infection and its common sequela in children*

Condition	Treatment
HIV infection	Zidovudine (Retrovir, AZT), younger than 13 years: 180 mg/ m^2/dose orally Q6H, older than 13 years: 100 mg/dose orally Q4H, 5 × /day
	Didanosine (ddl, Videx): 90–120 mg/m²/dose given orally 2 × /day
	Zalcitabine (ddC, HIVID 0.005–0.01 mg/kg/dose orally Q8h
Humoral immunodeficiency (with recurrent serious bacterial infections or	Immune globulin 400 mg/kg IV 1 × /month
documented functional antibody defect)	Zidovudine plus Lamivudine (Epivir, 3TC): 4 mg kg/dose orally Q12H (150 mg BID maximum)
Pneumocystis carinii pneumonia	
Prophylaxis	Trimethoprim/sulfamethoxazole (TMP-SMX) 150 mg TMP/m²/ day with 750 mg SMX/m²/day given orally divided BID 3 × /week on consecutive days (e.g., M-T-W). Other dosing schedules include: (1) once daily dose 3 × /week on consecutive days (e.g., M-T-W); (2) BID 7 × /week; (3) BID dose given on alternate days (e.g., M-W-F)
	Alternate regimens: (1) dapsone 2 mg/kg/dose orally 1 × /day not to exceed 100 mg/day; (2) aerosolized pentamidine (age 5 years or older) 300 mg/dose via Respirgard II 1 × /month; (3) if above not tolerated: IV pentamidine 4 mg/ kg/dose every 2 or 4 weeks
Treatment	Trimethoprim/sulfamethoxazole (TMP-SMX) 5 mg TMP/kg/ dose with 25 mg SMX/kg/dose IV Q6H
	or
	Pentamidine isethionate 4 mg base/kg/day IV daily
	Adjunctive: steroids
Candida	
Thrush	Nystatin suspension 2–6 cc swish in cheeks 3–5 × /day
	or
	Miconazole vaginal cream apply orally BID-QID
	or
	Terazol vaginal cream apply orally BID-QID
	or
	Clotrimazole troches, one troche in mouth 5 × /day
	or
	Fluconazole 2–8 mg/kg/day orally given once a day
	or
	Ketoconazole 5–10 mg/kg/day orally given once a day or BID
Esophagitis	Fluconazole loading dose of 10 mg/kg given orally then 3–8 mg/kg/day orally or IV given once a day
	or
	Ketoconazole 5–10 mg/kg/day orally given once a day or BID
	or
	Amphotericin B 0.25–1.5 mg/kg/day IV
Disseminated cryptococcosis	Induction: amphotericin B 0.25–1.5 mg/kg/day IV
	Maintenance: amphotericin B 1 mg/kg 1–2 × /week
	or
	Fluconazole 3–8 mg/kg/day orally 1 × /day

TABLE 4. *Continued*

Condition	Treatment
Disseminated cytomegalo-virus	Induction: ganciclovir 5 mg/kg/dose Q12H IV or 2–5 mg/kg/dose Q8H IV Alternative: foscarnet 60 mg/kg/dose Q8H IV Maintenance: ganciclovir 5 mg/kg/dose QD IV or 6 mg/kg/dose QD for 5 days/week or oral ganciclovir (investigational) Alternative: foscarnet 90–120 mg/kg QD IV (run over 2 hr)
Mycobacterium avium complex	Clarithromycin: 15 mg/kg/day divided Q12H OR Azithromycin: 10–40 mg/kg/day in combination with at least two of the following: rifabutin, ethambutol, ciprofloxacin, and clofazimine. Prophylaxis: Rifabutin 5 mg/kg/day (maximum 300 mg/day) or clarithromycin 5–15 mg/kg/day.
Lymphoid interstitial pneumonitis (LIP)	Steroids are indicated when LIP is associated with significant hypoxemia defined as a documented PaO_2 of less than 65 torr on three separate occasions over a 1-month period. Prednisone 2 mg/kg/day for 2–4 weeks or until there is an increase in PaO_2 of at least 20 torr, then gradually taper to 0.5 mg/kg every other day provided PaO_2 remains above 70; duration of steroid therapy is not established
Herpes simplex virus	Acyclovir 250 mg/m^2/dose IV Q8H or 600 mg/m^2/dose orally Q6H (in cases of visceral or disseminated infection use dose of 500 mg/m^2/dose IV Q8H) Alternative for acyclovir resistant herpes: foscarnet
Varicella zoster	Treatment: acyclovir 500 mg/m^2/dose IV Q8H or 900 mg/m^2/dose orally Q6H Exposure: varicella zoster immune globulin (VZIG) 125 units (one vial) for each 10 kg of body weight (maximum of 625 units) IM within 96 hours of exposure to varicella
Measles	All children should be immunized with measles vaccine Exposure: immune globulin 0.5 ml/kg (maximum dose of 15 ml) IM within 6 days of exposure Investigational therapy: ribavirin

important part of the differential diagnosis in children. Because of the importance of aggressive management, it is not necessary to make a definitive diagnosis of PCP to initiate treatment. Corticosteroids have been recommended as adjunctive therapy for adults with PCP and are being used by many clinicians to treat PCP in children based on data supporting its use in infants with primary infection.

Candida esophagitis is a common opportunistic infection in pediatric AIDS. It may be seen with or without oral candidiasis. The symptoms of dysphagia, odynophagia, substernal pain, and fever are similar to those in adults. Infants and children who are either unable to verbalize or cannot localize pain frequently present with a decrease in oral intake, weight loss, and failure to thrive. Unusual neck movements may be seen in a child who is attempting to relieve pain. The diagnosis is suggested by symptomatology and barium swallow, and is made definitively by endoscopy. Neurologic causes of dysphagia are an important part of the differential diagnosis in children.

Disseminated *Mycobacterium avium* complex (MAC) infection is associated with more severe immunocompromise and was the AIDS indicator disease in 7% of children diagnosed in 1993. Among 139 children with AIDS followed at Children's Hospital AIDS Program (CHAP) in Newark, New Jersey, between 1981 and 1991, 14 (10.1%) had evidence of disseminated MAC with an additional 6 (4.3%) having evidence of gastrointestinal colonization. The mean $CD4^+$ lymphocyte count at the time of diagnosis for this group was 29. The most common clinical signs and symptoms of disseminated MAC are anorexia, transfusion-dependent anemia, fever, malaise, weight loss, diarrhea, and abdominal pain. All of the children followed at CHAP had the additional sign of persistent failure to gain weight. A review of HIV-infected children followed at the Children's Hospital of Philadelphia between 1981 and 1991 revealed that 10% (including 18% of those with AIDS) had evidence of disseminated MAC infection, with an increasing incidence in those with $CD4^+$ lymphocyte counts less than 100. It is diagnosed chiefly by blood culture and also by means of culture of bone marrow or liver biopsy.

Recurrent Bacterial Infections

HIV infection is associated with significant abnormalities in B-cell–mediated immune responses. In infants, laboratory-documented B-cell dysfunction usually precedes T-cell abnormalities. This may be the result of an interference with normal B-cell maturation, as humoral immune responses are incomplete at birth. The normal maturation of B cells, including the ability to produce antigen-specific antibodies, requires lymphokines produced by functioning $CD4^+$ lymphocytes. Most adults with HIV infection were exposed to the common bacterial pathogens prior to becoming HIV infected; because of this, they tend to have circulating protective antibodies against them and circulating B cells with a retained anamnestic response to these pathogens. Thus, adults tend to get serious bacterial infections with common pathogens only late in the course of the disease, when they are severely immunocompromised. With improved survival in a more immunocompromised state, however, the problem of severe bacterial infections in adults is on the rise. In contrast, HIV-infected children have been shown to have defective primary and secondary antibody production to T-cell–dependent and –independent antigens; when children are exposed to common bacterial pathogens for the first time, these abnormalities result in severe manifestations of infection early in the course of their HIV infection. Since 1987, multiple or recurrent serious bacterial infections have been a part of the CDC case definition of AIDS for children. The most common infections that meet the case definition are bacteremia and pneumonia. The most common organisms include *Streptococcus pneumoniae*, *Haemophilus influenzae*, *Salmonella* spp., and *Staphylococcus aureus*. Clinicians should be aggressive in treating less-severe bacterial infections such as otitis or impetigo so as to prevent dissemination.

Lymphoid Interstitial Pneumonitis

Lymphoid interstitial pneumonitis is a diffuse lymphocytic infiltration of the interstitium of the lung that can interfere with gas exchange. It is an AIDS-defining condition only in children, and it has been the AIDS-defining condition in over 25% of cases of pediatric AIDS. It may result from dual infection with HIV and Epstein-Barr virus (EBV), but its etiology has not been definitively established. Hypoxemia, clubbing, and superimposed bacterial infections may be present, and long-standing LIP can progress to chronic bronchiectasis. Treatment is directed at the hypoxemia, which can be reversed with corticosteroids, the superimposed bacterial pneumonitis, and the chronic lung damage. Children with LIP often have other evidence of lymphoproliferative disease and tend to have significant lymphadenopathy, hepatomegaly, splenomegaly and relatively frequently, parotitis.

Central Nervous System Involvement

Central nervous system (CNS) involvement is a more common manifestation of HIV infection in infants and children than in adults, and although the exact incidence is unknown, it is felt to occur in the vast majority of those infected. The severity of CNS dysfunction may relate to when in the course of pregnancy or delivery the infant became infected. HIV is believed to enter the CNS through HIV-infected macrophages that can cross the blood-brain barrier. In infants, entry of HIV into the CNS may be facilitated by infection with HIV *in utero* prior to establishment of this barrier. It is unclear exactly how HIV causes neurologic dysfunction; direct HIV effects and indirect effects through cells of the macrophage lineage and the elaboration of toxic cytokines have been postulated.

There is a broad clinical spectrum of neurologic abnormalities seen in pediatric HIV infection. Most children have some degree of developmental delay, whether subtle or obvious, affecting both motor and cognitive milestones. The presentation of developmental delay is variable. There may be relatively normal development suddenly followed by either a loss of milestones or a failure to attain new milestones. The onset of developmental delay may be followed by periods of relative stability in neurologic function or a course of rapid neurodevelopmental deterioration. Pyramidal tract involvement may be seen, with resulting spastic paresis. Hypertonicity and hyperreflexia are common manifestations of motor involvement.

Static encephalopathy is seen in about one-quarter of children with HIV and is characterized by developmental delay of varying severity without loss of previously attained milestones. Children in this group can have improvement in neurologic function with continued acquisition of developmental skills, but usually in a delayed fashion. Progressive encephalopathy, characterized by progressive deterioration in cognitive, motor, or language skills and a loss of previously attained developmental milestones, is often seen in patients who also have opportunistic infections. Progressive encephalopathy, which is associated with a very poor prognosis, can be characterized by a plateau course without continued loss of milestones, a subacute progressive course associated with slow, continued losses in motor and nonmotor developmental milestones, or a rapidly progressive course. Neuroimaging studies of HIV infection in children include findings of ventricular enlargement, cerebral atrophy, white matter attenuation, and cerebral and basal ganglial calcification. The possibility of a CNS lymphoma must always be considered in the child who develops new neurologic signs and symptoms.

Antiretroviral therapy with zidovudine has been shown to improve the neurodevelopmental functioning of infants and children with HIV. Children can regain lost motor and developmental milestones with therapy. In some this is dramatic, with the reversal of incontinence, gait abnormalities, or lost cognitive milestones after initiation of therapy. In pediatric trials, as opposed to those in adults, improvements in neurodevelopmental outcome is a primary goal of antiretroviral therapy. Both didanosine (ddI) and zalcitabine (ddC) have more limited penetration into the central nervous system and their role in the treatment of HIV-related neurologic abnormalities is less well established.

PRESENTATION AND PROGNOSIS IN INFANTS AND CHILDREN

There are two general patterns of presentation of HIV infection in children. One of them, representing about one-third of all perinatally acquired infections, involves early onset of severe disease with rapid progression and poor prognosis. Infants in this group usually present with severe opportunistic infections (most often PCP) and/or encephalopathy, within the first 2 years of life. Many of these children become identified as HIV infected because of severe illnesses that arise abruptly. PCP in this group is seldom insidious; infants may be seen by a physician one week with some mild general symptoms and have fulminant, life-threatening PCP the next. It is because of the presentation of illness in this group of patients that early PCP prophylaxis is required. A natural history study of a French cohort of HIV-infected children revealed a bimodal presentation of illness with a 3-year survival of 48% in the group that presented with encephalopathy or opportunistic infection within the first 2 years of life, compared with 97% in the group that did not. Data from the Pediatrics Spectrum of Disease Project delineates the group of rapid progressors as those with early onset of disease manifestations and death prior to 48 months of age.

The second pattern of pediatric HIV infection involves later onset of disease symptomatology and is associated with a better prognosis. These children generally present after the first year of life with a more indolent disease course, consisting of a variety of the more general clinical manifestations discussed above. Relative to children diagnosed with AIDS in the first year of life, LIP is more common in this group, as are other signs of lymphoproliferation such as generalized lymphadenopathy and parotitis. It is not unusual for school-age children to be identified with perinatal HIV infection as a result of this type of presentation; some of these children are not diagnosed with AIDS or HIV infection until 10 or 11 years of age. One study has reported a median incubation period of over 6 years in this group, which is more comparable to the adult experience. In a cohort of 42 perinatally infected children ages 9 to 16 years followed at Children's Hospital AIDS Program in Newark, New Jersey, the mean age at diagnosis of HIV infection was 88 months. Although most of the children in this cohort have HIV-related symptomatology, many with significant disease, almost a quarter of the children remain asymptomatic with relatively intact immune systems. Children who present later in life may be clinically similar to asymptomatic adults or show only subtle HIV-related signs and symptoms before presenting with more obvious conditions such as thrush. Recurrent bacterial infections are likely to occur as AIDS-defining conditions in both the early- and late-onset presentations of HIV. Renal and cardiac involvement usually occur as later manifestations of illness after other significant HIV-related disease is diagnosed.

It is unclear why some children present early with fulminant disease and others present later. One can speculate that this is related to the timing of perinatal infection—early in gestation versus late in gestation. Most researchers feel that the group of rapid progressors are likely to represent infants infected during the early prenatal period. A recent analysis of 162 HIV-infected infants from the French Prospective Multicenter Cohort revealed that the infants' risk of opportunistic infection or encephalopathy in the first 18 months of life correlated directly with the degree of maternal HIV-related symptomatology and p24 antigen level and inversely with maternal CD4$^+$ lymphocyte count at the time of delivery. Fifty percent of infants in this study born to mothers with AIDS developed opportunistic infections (OIs) or encephalopathy by 18 months compared with 14% of infants born to mothers who were either asymptomatic or had only generalized lymphadenopathy.

Two major factors affect the prognosis of children with HIV infection: their specific HIV-related diseases and their age at presentation. A study of 172 perinatally infected children treated at a Miami hospital showed median survival rates from diagnosis of 1 month for those with PCP, 5 months for those with nephropathy, 11 months for those with encephalopathy, 12 months for those with *Candida* esophagitis, 50 months for those with recurrent bacterial infection, and 72 months for those with LIP. A study at the Children's Hospital of New Jersey showed a median survival rate following PCP of 2 months. PCP continues to be a leading AIDS indicator disease in infants under 1 year of age and carries a bad prognosis in this group. In addition, a study at a New York hospital showed a mean survival time for perinatally infected children of 67 months, while the survival time from infection for children over 2 years of age infected by transfusion averaged 90 months. Thus, both later presentation and later infection appear to be associated with longer survival.

It is important to note that an AIDS diagnosis, in and of itself, is not an accurate prognostic indicator for children. The variability in prognosis is a function of the conditions responsible for the AIDS diagnosis. While opportunistic infections, encephalopathy, LIP, and recurrent bacterial infections are all AIDS-defining conditions, the first two are associated with a significantly worse prognosis than the last two. In a cohort of children ages 9 to 16 years followed at Children's Hospital AIDS Program in Newark, New Jersey, those children with LIP as their only AIDS-defining diagnosis had $CD4^+$ lymphocyte counts comparable to the asymptomatic children. Therefore, information about the average survival time for adults after an AIDS diagnosis is not valid for children. While an AIDS diagnosis may be of epidemiologic interest and can be important in gaining access to care for children through eligibility for public entitlement programs, by itself it is of limited value in predicting survival time. Thus, contrary to the general impression held by many parents and caregivers, a diagnosis of AIDS does not mean that a child will die within a very short period of time; it is important for health care workers to discuss the prognosis for children in terms of specific conditions.

TREATMENT OF HIV AND RESULTING ILLNESSES IN CHILDREN

Medical management of children with HIV infection should begin with identification of those who are at risk prior to delivery, followed by careful monitoring to determine their HIV infection status. Primary HIV-specific treatment consists of specific antimicrobial prophylaxis for opportunistic infections and antiretroviral therapy. General supportive management includes psychosocial support, pain management, nutritional supplementation, developmental intervention, patient education, and advocacy. In addition, medical management should encompass general pediatric care, including childhood immunizations.

HIV-Specific Treatment

PCP Prophylaxis

PCP in children with HIV infection is associated with a high rate of morbidity and mortality. It often presents acutely with a peak incidence in the first 3 to 6 months of life. In March 1991, standards of care regarding PCP prophylaxis for children were endorsed by the CDC and published in the *Morbidity and Mortality Weekly Report* (*MMWR*). The recommendations for infants and children were based on age-dependent $CD4^+$ lymphocyte counts, which differ from values in adults. The guidelines called for the initiation of PCP prophylaxis for HIV-exposed children 1 to 11 months of age with $CD4^+$ lymphocyte counts under 1,500 cells/μl, for children 12 to 23 months of age with $CD4^+$ lymphocyte counts under 750, for those 24 months to 5 years of age with $CD4^+$ lymphocyte counts below 500, and for those greater than or equal to 6 years of age with $CD4^+$ lymphocyte counts below 200.

Since publication of those guidelines, data have been collected that indicate that a larger proportion of infected infants than previously thought develop PCP in the first year of life with $CD4^+$ lymphocyte counts greater than 1,500 cells/μl. This is particularly true for infants in the first 6 months of life with up to 25% of infants with PCP in that age group having $CD4^+$ lymphocyte counts greater than 1,500 cells/μl. In response to this and other data, the National Pediatric and Family HIV Resource Center in collaboration with the CDC convened an expert panel to reevaluate the 1991 guidelines. This meeting resulted in the publication of revised guidelines for PCP prophylaxis for HIV-infected infants and children in 1995. The most significant change in the revised guidelines involves the use of prophylaxis in the first year of life, during which time it is recommended that all HIV-infected infants be placed on prophylaxis regardless of $CD4^+$ lymphocyte values, beginning at 1 month of age. Since it is difficult to determine with certainty by 1 month of age which infants born to HIV-infected women are themselves infected, and especially which ones are uninfected, the new guidelines recommend initiating prophylaxis on all infants born to HIV-infected women at 1 month of age and continuing the prophylaxis until HIV infection can be reasonably excluded. HIV infection can be reasonably excluded with two negative HIV culture or PCR results, one obtained at greater than or equal to 1 month of age and the other at greater than or equal to 4 months of age. After the first year of life, the use of prophylaxis is advised in HIV-infected children based on $CD4^+$ lymphocyte values. See Table 5 for a summary of the 1995 PCP prophylaxis guidelines.

Antiretroviral Agents

Zidovudine (AZT)

Zidovudine was approved by the Food and Drug Administration (FDA) for use in children 3 years after it was approved for use in adults. Its approval for children was based on the results of efficacy trials in adults, pharmacokinetic and toxicity trials in children, and some efficacy data that were deduced from phase I and phase II studies in children. It is important that drug development in children proceed in parallel with development in adults, and not following that development. This situation is improving, with current research into promising therapeutics for children proceeding more in conjunction with adult research.

In asymptomatic and symptomatic adults with $CD4^+$ lymphocyte counts less than 500 cells/μl, the use of zidovudine has been shown to delay clinical progression, although its ability to prolong life is unproven. No placebo-controlled efficacy studies have been completed in children. However, children with advanced HIV disease involved in ACTG protocol 043 (an open label trial of zidovudine) experienced weight gain and improvement in cognitive function as measured by neuropsychological testing. The observed gains in cognitive function were similar to the results of phase I and II studies of zidovudine conducted by Pizzo et al.

TABLE 5. *Recommendations for PCP prophylaxis and CD4$^+$ monitoring for HIV-exposed infants and HIV-infected children, by age*

Age	PCP prophylaxis	CD4$^+$ monitoring
Birth to 4–6 weeks, HIV exposed	No prophylaxis	1 month
4–6 weeks to 4 months, HIV exposed	Prophylaxis	3 months
4–12 months		
HIV infected or indeterminate	Prophylaxis	3, 9, 12 months
HIV infection reasonably excluded[a]	No prophylaxis	None
1–5 years, HIV infected	Prophylaxis if CD4$^+$ count is <599 or CD4$^+$ percent is <15%[b,c]	Every 3–4 months[d]
6–12 years years, HIV infected	Prophylaxis if CD4$^+$ count is <200 or CD4$^+$ percent is <15%[c]	Every 3–4 months[d]

[a]HIV infection can be reasonably excluded among children who have had two or more negative HIV diagnostic tests (e.g., culture or PCR), both of which are performed at ≥1 month of age and one of which is performed at ≥4 months of age, or two or more negative HIV IgG antibody tests performed at >6 months of age among children who have no clinical evidence of HIV disease.

[b]Chidren 1–2 years of age who were on PCP prophylaxis and had a CD4$^+$ count of <750 at <12 months of age should continue on prophylaxis.

[c]Prophylaxis should be considered on a case-by-case basis for children who may otherwise be at risk for PCP, such as children with rapidly declining CD4$^+$ counts or percents, or children with category C conditions. Children who have had PCP should receive lifelong PCP prophylaxis.

[d]More frequent monitoring (e.g., monthly) is recommended for children whose CD4$^+$ counts or percents are approaching the threshold for prophylaxis.

Improvements in neurodevelopmental function are particularly important in pediatric HIV infection, since neurodevelopmental abnormalities occur in the vast majority of patients.

Children in ACTG protocol 043 had reductions in serum and cerebrospinal fluid (CSF) levels of p24 antigen. In addition, HIV could no longer be grown from CSF of the vast majority of children who had had a positive viral culture at entry into the protocol. Finally, changes in the CD4$^+$ lymphocyte count of children in the protocol were consistent with those seen in adults: an increase during the first 12 weeks of therapy, followed by a subsequent decline by 24 weeks to counts at or above baseline.

The toxicity of zidovudine in children is similar to that in adults and is primarily hematologic. In protocol 043, one or more episodes of hematologic toxicity occurred in 61% of the children, with anemia in 26% and neutropenia in 48%. Blood transfusions or dose modifications were required in 34% of the children because of hematologic toxicity. As noted above, children in the protocol had advanced disease: 57% of them were anemic at entry into the trial. Experience with zidovudine in adults has shown that those whose disease is less advanced when they begin taking the medication have a lower incidence of hematologic toxicity. Thus it is likely that the toxicity seen in protocol 043 represents the worst-case scenario.

Zidovudine is available in a syrup formulation and is currently recommended for children in a dose of 180 mg/m^2 every 6 hours, comparable to the high dose originally used in adults. A lower dose of zidovudine has become the standard of care in adults. The results of ACTG 128, comparing the effects of the recommended dose with a dose half its size (90 mg/m^2), revealed that there was no difference in toxicity between the groups. From a clinical standpoint, the two dosages were also equivalent in that study, with the exception that those children with neurologic disease fared better on the higher dose.

A major limitation of drug therapy with zidovudine is the development of viral resistance. Three of eight children studied whose viral isolates were susceptible to zidovudine prior to starting therapy developed resistant strains after a median of 11 months on therapy. Development of zidovudine resistance is associated with disease progression and poor clinical outcome in children on chronic therapy. A regimen of alternating zidovudine and zalcitabine therapy in children has not been shown to prevent the development of resistance to zidovudine.

Didanosine (ddI)

Didanosine is an antiretroviral medication whose mechanism of action is similar to that of zidovudine. Didanosine was simultaneously approved for adults and children in October 1991 for individuals who are intolerant to, or develop disease progression while on, zidovudine therapy. Evidence of the immunologic efficacy of didanosine in children was seen in the phase I and II trials conducted at the National Cancer Institute (NCI), with a sustained increase in CD4$^+$ lymphocyte counts throughout the 24 weeks of the trials and for up to 3 years in some of the more immunocompetent patients. A decrease in p24 antigen levels has also been demonstrated with ddI use. There is some indication of improvement in neurodevelopmental function of children on ddI; whether these preliminary observations are accurate will be determined with further pediatric experience with the drug. There appears to be variability of absorption of ddI in children, which may be related to gastric acidity. Improvement with ddI correlated with serum levels of the drug; those children with higher levels experienced more significant improvement. In phase I and II pediatric trials with ddI, the main toxicity was hyperamylasemia, with pancreatitis occurring in 2 of 43 patients studied. Of 95 children on ddI for a mean of 56 weeks, 7 developed pancreatitis, which resolved after stopping the medication. Pancreatitis occurred in the patients receiving the two highest doses in these trials, suggesting that this complication is dose related. Although peripheral neuropathy has been reported in adults on ddI, this toxicity was not appreciated in any of the children in phase I and II trials. However, it is generally the patient who reports symptoms of neuropathy, which may account for its being underreported in children who cannot verbalize. Five of 34 children followed in a comparative dosing study of didanosine developed elevation of hepatic alkaline phosphatase requiring interruption of therapy after being on drug for a minimum of 6 months. Peripheral retinal depigmentation is another potential side effect of ddI that has been reported in approximately 5% of children. Although the optimal dosing schedule for didanosine remains to be determined, the currently recommended dosage ranges between 90 and 120 mg/m^2 orally every 12 hours. As with zidovudine, resistance to didanosine has been documented to emerge with chronic usage, although its clinical relevance is less well understood.

Zalcitabine (ddC)

Zalcitabine has been approved for use in HIV-infected adolescents and adults in combination with zidovudine. Its mechanism of action is similar to that of zidovudine, but like ddI, it does not cause significant hematologic toxicity. There are very limited published data available on the use of ddC in children. In a small pilot study in HIV-infected children, ddC was shown to decrease p24 antigen levels and raise CD4$^+$ lymphocyte counts. A dose-dependent toxicity of ddC seen in adults, painful peripheral neuropathy, has yet to appear in the limited-time trials at lower doses in children. Rashes and mouth sores have been the main side effects seen in children. ACTG protocol 138 is examining efficacy and toxicity of ddC in children who are intolerant of zidovudine or show evidence of disease progression while on zidovudine. Since ddC is only available in 0.375 and 0.75 mg tablets, use in infants and small children at the dose of 0.1 mg/kg orally every 8 hours is difficult.

Institution of Antiretroviral Therapy

Guidelines for the use of antiretroviral therapy in infants, children, and adolescents were published in 1993 as a result of a multidisciplinary meeting of researchers, health care providers, and parents coordinated by the National Pediatric and Family HIV Resource Center. These guidelines call for the initiation of antiretroviral therapy in children with (a) symptomatic HIV infection, regardless of CD4$^+$ lymphocyte count, as described in Table 6, or (b) evidence of immunosuppression as described in Table 7. Information currently available does not support the use of antiretroviral therapy in asymptomatic children (including those with lymphadenopathy or hepatomegaly only) with relatively intact immune systems.

The 1993 guidelines called for the use of zidovudine for initial therapy of HIV-infected children. Disease progression as outlined in Table 8, and intolerance, as manifested by significant and persistent toxicity, were given as indications for changing to another antiretroviral regimen. Didanosine, recommended as the agent for children who are intolerant of, or have disease progression while on, zidovudine. Use of zalcitabine in combination with zidovudine for adolescents was also listed as an approved alternative. Since publication of the 1993 guidelines, there has been a great deal of new information regarding the use of antiretroviral therapy in HIV-infected individuals. Results of the two adult studies, ACTG 175 and the European Delta Study, indicate that combination therapy (zidovudine plus didanosine and zidovudine plus zalcitabine) or didanosine monotherapy is superior

TABLE 6. *Initiating antiretroviral therapy: clinical criteria*

Clinical conditions that definitively warrant initiation of antiretroviral therapy
  AIDS-defining opportunistic infection
  Wasting syndrome
  Failure to thrive: crossing two percentiles or below the fifth percentile for age and falling off of
    curve
  HIV-related encephalopathy
  HIV-associated malignancy
  Recurrent septicemia or meningitis (two or more episodes)
  Thrombocytopenia (platelet count <75,000/mm^3 on two or more occasions)
  Hypogammaglobulinemia (total IgG/IgM/IgA <250/mm^3)
Clinical conditions that may warrant initiation of antiretroviral therapy depending on the overall
    clinical profile and judgment of health care provider
  Lymphoid interstitial pneumonitis
  Parotitis
  Splenomegaly
  Recurrent oral candidiasis
  Recurrent or persistent diarrhea
  Symptomatic HIV-related cardiomyopathy
  HIV-related nephrotic syndrome
  Severe hepatic transaminitis (>5-fold normal)
  Chronic bacterial infections (sinusitis or pneumonia)
  Recurrent herpes simplex or varicella zoster
  Neutropenia (<750/mm^3) or age-corrected anemia on at least two occasions over 1 week

TABLE 7. *CD4$^+$ lymphocyte values for the initiation of antiretroviral therapy*

	Criteria for antiretroviral therapy
CD4$^+$ percentage	
<1 year	<30
1–2 years	<25
>2 years	<20
CD4$^+$ lymphocyte count (cells/μl)	
<1 year	<1750
1–2 years	<1000
2–6 years	<750
>6 years	<500

TABLE 8. *HIV disease progression*

Clinical conditions that warrant alternative antiretroviral therapy
  Growth failure: crossing two percentiles or sustained deviation from a parallel curve for chil-
    dren who are below the fifth percentile (remediable causes should be ruled out and
    treated)
  Neurodevelopmental deterioration (should have at least two of the following)
    Impairment of brain growth (for children >2 years neuroimaging is necessary to confirm
      atrophy)
    Decline of cognitive function (sustained decline as defined by standardized testing)
    Clinical neurologic deterioration
Clinical conditions that merit consideration of a change in antiretroviral therapy
  Development of a new opportunistic infection
  Symptomatic cardiomyopathy
  HIV-related nephrotic syndrome
  Severe transaminitis (>5-fold normal)

to zidovudine monotherapy in terms of disease progression. The inferiority of zidovudine monotherapy to didanosine monotherapy and zidovudine plus didanosine combination therapy was confirmed in the pediatric age group with the results of ACTG 152. It seems to be clear at this time that zidovudine monotherapy is not the most effective antiretroviral regimen. Clinicians are considering other regimens such as didanosine monotherapy and various combinations including didanosine plus zidovudine, zidovudine plus zalcitabine, and the recently approved combination of zidovudine plus lamivudine (3TC).

Intravenous Immune Globulin Therapy

Intravenous immune globulin (IVIG) is standard therapy for children and adults with primary humoral immunodeficiency disorders such as Bruton's agammaglobulinemia. Passive immunotherapy in the form of IVIG provides protection against a wide range of bacterial and viral pathogens. As discussed above, children with HIV infection often have functional abnormalities of their B-cell–mediated immune system that place them at risk for infections that require an intact humoral immune response. Although most children with HIV infection have elevated immunoglobulin levels, this is believed to represent nonspecific polyclonal B-cell activation. Many children fail to mount an antibody response to routine childhood immunizations, indicating a functional immunodeficiency.

Pediatric immunologists have been administering IVIG to HIV-infected children with B-cell immunodeficiency since early in the epidemic. Uncontrolled studies have suggested that IVIG therapy is efficacious in reducing the frequency of sepsis and other clinical symptomatology. Improvements in mitogen-induced lymphoproliferative responses and a decrease in the concentration of circulating immune complexes has also been shown to occur in some children on IVIG. Other researchers have been skeptical regarding the effectiveness of IVIG relative to other modalities, such as prophylactic antibiotics. The National Institute of Child Health and Human Development (NICHD) recently completed a placebo-controlled trial using IVIG in HIV-infected children. The trial found that IVIG prolonged the time free from serious laboratory-proven bacterial or clinically diagnosed serious or minor bacterial and viral infections in symptomatic HIV-infected children with CD4 counts greater than 200, and was also associated with a slowing of $CD4^+$ lymphocyte count decline. Unfortunately, this trial did not separately evaluate the efficacy in those children with documented B-cell defects but looked only at groups based on CD4 counts. The results of the placebo-controlled National Institute of Allergy and Infectious Diseases (NIAID)/ACTG study 051 did not demonstrate additional protection against laboratory-proven severe bacterial infections in children receiving trimethoprim-sulfamethoxazole prophylaxis. Neither study showed an effect by IVIG on overall survival.

Based on clinical experience in treating children with humoral immunodeficiency and HIV with IVIG and the results of the above reports, a group of pediatric HIV specialists has agreed that IVIG should be considered for use in HIV-infected children with the following conditions: (a) evidence of humoral immunodeficiency as defined by severe recurrent bacterial infections, hypogammaglobulinemia, poor functional antibody responses to documented infections, or a lack of response to immunizations; (b) thrombocytopenia; or (c) chronic bronchiectasis.

Childhood Immunizations

Immunizations represent the cornerstone of preventive medicine for children. Immunization schedules for HIV-infected children must take into account the potential for complications secondary to live or attenuated viral vaccines. Paralytic poliomyelitis is a potential complication of the oral polio vaccine (OPV) for both the immunocompromised patient and immunocompromised family members through excreted virus in stool. There is also a potential for serious complications from other attenuated viral vaccines such as measles. However, no serious side effects have been documented in immunized HIV-infected children. The use of inactivated polio vaccine (IPV) instead of OPV is recommended for these children. In the case of measles, where no alternative is available, the use of measles-mumps-rubella (MMR) vaccine is recommended routinely for HIV-infected children. Despite vaccination, many children continue to be susceptible to the immunized organisms; inadequate antibody responses have been documented in some children. Current recommendations for immunization of HIV-infected children are listed in Table 9.

EARLY IDENTIFICATION OF HIV-INFECTED AND AT-RISK INFANTS

Although there is currently no cure for HIV infection, there are several available interventions, as discussed above, that can reduce morbidity, delay progression of

TABLE 9. *Immunizations for HIV antibody-positive children*

Immunization	Schedule
Diphtheria-tetanus-pertussis	Normal schedule[a]
Inactivated polio virus[b]	Normal schedule
Hepatitis B vaccine	New normal schedule
Haemophilus influenzae type B conjugate	Normal schedule
Measles-mumps-rubella	Normal schedule
Pneumococcal vaccine	2 years of age; second dose 3 to 5 years after initial dose (3)
Influenza vaccine	Annually (from 6 months)

[a]As recommended by the American Academy of Pediatrics Commitee on Immunizations.
[b]Instead of the polio virus; should continue to be given to seroreverters and all household members where an individual with HIV infection is in residence.

disease, and reduce perinatal transmission. New treatments directed at both HIV and the opportunistic infections secondary to HIV infection are increasingly being investigated. A delay in disease progression may in fact enable an individual to have access eventually to a medication that will be life-saving. It is because of this that adults are encouraged to have confidential and voluntary HIV testing with informed consent. It has become increasingly obvious that knowledge of the HIV status of a pregnant woman has implications for the health of both the woman and her newborn infant. As with other HIV-infected adults, pregnant women with HIV infection may directly benefit from antiretroviral therapy and prophylactic antimicrobial regimens. The results of ACTG protocol 076, which indicate that the use of antiretroviral therapy in specific situations lowers the rate of perinatal transmission, provide impetus for knowing the HIV status of every pregnant woman. The U.S. Public Health Service Task Force on the Use of Zidovudine to Reduce Perinatal Transmission of Human Immunodeficiency Virus recently published recommendations calling for either the use of or the consideration of the use of zidovudine in HIV-infected pregnant women in various clinical situations within the context of a risk-benefit discussion.

Given the peak incidence of PCP in infancy of 3 to 6 months and the rapid onset of fulminant illness in this age group, it may be impossible to prevent PCP in infants during the first year of life without initiating prophylaxis in at-risk infants by 1 month of age. This cannot be done without knowledge of the HIV status of pregnant women or identification of the HIV status of infants at birth. In addition, only through knowing the HIV status of a pregnant woman can the clinician offer appropriate counseling with regard to breast-feeding in the immediate postnatal period. Knowledge of the HIV status of pregnant women or voluntary testing of newborns would also be sensible from a medical standpoint so that those infants who are at risk can be identified for (a) early initiation of antiretroviral therapy when appropriate, (b) change in immunization schedule from the use of OPV to IPV and inclusion of pneumococcal and influenza vaccines, and (c) access to social service benefits to assure better access to health care. Along with voluntary testing of infants and women, there must be assurance of confidentiality, protection against discrimination, and access to state-of-the-art health care.

Nutritional Issues in Children with HIV Infection

Pediatric HIV infection frequently results in nutritional deficiencies and growth failure. Weight loss and failure to gain weight can occur as early as the first 4 months of life as well as in children who become symptomatic at an older age. Failure to thrive and malnutrition may be due to a number of factors including (a) decreased intake resulting either from oral and gastrointestinal pathology that cause nausea, anorexia, pain, and decreased taste, or from neurologic complications that cause ineffective swallowing mechanisms; (b) impaired absorption due to HIV-related enteropathy and gastrointestinal infections; (c) increased metabolic requirements secondary to chronic HIV-related inflammatory illness; and (d) decreased intake resulting from side effects and toxicities (such as nausea, anorexia, vomiting, hepatitis, and pancreatitis) of various medications used to treat HIV infection and its complications. Particularly in children in end-stage disease it is important for the clinician to consider these adverse reactions within the risk versus benefit ratio of therapy with a specific agent. These physical complications of HIV infection further contribute to the marginal nutritional balance frequently seen in children living in communities affected by poverty. Besides protein and caloric deficiencies, there are a number of trace element and vitamin deficiencies that may complicate the clinical course of HIV infection. Specific nutritional deficiencies of selenium, iron, zinc, vitamin B_6, vitamin A, and vitamin E may result in neurologic or cardiac abnormalities and contribute to the rashes and cytopenias commonly seen in HIV infection. In young infants, when CNS growth is still occurring, nutritional deficiencies may have profound long-term effects.

Based on these considerations, there should be an aggressive approach to nutritional support for HIV-infected infants and children that includes (a) proactive nutritional assessment including anthropometric measurements and dietary intake history with each physician visit, and periodic selected laboratory parameter monitoring; (b) diagnosis and treatment of oral-gastrointestinal disease, with special attention to pain management; (c) aggressive replacement and nutritional supplementation beginning with oral supplementation, and progressing as necessary to nasogastric/gastrostomy tube feeding, and in advanced disease with malabsorption to total parenteral hyperalimentation; and (d) use of appetite stimulants and hormone replacements such as megestrol acetate (megace), growth hormone, cyproheptadine (Periactin), and dronobinol (marinol). Nutritional care of HIV-infected children needs to receive the attention of the research community as well as those providing direct care.

Pain Management

Pain management is an especially important but frequently undertreated clinical problem in HIV-infected infants. Children with AIDS suffer from two types of pain—pain of the disease, both acute and chronic, and pain of the multiple diagnostic and therapeutic procedures these children need. Physicians in general are poorly trained in the control of pain by medication, and many do not appreciate that newborns and infants experience pain. While many fear that they will make their patients drug addicts, only 0.4% of patients given narcotics in hospitals ever have a problem with opiate dependence.

A much more aggressive approach must be taken to controlling pain in children. Specific barriers to the management of pain in HIV-infected children include (a) the difficulty of assessing pain in young children; (b) the difficulty of assessing pain in children with neurologic impairment; (c) parental denial of their children's disease; (d) resistance to the use of narcotics by families who have a history of drug use; and

(e) resistance by clinicians to treating pain in children because of myths, such as that children lie about pain to get attention, that if children deny pain or do not complain they are not in pain, and that children who can fall asleep or who can play cannot be in pain. Vigorous and proactive use (preferably before the onset of anticipated pain) of appropriate pain medications using weight-adjusted dosages, including aspirin, acetaminophen, codeine, ibuprofen, morphine, and methadone, is essential to the overall quality of life for HIV-infected children (Table 10). At Children's Hospital AIDS Program in Newark, New Jersey, a combination of methadone and diazepam is used in children with chronic end-stage pain. Both health care providers and families need to be educated as to the appropriate use of these medications. Non-pharmacologic approaches to pain management (including relaxation, hypnosis,

TABLE 10. *Pain management for HIV-infected infants and children*[a]

	Medication	Dose,[b] route, and frequency
Mild pain	Acetaminophen	10–15 mg/kg po Q4h
		15–20 mg/kg rectally Q4h
	Choline-magnesium salicylate	10–15 mg/kg po Q6–8h
	Aspirin	10–15 mg/kg po Q6h
	Ibuprofen	4–10 mg/kg po Q6–8h
	Naproxen	5–7 mg/kg po Q8–12h
	Assess pain relief; if not relieved, go to Moderate pain	
Moderate pain	Continue above and add weak opioid	
	Codeine	0.5–1 mg/kg po Q4h
	Assess pain relief; if not relieved, go to Severe pain	
Severe pain	Continue nonopioid medication if tolerated and add stronger opioid	
	Morphine	0.2–0.4 mg/kg po Q4h
		0.1–0.15 mg/kg IM or SC Q3–4h
		0.08–0.1 mg/kg IV Q2h
		0.05–0.06 mg/kg/hr IV continuous infusion
	Morphine timed release (MS-Contin)	0.3–0.6 mg/kg po Q12h
	Methadone	0.1 mg/kg IV or po Q4h initially for 2–3 doses, then Q6–12h (titrate carefully)
Assess pain relief; if inadequate, increase dosages of opioids until comfort is achieved or limited by side effects; consider adding adjunctive medications such as tricyclic antidepressants for neuropathic pain and sleep disorders		
Monitor for side effects of pain mediciations including nausea and vomiting, constipation, pruritus, urinary retention, and respiratory depression; treat side effects when appropriate (i.e., phenothiazines for nausea and vomiting)		

[a]Adapted from Report of the subcommittee on disease-related pain in childhood cancer. *Pediatrics* 1990;86:818–825 and Pain Management Protocol Children's Hospital AIDS Program, Children's Hospital of New Jersey.

[b]All dosages should be modified based on individual circumstances. These represent starting dosages. Opioid doses can be increased steadily dependent upon need until pain is relieved or dose limited by side effects. For infants less than 3 months of age initial dosages of opioids should be ¼–⅓ the doses listed above.

play therapy, visualization, and distraction) should also be applied in the control of pain, especially for pain related to procedures.

Social Issues in the Delivery of Care

Epidemiologic data on pediatric HIV disease make it clear that in the United States there has been a disproportionate impact upon the poor and people of color, particularly those with histories of injecting drug use. The health care needs of these people have traditionally been underserved, and previous contact with public agencies may dispose them toward distrust and discourage them from seeking timely medical care. Often one of the first relationships of trust that affected families develop is with the health care providers who treat their children. Health care professionals should attempt to establish a partnership with the family rather than reinforcing the more traditional role of passivity and dependence.

The conditions of poverty, including inadequate housing, may interfere with the delivery of optimal health care. Mothers are typically the strongest advocates for their children, but this advocacy may be hindered by the fact that the mothers of HIV-infected children are often single parents and poor. In some cases, symptomatic HIV infection or drug use may interfere with a mother's ability to care properly for her child; more often, however, mothers are assertive in seeking care for their children while neglecting their own care needs. The general shortage of openings in drug treatment programs is especially severe for women who are HIV-infected, pregnant, or have children. All of these socioeconomic conditions have to be addressed in designing effective health care systems for families with HIV infection.

Families can also benefit from psychosocial support in dealing with many aspects of an HIV diagnosis in a child. The diagnosis may be the first evidence that a parent is infected and may give rise to guilt or anger leading to further disruption of the family unit. Apparently resolved emotional issues may require periodic reexamination, as for example when parents are confronted repeatedly by the differences between a child who is developmentally delayed and healthy peers. Decisions about the disclosure of an HIV diagnosis may arise on multiple occasions as different audiences are encountered such as family, friends, siblings of the infected child, the child himself, day care workers, school nurses, and teachers. Many parents choose to disclose the diagnosis on a need-to-know basis. However, children and their siblings often find it less stressful to know the diagnosis than to be left in the dark about something unnamed but apparent. Counseling may help parents decide whether to disclose the diagnosis and how to do so in a developmentally appropriate way. Clinical experience suggests that under the proper circumstances it is beneficial for children with normal cognitive development to have the opportunity to discuss aspects of their illness with trusted adults. The issue of disclosure of diagnosis is particularly pressing as perinatally infected children live into mid- and late adolescence. In a cohort of 42 perinatally infected children ages 9 to 16 years followed at Children's Hospital AIDS Program in Newark, New Jersey, less than 60%

were specifically told their diagnosis. Uninfected but HIV-affected siblings often have mental health needs as well, especially when they face the eventual loss of siblings and one or both parents. Failure to deal successfully with psychosocial issues may impede families from seeking optimal medical care for their children.

The Challenge of HIV Infection in Adolescents

Like other HIV-infected individuals, adolescents with HIV infection come disproportionately from minority communities. The exception to this generalization is the now decreasing epidemic experienced by adolescent hemophiliacs infected through contaminated blood product–derived clotting factors prior to screening programs implemented in 1985. As a group, adolescents are at high risk of acquiring HIV infection by nature of their developmental stage. The Agency for Health Care Policy and Research (AHCPR) guidelines on Evaluation and Management of Early HIV Infection details the unique set of issues in caring for adolescents with HIV infection. These include (a) differences in epidemiology of HIV infection among youth; (b) special barriers to youth both in receiving care for their HIV infection and in preventive services including counseling and testing, resulting from variable laws regarding consent and confidentiality for those under 18 years of age; (c) lack of HIV-specific clinical services for adolescents; and (d) the limitation on youths participating in clinical trials.

One of the major challenges facing those caring for adolescents is the prevention of HIV transmission, both primary and secondary. In general, preventive programs have relied on incomplete or limited information services not linked to care, or programs that teach and encourage behavioral change. Successful adolescent-HIV programs have employed voluntary, confidential or anonymous counseling and HIV testing with direct linkage to adolescent specific care. Although specifics of medical management of HIV-infected adolescents, in terms of medication usage and disease assessment, are similar to that used for adults, many aspects do differ from that which is appropriate for children and adults. The history and physical examination need to be interpreted in the context of age-specific differences. History-taking from adolescents needs to detail sexual and drug using behavior while recognizing the psychosocial and cognitive-developmental stage that may influence the accuracy of the information obtained, and incorporate counseling and coping mechanisms employed by adolescents. There should be an awareness of the potential for other sexually transmitted diseases. Perhaps most importantly, services for adolescents need to be provided by an experienced physician comfortable in dealing with youth and issues of adolescent sexuality within the context of a developmentally appropriate environment.

Developing Standards of Care for Children with HIV

Twenty years ago, 95% of children with leukemia died; today, up to 85% are cured. The intensity of effort put into controlling childhood leukemia should serve as a template for efforts to treat HIV-infected children. Efforts to improve quality of life while working toward a cure for HIV infection will require a multidisciplinary approach, calling on the skills of physicians, nurses, social workers, nutritionists, pharmacists, dentists, and developmental specialists. The child's entire family must be taken into consideration, whether it be the family of birth or a foster family. At Children's Hospital AIDS Program in Newark, New Jersey, 40% of the children with HIV infection are in foster or adoptive care, often provided by a member of the extended family. These families need supportive services, like any family caring for a multiply handicapped fragile baby.

Symptomatic care of HIV-infected children serves both to prolong life and to improve its quality. The challenge to pediatric HIV treatment centers is to make investigational antiretroviral, immunomodulating, and antimicrobial therapies available rapidly. Research programs and those providing clinical care should be linked synergistically. Potentially useful investigational drug studies for HIV-infected infants and children should be pursued in parallel to studies in adults.

SUGGESTED READING

Blanche S, Mayaux MJ, Rouzioux C, et al. Relation of the course of HIV infection in children to the severity of the disease in their mothers at delivery. *N Engl J Med* 1994;330:308–312.

Blanche S, Tardieu M, Duliege AM, et al. Longitudinal study of 94 symptomatic infants with perinatally acquired human immunodeficiency virus infection: evidence for a bimodal expression of clinical and biological symptoms. *AJDC* 1990;144:1210–1215.

Boyer PJ, Dillon M, Navaie M, et al. Factors predictive of maternal-fetal transmission of HIV-1. *JAMA* 1994;271:1925–1930.

Centers for Disease Control and Prevention (CDC). 1994 revised classification system for human immunodeficiency virus infection in children less than 13 years of age. *MMWR* 1994;43(RR-12):1–10.

Centers for Disease Control and Prevention (CDC). Recommendations of the U.S. Public Health Service Task Force on the use of zidovudine to reduce perinatal transmission of human immunodeficiency virus. *MMWR* 1994;43(RR-11):1–20.

Centers for Disease Control and Prevention (CDC). U.S. Public Health Service recommendations for HIV counseling and testing for pregnant women. *MMWR* 1995;44(RR-7):1–15.

Centers for Disease Control and Prevention (CDC). 1995 revised guidelines for prophylaxis against *Pneumocystis carinii* pneumonia for children infected with or perinatally exposed to human immunodeficiency virus. *MMWR* 1995;44(RR-4):1–11.

Connor EM, Sperling RS, Gelber R, et al. Reduction of maternal-infant transmission of human immunodeficiency virus type 1 with zidovudine treatment. *N Engl J Med* 1994;331:1173–1180.

Dunn DT, Newell ML, Ades ED, Peckham CS. Risk of human immunodeficiency virus type 1 transmission through breast feeding. *Lancet* 1992;340:585–588.

El-Sadr W, Oleske JM, Agins BD, et al. *Evaluation and management of early HIV infection.* Clinical Practice Guideline No. 7. AHCPR Publication No. 94-0572. Rockville, MD: Agency for Health Care Policy and Research, Public Health Service, U.S. Department of Health and Human Services, January 1994.

Grubman S, Gross E, Lerner-Weiss N, et al. Older children and adolescents living with perinatally acquired human immunodeficiency virus infection. *Pediatrics* 1995;95:657–663.

Gwinn M, Pappaionaou M, George JR, et al. Prevalence of HIV infection in childbearing women in the United States: surveillance using newborn blood samples. *JAMA* 1991;265:1704–1708.

McIntosh K, Pitt J, Brambilla D, et al. Blood culture in the first 6 months of life for the diagnosis of vertically transmitted human immunodeficiency virus infection. *J Infect Dis* 1994;170:996–1000.

Report of a Consensus Workshop, Siena, Italy, January 17–18, 1992. Early diagnosis of HIV infection in infants. *J Acquir Immun Defic Syndr* 1992;5:1169–1178.

Scott GB, Hutto C, Makuch RW, et al. Survival in children with perinatally acquired human immunodeficiency virus type 1 infection. *N Engl J Med* 1989;321:1791–1796.

Simonds RJ, Lindegreen ML, Thomas P, et al. Prophylaxis against *Pneumocystis carinii* pneumonia among children with perinatally acquired HIV infection in the United States. *N Engl J Med* 1995; 332:786–790.

Tovo PA, DeMartino M, Gabiano C, et al. Prognostic factors and survival in children with perinatal HIV-1 infection. *Lancet* 1992;339:1249–1253.

Working Group on Antiretroviral Therapy: National Pediatric HIV Resource Center. Antiretroviral therapy and medical management of the human immunodeficiency virus-infected child. *Pediatr Infect Dis J* 1993;12:513–22.

A Clinical Guide to AIDS and HIV,
edited by Gary P. Wormser.
Lippincott-Raven Publishers, Philadelphia © 1996.

5

Pulmonary Complications of HIV Infection

Emily J. Erbelding, Richard E. Chaisson, and *Joel E. Gallant

*Department of Medicine, *Division of Infectious Diseases, The Johns Hopkins University
School of Medicine, Baltimore, Maryland 21205*

The lungs have been recognized as a major target for opportunistic infections in patients with HIV infection since the first descriptions of AIDS in 1981. Since that time, *Pneumocystis carinii* pneumonia (PCP) has remained a common AIDS-related respiratory infection, and experience with other respiratory complications, both infectious and noninfectious, has grown. In this chapter we discuss the pulmonary complications of HIV infection with an emphasis on distinctive clinical features, diagnosis and treatment, and prevention.

The occurrence of opportunistic disease in patients with HIV infection is a function of underlying host immunocompetence, exposure to potential pathogens, pathogen virulence, and other modifying factors. Cigarette smoking may increase the likelihood of pulmonary infections, for example, while use of chemoprophylaxis may decrease risk. Thus, the spectrum of pulmonary infections in patients with HIV infection may vary over time or between populations.

Of the diseases listed in Table 1, those that the clinician should expect to encounter in an individual patient depend upon the degree of immunosuppression at the time of presentation. The CD4 cell count remains the best surrogate marker for assessing host immunocompetence. In the early stages of HIV infection, with CD4 cell counts greater than $500/mm^3$, there is an increased risk for infections with more virulent organisms capable of causing disease in persons with intact immune systems, such as *Streptococcus pneumoniae* or *Mycobacterium tuberculosis*. As the circulating number of CD4 cells declines to less than $200/mm^3$, the HIV-infected patient remains susceptible to infection from these virulent organisms, but also becomes increasingly susceptible to opportunistic pathogens, such as *P. carinii*.

APPROACH TO DIAGNOSIS

An algorithm for the stepwise evaluation of the HIV-infected patient with respiratory symptoms and a CD4 count less than $200/mm^3$ is depicted in Fig. 1. Pulmonary abnormalities are first confirmed, either by chest radiograph or by nonspecific test-

TABLE 1. *Common respiratory pathogens in HIV infection
listed in relation to CD4 count*

Pathogen	CD4 count
Bacteria	
Streptococcus pneumoniae	Any
Haemophilus influenzae	Any
Pseudomonas aeruginosa	Any, usually <50
Rhodococcus equi	<100
Nocardia species	<100
Mycobacterium tuberculosis	Any
Nontuberculous mycobacteria	<100
Protozoa	
Pneumocystis carinii	<200
Toxoplasma gondii	<100
Fungi	
Cryptococcus neoformans	<100
Histoplasma capsulatum	<200
Coccidioides immitis	<200
Aspergillus fumigatus	<100
Viruses	
Cytomegalovirus	<50

ing documenting either defects in gas exchange or lung inflammation. Sputum induction is performed with analysis of the specimen for *P. carinii* along with mycobacterial smear and culture. Because the negative predictive value of sputum induction for PCP is low (50–60%) and PCP is not ruled out by a nondiagnostic sputum induction, bronchoscopy with bronchoalveolar lavage (BAL) is undertaken in patients with no pathogen identified after sputum induction. Transbronchial biopsy may improve the yield for certain pathogens, but because of the higher complication rate, biopsy is usually not done unless a specific diagnosis is not made after BAL. Open lung biopsy is considered for patients with pulmonary abnormalities on chest radiograph and progressive symptoms in whom other testing fails to yield a diagnosis.

PROTOZOAL INFECTIONS

Pneumocystis carinii

Epidemiology

P. carinii will be treated here as a protozoan under its traditional taxonomic group, although ribosomal RNA analysis places it within the fungal group of organisms. Although the organism cannot be cultured and thereby identified anywhere in the environment, it is presumed to be ubiquitous. Exposure occurs early in life with nearly 100% of children having specific antibody by age 2. PCP occurs in a variety

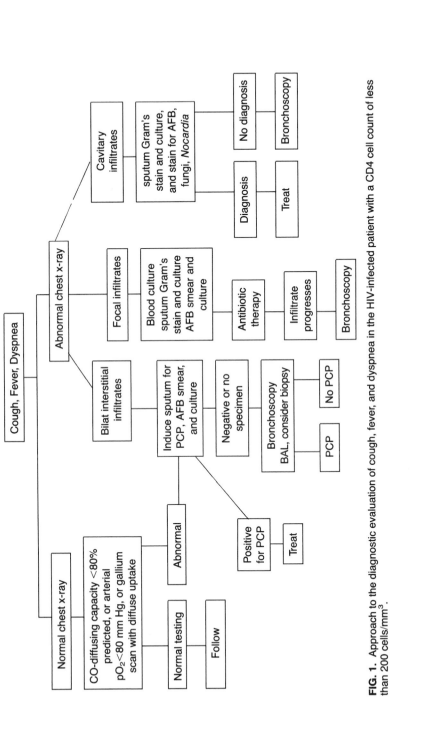

FIG. 1. Approach to the diagnostic evaluation of cough, fever, and dyspnea in the HIV-infected patient with a CD4 cell count of less than 200 cells/mm^3.

of conditions accompanied by defects in cell-mediated immunity, but the unique susceptibility of patients with HIV to this organism is remarkable. Since the first conclusive report of human disease in 1951, cases were noted sporadically in premature infants and in patients receiving cytotoxic drugs or steroids for malignancy or organ transplants. The clusters of PCP reported in 1981 in Los Angeles, San Francisco, and New York marked the beginning of the AIDS epidemic. In the following decade, PCP was the presenting manifestation of HIV infection for 60% of all AIDS patients. The proportion of AIDS patients with an initial diagnosis of PCP fell to 45% by 1992, reflecting the widespread use of prophylaxis. Nonetheless, PCP remains the most common AIDS-defining opportunistic disease in the United States. Thus PCP, formerly regarded as a rare complication of immunosuppression, has moved into the realm of primary care medicine.

Clinical and Laboratory Manifestations

In the HIV-infected patient, the time course of PCP symptoms is typically indolent or subacute, with respiratory complaints such as dyspnea and nonproductive cough progressing over weeks to months. This presentation contrasts with that described in other immunocompromised groups, where symptoms tend to have a more acute onset. It is important to bear in mind that the presenting symptoms and time course in AIDS are variable and dyspnea may be progressive over several days. Other common symptoms are fever, fatigue, anorexia, and weight loss. An abrupt onset of symptoms or the presence of rigors would be atypical of PCP and more suggestive of bacterial infection. The physical examination may document fever and tachypnea, as well as other signs of advanced HIV infection, such as oral thrush or oral hairy leukoplakia. The presence of such signs is of particular significance when facing a patient not yet known to be HIV seropositive, or with an unknown CD4 count. The chest examination is often normal.

Laboratory findings in PCP are generally nonspecific. The blood count usually reveals the mild anemia commonly encountered in the later course of HIV infection. The white blood cell count is typically normal or reduced, with a marked lymphopenia. If a leukocytosis is present and the white cell differential is shifted to the left, the clinician should be suspicious of the possibility of a pyogenic bacterial process, either alone or in combination with PCP. Lactate dehydrogenase (LDH) levels are typically elevated, and the degree of elevation may correlate with the severity of disease and outcome. LDH elevation is a sensitive but not specific marker for PCP, and many other pulmonary infections can be associated with a similar rise in LDH. Arterial blood gas measurements usually show a respiratory alkalosis, hypocarbia, and a widened alveolar-arterial oxygen gradient.

The chest radiograph can be variable in PCP (Figs. 2A and 3A). The pattern most typical is that of bilateral diffuse infiltrates in an interstitial or interstitial-alveolar pattern, reported in approximately 80% of cases. Less frequently, PCP may manifest radiographically as unilateral or focal infiltrates, cystic lesions, nodular densi-

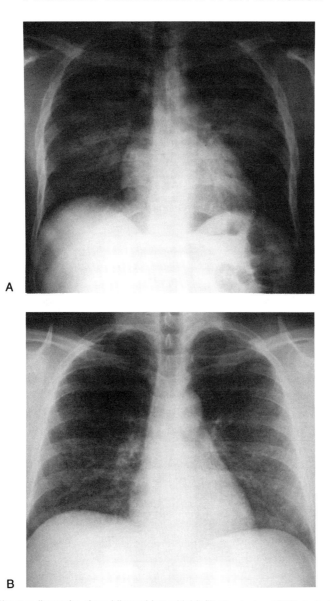

A

B

FIG. 2. Chest radiographs show bilateral intersitial infiltrates in two HIV-infected patients presenting in a similar manner with fever, fatigue, and a CD4 count of less than 100/mm^3. Bronchoalveolar lavage yielded *Pneumocystis carinii* in patient 2A, while bronchoscopy revealed no pathogens in patient 2B, but blood cultures grew *Histoplasma capsulatum*.

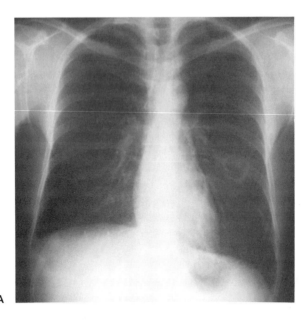

A

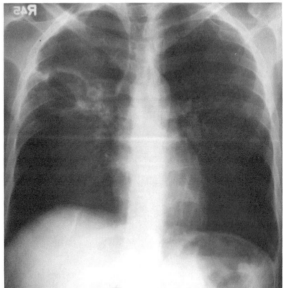

B

FIG. 3. Chest radiographs show cavitary processes in two HIV-infected patients presenting with fever and cough. Bronchoalveolar lavage fluid yielded *Pneumocystis carinii* in patient 3A. Bronchoalveolar lavage revealed purulent respiratory secretions with small gram-negative bacilli in patient 3B. Culture grew *Pseudomonas aeruginosa* and no other pathogens.

ties, or pneumothoraces. Adenopathy and pleural effusions are reported only rarely, and when present should raise concern for mycobacterial or fungal disease. Atypical radiographic features, particularly apical infiltrates, are seen more commonly in patients who have received aerosolized pentamidine as PCP prophylaxis. The radiographic appearance may be normal in 10–15% of confirmed cases of PCP, usually reflecting mild disease.

In the face of a normal chest radiograph and relatively normal oxygenation at rest, other specialized testing may provide further supporting evidence for the presence of PCP in the evaluation of a patient presenting with unexplained fevers or fatigue. The documentation of oxygen desaturation with exercise is 80% sensitive in identifying early PCP. A reduced diffusion capacity for carbon monoxide (DLCO), as well as a diffuse bilateral pattern of uptake on gallium citrate scanning, have also been shown to be sensitive.

Diagnostic Testing

Empiric antipneumocystis therapy should be initiated in patients with suspected PCP as the evaluation proceeds. Because a number of other respiratory pathogens can present in a manner similar to PCP, and because adverse reactions to anti-PCP therapy occur frequently, the diagnosis should be confirmed by visualization of *P. carinii* in respiratory specimens. While the organisms can, on occasion, be identified in expectorated sputum samples, PCP is characteristically associated with a dry, nonproductive cough, and therefore this procedure does not produce a reliable specimen for laboratory analysis. Sputum induction by nebulized hypertonic saline is the initial step in the diagnostic evaluation. The reported sensitivity of sputum induction for PCP varies greatly, but approaches 90% at some centers with experienced personnel. Traditional stains used to identify PCP include toluidine Blue-O and methenamine silver, which stain the cyst wall. Giemsa stains identify trophozoite forms and have proved especially useful in identifying PCP in sputum specimens. Direct and indirect immunofluorescence stains utilize monoclonal antibodies and are rapid, sensitive, and specific. The application of more advanced technology such as polymerase chain reaction may have a role in the future in the routine diagnosis of PCP.

When a diagnosis is not established by the examination of induced sputum, fiberoptic bronchoscopy should be performed. Bronchoalveolar lavage (BAL) is well tolerated and has a high yield for diagnosing PCP in AIDS patients, with sensitivities ranging from 79% to 98%. When BAL is combined with transbronchial biopsy, the sensitivity is increased to 94% to 100%, although pneumothorax may occur in up to 10% of patients. Either repeat bronchoscopy with biopsy or open lung biopsy is considered for patients who have no confirmed diagnosis after BAL and have clinically progressive disease. Repeat bronchoscopy is rarely helpful in patients with confirmed PCP who are failing therapy.

Treatment

Trimethoprim-sulfamethoxazole (TMP-SMX) given orally or intravenously (as 15 mg/kg TMP and 75 mg/kg SMX daily) is well established as highly effective treatment for PCP and is the agent of choice for initial therapy (Table 2). AIDS patients, however, have a high incidence (30%) of adverse reactions to this drug. Common reactions include fever, rash, bone marrow suppression, and elevation of liver enzymes. Intravenous pentamidine (4 mg/kg/day) is an alternative agent to TMP-SMX as initial therapy. Pentamidine is also associated with a high incidence of adverse reactions. These include azotemia, hyper- and hypoglycemia, pancreatitis, hypotension, and bone marrow suppression. In efficacy trials comparing the two agents, TMP-SMX and pentamidine have similar rates of efficacy and a similar incidence of adverse reactions, with 60% to 90% of patients surviving the episode of PCP and 25% to 60% experiencing severe adverse reactions.

A growing number of alternative regimens are available for treating patients with PCP and intolerance to TMP-SMX. Trimethoprim (15 mg/kg/day) in combination with dapsone (100 mg/day) is as effective in mild to moderate PCP and may be better tolerated than TMP-SMX. Adverse reactions include hemolytic anemia in patients with glucose-6-phosphate dehydrogenase (G-6-PD) deficiency, methemoglobinemia, and hepatotoxicity. Dapsone alone in the treatment of PCP has a high rate of treatment failure. Oral or intravenous clindamycin (1800–2400 mg/day) combined with oral primaquine (15–30 mg base/day) is also effective in the treatment of mild to moderate PCP. Common adverse reactions include fever, rash, methemoglobinemia, and diarrhea. Primaquine is contraindicated in individuals with G-6-PD deficiency.

Atovaquone is a hydroxynaphthoquinone that is safe and well tolerated. In a randomized double-blind study of 322 patients with mild to moderate PCP, 82% of patients receiving atovaquone (750 mg orally three times daily) responded to therapy compared with 94% of those receiving TMP-SMX, and significantly more patients on atovaquone died. The TMP-SMX group had more treatment-limiting adverse reactions (20% vs. 7%). The bioavailability of atovaquone is variable and is enhanced if the drug is taken with food, particularly fatty foods. This unpredictable bioavailability limits the usefulness of atovaquone in more seriously ill patients whose oral intake may be compromised. Treatment failures on atovaquone have been associated with low serum levels and the presence of diarrhea. The bioavailability of the new oral suspension formulation of atovaquone is greater and the dose has been reduced to 750 mg twice daily.

Trimetrexate (TMTX) is an inhibitor of folate metabolism that has recently been approved in the United States as second-line antipneumocystis therapy. Leucovorin (folinic acid) must be given to limit toxicity because of severe inhibition of dihydrofolate reductase in host cells. In a randomized trial of patients with moderate to severe PCP, the group receiving TMTX and leucovorin had a higher failure rate than the group receiving TMP-SMX (38% vs. 20%) but fewer adverse reactions. The recommended dose of TMTX is 45 mg/m^2/day intravenously as a single dose, along with leucovorin 20 mg/m^2 every 6 hours. Toxicities include rash, bone marrow sup-

TABLE 2. *Management of common respiratory infections in patients infected with HIV*

Organism	Treatment options	Comments
Parasites		
P. carinii	Trimethoprim (15 mg/kg/day) and sulfamethoxazole (75 mg/kg/day) po/iv in 3–4 divided doses × 21 days	TMP-SMX preferred therapy for PCP of any severity
	Pentamidine 4 mg/kg/day iv × 21 days	Drug of choice in severe PCP for those intolerant of TMP-SMX
	Trimethoprim (15 mg/kg/day) po/iv in 3 divided doses and dapsone (100 mg/day) × 21 days	Effective therapy in mild or moderate PCP
	Clindamycin (600 mg iv Q6–8hr or 300–450 mg po Q6h) and primaquine 15–30 mg base po/day × 21 days	Effective therapy in mild or moderate PCP
	Atovaquone (750 mg po bid with food) × 21 days	Effective therapy in mild or moderate PCP
	Trimetrexate (45 mg/m^2) iv/day) and leucovorin (20 mg/m^2 po/iv/day) × 21 days	Effective in moderate or severe PCP for those intolerant of other options
	If pO$_2$<70 mm Hg, or if A-a gradient>35, add corticosteroids:	
	Prednisone 40 mg po (or iv equivalent), bid × 5 days, then 20 mg po bid × 5 days, then 20 mg po daily to completion of therapy	
T. gondii	Pyrimethamine (100–200 mg po load, then 50–100 mg/day) and folinic acid (10 mg po/day) and sulfadiazine (4–8 g po/day) × 6 weeks	Lifelong maintenance with pyrimethamine (25–50 mg/day) and sulfadiazine (2–4 g/day) and folinic acid (5 mg/day) required
	Pyrimethamine and folinic acid (as above) and clindamycin (600 mg iv Q6h or 300–450 mg po/day) × 6 weeks	Life-long maintenance with pyrimethamine and folinic acid (as above) and clindamycin (300–450 mg po Q6–8h) required
Bacteria		
S. pneumoniae	Penicillins or erythromycin (250–500 mg po qid) or cephalosporins	Response to traditional therapy usually good
H. influenzae	Cefuroxime (500 mg po bid or 750 mg iv Q8h) or trimethoprim-sulfamethoxazole (DS po bid) or amoxicillin-clavulanate (250–500 mg po tid)	Response to traditional therapy usually good
P. aeruginosa	Antipseudomonal penicillin or cephalosporin and an aminoglycoside	Antibiotic choice should be guided by sensitivity in culture
Nocardia sp.	Sulfadiazine 4–8 g po/iv daily × ≥6 months Trimethoprim-sulfamethoxazole	Relapse common; lifelong suppressive therapy recommended
R. equi	Vancomycin 15 mg/kg iv/Q12h (optional: addition of rifampin 600 mg po daily) or erythromycin 2–4 g daily or ciprofloxacin 1–1.5 g daily	Relapse common

TABLE 2. *Continued*

Organism	Treatment options	Comments
Fungi		
C. neoformans	Amphotericin B 0.5–1.0 mg/kg/ day iv for 2 weeks, or to total dose of 0.5–1.0 g (optional: add flucytosine 100 mg/kg/day in 4 divided doses) Fluconazole 400 mg/day × 6–10 weeks	Lifelong maintenance with fluconazole 200 mg daily required
H. capsulatum	Amphotericin B 0.5–1.0 mg/kg/ day iv × 6–8 weeks (1.0–2.0 g total dose) Itraconazole (200 mg po tid × 3 days, then bid)	Lifelong maintenance therapy required
C. immitis	Amphotericin B (0.5–1.0 mg/kg/ day iv) × 6–8 weeks (1.0–2.0 g total dose)	Lifelong maintenance therapy required
B. dermatidis	Amphotericin B (0.5–1.0 mg/kg/ day iv to 1.0–2.0 g total dose)	Lifelong maintenance therapy required
Aspergillus sp.	Amphotericin B (0.7–1.5 mg/kg/ day iv) or itraconazole (200 mg po tid × 3 days, then bid)	
Viruses		
Cytomegalovirus	Ganciclovir (5 mg/kg iv bid) × 14– 21 days or foscarnet (60 mg/kg iv Q8h or 90 mg/kg Q12h) × 14–21 days	Maintenance therapy not recommended unless ocular disease demonstrated

pression, hepatitis, azotemia, and mucositis. Fever and rash are also associated with leucovorin use.

Adjunctive corticosteroids are recommended in the treatment of moderate-to-severe PCP (pO_2 <70 mm Hg or A-a gradient >35). Three controlled trials documented that the addition of corticosteroids significantly reduces short-term mortality and progression to respiratory failure in AIDS-related PCP. Adverse effects of steroids include exacerbation of mucocutaneous candidal and herpetic infections. The recommended regimen is prednisone 40 mg orally twice daily for 5 days, then 20 mg twice daily for 5 days, then 20 mg daily for the duration of PCP therapy, or the equivalent parenteral dose of methylprednisolone.

Common Problems in Management

The clinical response to effective anti-PCP therapy may be slow. On average, HIV-infected patients with PCP who do not receive adjunctive corticosteroids defervesce 5 to 9 days after the initiation of therapy and may require supplemental oxygen for several weeks. Chest radiograph improvement occurs slowly. Steroids accelerate improvement by clinical parameters. If a patient with confirmed PCP is deteriorating on TMP-SMX or pentamidine, there is no evidence that either switching or combining agents will improve outcome, but switching from a failing regimen is commonly done. Additional treatable conditions, such as a second respiratory infection or fluid overload, should be considered and therapy instituted.

If a patient is slow to respond to anti-PCP therapy and remains on supplemental oxygen or has residual respiratory symptoms at the end of 21 days of treatment, the treatment course should be lengthened to 4 to 5 weeks. Repeat bronchoscopy at the completion of therapy frequently demonstrates the presence of *P. carinii*, even in patients who have responded clinically; this finding is not predictive of a group more likely to relapse, and if a patient is doing well clinically, is not an indication for the continuation of therapy beyond 3 weeks.

The decision to use mechanical ventilation in a patient with PCP and respiratory failure may be a difficult one. Data from early in the AIDS epidemic suggested that this intervention was medically futile, with no survivors in a group of 16 patients who required mechanical ventilation for PCP. Later reports showed survival rates of 20% to 40%, probably reflecting earlier diagnosis of PCP and the use of adjunctive corticosteroid therapy. Some investigators have tried to define the unique characteristics of survivors and nonsurvivors in order to identify prospectively those AIDS patients likely to benefit from the invasive and sometimes painful manipulations of a course in the intensive care unit (ICU). Multi–organ system failure identified nonsurvivors in one group of AIDS patients with PCP in an ICU. In another series reviewing 14 AIDS patients with PCP admitted to an ICU, all patients who ultimately survived the ICU experience demonstrated improvement in the level of respiratory support required by day 4 to 5 of their ICU stay. Either worsening or unchanged ventilatory status at day 4 to 5 were associated with ICU death. No clinical or laboratory parameter documented prior to intubation was predictive of ICU survival. Another clinical feature identifying nonsurvivors in a retrospective review of 33 patients with AIDS-related PCP was the onset of respiratory failure in relation to the start of anti-PCP therapy; if mechanical ventilation was required early in the treatment course (<5 days), survival was 50%, but if it was required late (>5 days after the start of therapy) mortality approached 100%.

Prevention

Because PCP contributes significantly to morbidity and mortality in advanced HIV infection, identifying those at risk for PCP and preventing its occurrence is a high priority in the care of HIV-infected persons. The risk for PCP is elevated in individuals with HIV infection and a prior history of PCP, in patients with a CD4 count of less than 200 cells/mm^3, and patients with more than 2 weeks of unexplained fevers, diarrhea, or oral candidiasis. Prior to the AIDS epidemic, TMP-SMX was shown to be effective PCP prophylaxis in children undergoing treatment for leukemia. Multiple trials have since demonstrated that various regimens of PCP prophylaxis are effective in reducing the incidence of PCP and reducing AIDS mortality. The first such trial was conducted by Fischl and colleagues in 1988. Sixty patients with Kaposi's sarcoma were randomized to receive either TMP-SMX (160 mg TMP/800 mg SMX twice daily) with folinic acid or no therapy. Adverse reactions required discontinuation of TMP-SMX in 17% of patients, but none of the patients who were able to tolerate therapy developed PCP; in contrast, 53% of the patients receiving placebo developed PCP. TMP-SMX prophylaxis was associated with longer median survival (23 months vs. 13 months in the untreated group). Many studies done subsequently have confirmed the benefits of TMP-SMX in PCP prevention. Aerosolized pentamidine, developed in an effort to target drug delivery and minimize systemic toxicity, has also been shown to be effective in reducing the incidence of PCP with fewer associated adverse effects than TMP-SMX. Extrapulmonary pneumocystosis and pneumothorax have been associated with its use. Oral dapsone is likewise an effective alternative for PCP prophylaxis in patients unable to tolerate TMP-SMX.

Clinical trials comparing the efficacy of TMP-SMX, aerosolized pentamidine, and dapsone in PCP prophylaxis have demonstrated that TMP-SMX is the superior agent and the preferred therapy in patients who can tolerate it. Not only has it been shown to be the most effective of the three agents in preventing PCP, it also protects against other bacterial infections and against toxoplasmic encephalitis. Dose regimens with established effectiveness include one double-strength tablet three times weekly, one single-strength tablet daily, or one double-strength tablet daily. Dapsone (100 mg orally daily) has been shown to be second to TMP-SMX as an effective agent of PCP prophylaxis and superior to aerosolized pentamidine. There are fewer data documenting the efficacy of lower dapsone doses (50 mg daily or 100 mg twice weekly). Aerosolized pentamidine (300 mg via Respiragard nebulizer) should be reserved for patients who cannot tolerate TMP-SMX or dapsone. Regimens employing atovaquone and clindamycin-primaquine have not been evaluated for efficacy.

Management of Adverse Reactions to TMP-SMX

Although TMP-SMX is the preferred therapy for acute episodes of PCP and the best agent for PCP prophylaxis, adverse reactions often limit its use. Cutaneous eruptions, pruritis, fever, hepatic transaminase elevation, and nephritis are common reasons for discontinuation of TMP-SMX therapy. Anaphylaxis and rashes that progress to life-threatening bullous eruptions are rare, although they do occur in HIV-infected patients. Some reports suggest a lower incidence of adverse reactions to TMP-SMX with concurrent use of corticosteroids in PCP therapy, and a higher frequency of adverse reactions in those patients with higher CD4 cell counts, but these associations are unclear. There is also evidence that adverse reactions to TMP-SMX are less frequent with the lower doses required for PCP prophylaxis than with the higher doses required for treatment.

Adverse cutaneous reactions to TMP-SMX occurring during therapy for PCP that are not life threatening have been successfully managed with antihistamines and antipyretics, allowing for continuation of therapy. For those patients who have re-covered from an adverse reaction to TMP-SMX, later rechallenge after several months with the low doses of TMP-SMX required for prophylaxis appears to be a safe option and well tolerated in approximately half of patients studied. Of the patients enrolled in the AIDS Clinical Trial Group study of secondary prophylaxis for PCP, rates of adverse reactions to TMP-SMX were similar in those reporting an adverse reaction in the past compared with those without such a history (68% vs. 74%).

Oral desensitization with increasing doses of TMP-SMX has been reported as a successful management option in those with a past adverse reaction to TMP-SMX. However, given the high proportion of patients in other studies who tolerate re-challenge well, it is not clear that oral desensitization with TMP-SMX provides any additional benefit over simply rechallenging. No trials have been conducted to com-pare these two alternative management options.

Toxoplasma gondii

The central nervous system is the most common site of toxoplasmosis in the setting of HIV infection. The lung is the second most common site of infection, although the incidence of toxoplasmic pneumonitis varies widely with geographic setting. In France, where there is a high risk of environmental exposure, 4% of HIV-infected patients requiring bronchoscopy were found to have toxoplasmosis. Similar studies based upon bronchoscopy data in U.S. centers report a diagnosis of *T. gondii* in less than 0.5% of cases. The clinical presentation of pneumonitis due to *T. gondii* may mimic PCP, with a subacute course of dyspnea, dry cough, and diffuse interstitial infiltrates on chest radiograph. The diagnosis requires visualiza-tion of tachyzoites with Giemsa stain of respiratory specimens, usually obtained at bronchoscopy. Serologic testing may document prior exposure but does not confirm the diagnosis. As is the case with suspected CNS disease, negative serology makes the diagnosis of toxoplasmosis less likely but does not exclude the diagnosis. Trials evaluating therapies for toxoplasmosis in HIV infection have focused on encepha-litis, and patients with toxoplasma pneumonitis should be treated with these estab-lished regimens. Pyrimethamine together with either sulfadiazine or clindamycin are recommended therapies (Table 2).

BACTERIA

Pyogenic Bacterial Pneumonia

Due to defects in both cell-mediated and humoral immunity, individuals with HIV infection are more susceptible to bacterial infections, particularly those due to encapsulated organisms. The most common bacterial pathogens in HIV are the pneumococcus and *Haemophilus influenzae*. The risk of developing bacterial pneumonia has been reported to be higher among certain groups; Witt and colleagues found a higher incidence of bacterial pneumonia among injection drug users than among homosexual or bisexual men. Recent studies suggest that cigarette or other drug smoking greatly increases the risk of bacterial pneumonia. Bacteremia with pneumonia also appears to be more common in HIV-infected patients than in HIV-seronegative hosts, particularly in cases of pneumococcal pneumonia. At the Johns Hopkins Hospital, 46% of HIV-infected patients with pneumococcal pneumonia had bacteremia. This represented an eightfold increase over that reported in series prior to the AIDS epidemic. Other isolates causing lower respiratory tract infection include *Pseudomonas aeruginosa, Staphylococcus aureus, Moraxella, Legionella*, and other *Haemophilus* species. Several investigators have reported a rising incidence of infections due to *P. aeruginosa*, including infections of the lower respiratory tract. The majority of affected patients had advanced HIV disease (CD4 <50/mm^3). Most of the infections were community-acquired. Risk factors included neutropenia, prior antibiotic use, and steroid therapy.

Clinical Manifestations

Bacterial pneumonia in patients infected with HIV present with symptoms similar to those in patients without HIV. Fever, rigors, cough productive of purulent sputum, pleurisy, and dyspnea are reported, and the duration of symptoms is shorter than the average duration of symptoms of PCP. An indolent course has been described, however, in a subset of HIV-infected patients with certain bacterial pathogens such as *H. influenzae* and *P. aeruginosa*. The physical examination may reveal fever, tachypnea, and evidence of consolidation on examination of the chest. Other systemic features of sepsis may be present on physical examination as well, but it is unlikely that a specific etiologic agent will be identified by the clinical presentation.

Laboratory Testing

The laboratory abnormalities found in patients with HIV-related bacterial pneumonia may be similar to those encountered in other hosts and are nonspecific. The white blood cell count may be elevated with a predominance of neutrophils and immature forms. The chest radiograph is variable. Focal segmental or lobar consolidation is common, particularly with pneumococcal pneumonia. Radiographic patterns observed with pneumonia due to *H. influenzae* are more variable and may include that of diffuse bilateral interstitial infiltrates, which is also typical of PCP. Cavitary lesions have been reported with a number of organisms, including *S. pneumoniae, Rhodococcus equi, P. aeruginosa*, and other gram-negative bacilli (Fig. 3B).

Diagnosis

Analysis of Gram-stained sputum, followed by the identification of a predominant organism by sputum culture, is useful in the identification of an etiologic agent. Because of the relatively high rate of bacteremia seen in HIV-infected patients with pneumonia, blood cultures should also be sent in the initial evaluation of a patient with pneumonia.

Treatment

Management of bacterial pneumonia is similar to the approach applied in HIV-seronegative individuals (Table 2). Initial empiric antibiotic therapy should be guided, whenever possible, by the results of the sputum Gram stain. If *S. pneumoniae* is suspected from the sputum analysis, penicillin or erythromycin are suitable choices; if sputum studies are unrevealing, or if *H. influenzae* is suspected, a second-generation cephalosporin such as cefuroxime, an extended spectrum macrolide, or amoxicillin-clavulinate are appropriate. If the features of the clinical presentation and chest radiograph are compatible with PCP as well, high-dose TMP-SMX is a good empiric choice while the diagnostic evaluation proceeds. Alternatively, if the clinical presentation is mild and could be compatible with either PCP or pyogenic bacterial pneumonia, a trial of a β-lactam antibiotic followed by close observation for symptomatic improvement may help the clinician distinguish between PCP and a bacterial process. HIV-infected patients with community-acquired bacterial pneumonia usually respond rapidly to appropriate antibiotic therapy. If a patient deteriorates on standard therapy for the common organisms, alternative or coexistent processes, such as PCP, fungal infection, or endocarditis, should be considered, and the appropriate diagnostic tests performed.

Other Bacterial Pathogens

Nocardia

Nocardia species have long been recognized as a pathogen causing disease in groups with compromised cellular immunity. Nocardiosis was not described in association with HIV infection until recently, however, and is not an opportunistic infection included in the AIDS surveillance case definition. In most reported cases, nocardiosis occurs later in the course of immunodeficiency (CD4 count $<200/mm^3$). As in HIV-seronegative patients, the lung is the most common site of involvement. Patients typically present with a chronic or subacute onset of constitutional symptoms; cough, fevers, and weight loss are prominent. A variety of radiographic patterns are described, including alveolar infiltrates, mixed reticulonodular infiltrates, and cavities. Gram stain of respiratory specimens shows branching or beaded gram-positive bacilli; modified acid fast stains reveal acid fast bacilli. Sputum analysis may lead to an early presumptive diagnosis if nocardia is considered, but more often diagnosis is delayed several weeks due to the characteristically slow growth of the organism in culture. Culturing respiratory pathogens for mycobacteria and fungi will improve the chance of identifying *Nocardia.*

Sulfonamides are considered first-line therapy for nocardiosis (Table 2). For patients intolerant of sulfa drugs, minocycline has also been proven to be successful therapy in several case reports in HIV-infected hosts. Cefotaxime, ceftriaxone, imipenem, and amikacin are effective *in vitro* as well. The optimum duration of therapy is uncertain, but at least 6 to 12 months is recommended for pulmonary disease. Because of the high risk of relapse, chronic suppressive lifetime therapy has been recommended in AIDS cases.

Rhodococcus

Rhodococcus equi (formerly *Corynebacterium equi*) is a common cause of pneumonia in farm animals and a relatively rare cause of pneumonia in immunocompromised hosts, including HIV-infected patients. The organism is an acid-fast, gram-positive, pleomorphic bacillus. Pneumonia clinically presents with an indolent course of fever, productive cough, and dyspnea. The chest radiograph typically shows focal or lobar infiltrates that often progress to cavity formation. The diagnosis can be made by sputum or BAL analysis and culture, or by blood culture. Effective antibiotics are erythromycin or vancomycin, in combination with rifampin to provide synergy (Table 2). Resistance to β-lactam antibiotics evolves rapidly. Long courses of therapy are required and surgical intervention may be of benefit in some cases. Relapse is common after cessation of antibiotics.

Prevention

Immunization and prophylactic antibiotics are the two primary strategies employed in order to prevent bacterial respiratory infections. Because of the high rates of pneumococcal pneumonia, vaccination with the 23-valent pneumococcal polysaccharide vaccine is recommended for all HIV-infected individuals, although there are reports of vaccine failure. Pneumococcal vaccine is less effective in patients with advanced immunodeficiency, although there is no CD4 cell level below which the vaccine can be said to be completely ineffective. Vaccination with the protein-conjugated *H. influenzae* type B vaccine is recommended in all HIV-infected children, but because of the low rate of type B infections in HIV-infected adults, it is not routinely recommended for them.

Antibiotic prophylaxis with TMP-SMX is recommended for adults at risk for PCP (CD4 count $<200/mm^3$). There is good evidence to suggest that AIDS patients receiving TMP-SMX for PCP prophylaxis have a lower incidence of bacterial infections compared with those receiving aerosolized pentamidine. Passive immunotherapy with immune globulin has been used in children with symptomatic HIV infection to reduce the incidence of bacterial infections, although it has been shown to be no more effective than TMP-SMX, and there is no evidence to support its use in adults. Patient counseling and clinical interventions to alter behavior (e.g., smoking cessation) are additional preventive measures.

Mycobacteria

Mycobacterium tuberculosis

The AIDS epidemic has contributed to a rising incidence of tuberculosis (TB) in the Western world and in the United States, where the rate of tuberculous disease had been declining. *M. tuberculosis* infection is a relatively virulent pathogen and can cause disease at any stage of immunosuppression in HIV infection. The lung is the most frequently involved organ, and the features of pulmonary infection will be discussed here.

Clinical and Radiographic Manifestations

The presenting clinical features of tuberculosis (TB) depend upon the degree of immunosuppression. Those HIV-infected patients with normal or only modestly depleted CD4 cell counts have presentations typical of TB in HIV-seronegative patients. Disease is usually confined to the lungs, and chest radiographs show lower or upper lobe disease, sometimes with cavity formation. At more advanced stages of immunosuppression, the radiographic findings are atypical and may resemble primary or progressive primary disease. Reticular and nodular opacities, lymphadenopathy, and pleural effusions are all common radiographic findings. Normal chest radiographs have been described in patients with smear-positive TB. Up to 70% may have extrapulmonary disease with the organs of the lymphatic system most commonly involved.

Diagnosis

The diagnosis of pulmonary tuberculosis is made by identification of acid-fast bacilli in respiratory secretions, followed by growth in culture. The yield of sputum smear in early stages of immunosuppression is comparable to that found in seronegative individuals; the sensitivity is lower in more advanced stages of immunosuppression. The sensitivity of smear and culture may be improved by BAL. Bacteremia occurs in 26% to 42% of HIV-infected patients.

Patients with acid-fast bacilli found on smear (or culture, if clinically appropriate) should be treated presumptively for TB until speciation is definite.

Nontuberculous mycobacteria

M. avium complex (MAC) is a common mycobacterial isolate from body secretions in the setting of HIV disease. Although it is a common cause of disseminated disease in advanced HIV infection, MAC rarely causes disease in the lung. The isolation of MAC from respiratory secretions without clinical evidence of MAC disease in the lungs is not an indication for therapy. MAC colonization of the respiratory tract does increase the probability of disseminated disease subsequently.

M. kansasii can cause significant pulmonary morbidity in patients with AIDS. *M. kansasii* occurs more commonly in advanced stages of immunosuppression (CD4 cell count less than 100/mm^3). Of 19 cases of *M. kansasii* infection reviewed at the Johns Hopkins Hospital, 17 had pulmonary disease. Typical radiographic features included upper lobe or diffuse interstitial infiltrates. Cavities were present in over half of the patients with pulmonary involvement. This finding contrasted with that reported in a smaller series from Parkland Hospital in which none of the patients with infiltrates had cavity formation. Response to therapy with isoniazid, rifampin, and ethambutol is good.

FUNGI

Cryptococcus neoformans

Of the organisms traditionally classified as fungi, *C. neoformans* is the most common pathogen causing deep-seated fungal infection in patients with HIV infection. The organism is widespread in the environment, and there is no clear-cut regional risk for infection, as with the endemic mycoses. Infection occurs after inhalation of the encapsulated yeast. Respiratory symptoms may evolve, or, more commonly, the infection disseminates. Meningitis is the most common life-threatening manifestation of cryptococcal infection. Of all cases of cryptococcosis, a quarter to a third will present with respiratory complaints. A minority of these will have isolated pulmonary infection.

Clinical Features

Typical presenting symptoms of cryptococcal pneumonia are cough, fevers, sweats, and fatigue over an indolent course. Headache and mental status decline may be present if pulmonary and CNS involvement coexist. An interstitial pattern on chest radiograph is the most common radiographic finding, although nodules, focal consolidation, cavities, and adenopathy have also been reported.

Diagnosis

The diagnosis of cryptococcal pneumonia rests on isolation of *C. neoformans* from respiratory secretions or the visualization of the typical encapsulated yeast forms in pulmonary specimens. Isolation from blood culture documents disseminated disease but does not indicate involved sites. Cryptococcal polysaccharide antigen testing can be performed on serum, cerebrospinal fluid, sputum, or urine, and is sensitive and specific for cryptococcal infection. Pulmonary cryptococcosis often occurs prior to dissemination, however, and a negative serum and/or spinal fluid antigen test does not rule out cryptococcal pneumonia. Examination of cerebrospinal fluid for evidence of cryptococcal meningitis is essential if pulmonary or other systemic disease is diagnosed.

Treatment

Most large studies comparing strategies of treatment of cryptococcal disease have enrolled patients with meningitis. Standard therapy consists of amphotericin B during the acute episode and lifelong maintenance with a triazole (Table 2). The dose of amphotericin B is gauged by clinical response and adverse reactions, and may vary between 5 and 15 mg/kg, or a total dose of 0.5 to 1.0 g. Flucytosine may be added during the acute phase for more clinically severe disease. Adverse reactions to flucytosine, especially bone marrow suppression, may require stopping the drug. Fluconazole is the most well-studied azole for lifelong maintenance therapy; the recommended dose is 200 mg daily. It may be reasonable to treat mild-to-moderate pulmonary cryptococcosis with fluconazole alone.

Endemic Mycoses

Histoplasmosis, coccidioidomycosis, blastomycosis, and paracoccidiomycosis are all fungal diseases linked to well-delineated geographic regions, and all require cellular immunity to contain infection following primary exposure. All may have respiratory involvement as part of their clinical presentation as well. As HIV infection has become increasingly prevalent in regions where these infections are endemic, experience has accumulated in treating these infections in patients with AIDS. The regional mycoses seen in the United States will be discussed in further detail.

Histoplasmosis

Disease due to *Histoplasma capsulatum* occurs throughout the Ohio, Mississippi, and St. Lawrence river basins in the United States, as well as Puerto Rico, southern Mexico, and Central America. Outbreaks of disease in endemic areas are linked to events that disturb the soil, such as building demolition or construction, leading to clouds of particles and inhalation of viable spores or micronidia. Rapid conversion to the yeast phase occurs in the pulmonary airspaces; the yeast is engulfed by pulmonary macrophages and continues to multiply and disseminate. Progressive disseminated histoplasmosis rarely occurs in immunocompetent individuals, but is the most common presenting manifestation in HIV-infected patients with advanced immunosuppression. Disseminated infection can be due to either newly acquired infection or reactivation of latent infection.

Clinical Manifestations

The clinical presentation of histoplasmosis is usually subacute or chronic with constitutional symptoms such as fevers, sweats, and weight loss predominant. Isolated pulmonary disease is unusual, but respiratory symptoms are common in the disseminated syndrome. Physical examination may reveal mucocutaneous lesions and hepatosplenomegaly. Laboratory evaluation often reveals pancytopenia. Approximately 10% of patients present with a severe, sepsis-like syndrome, in which case there may be laboratory evidence of disseminated intravascular coagulation or multi–organ system failure. Pulmonary infiltrates are present in approximately 50% of patients with disseminated disease; radiographic patterns are variable and include interstitial, alveolar, and nodular densities (Fig. 2B). Mediastinal adenopathy and calcifications, while common in immunocompetent individuals with histoplasmosis, appear to be rare in HIV-infected patients.

Diagnosis of histoplasmosis is confirmed by culture of *H. capsulatum* from blood or other tissues, or by visualization of characteristic yeast forms in tissue stained with silver or periodic acid-Schiff stains. Body fluids suitable for culture include blood, bone marrow aspirate, and bronchoalveolar lavage fluid if there is evidence of pulmonary involvement. Blood culture by the lysis centrifugation method may improve the sensitivity over standard radiometric methods. Procedures having a high yield in confirming disease include transbronchial biopsy (69%) and bone marrow biopsy (49–69%). Organisms can sometimes be visualized on peripheral blood smears or in skin biopsy specimens, representing a less-invasive means for confirmatory diagnosis. The demonstration of *Histoplasma* polysaccharide antigen in serum or urine (available through the Histoplasmosis Reference Laboratory, Indianapolis, IN) establishes the diagnosis presumptively in new cases and predicts relapse in patients on chronic suppressive therapy.

Treatment for histoplasmosis in HIV-infected patients requires induction therapy followed by lifelong maintenance (Table 2). During the induction phase, amphotericin B is given to a total dose of 1.0 to 2.0 g over 4 to 6 weeks. Itraconazole is also effective for initial treatment of patients with milder disease. Maintenance therapy with itraconazole (200 mg twice daily) is highly effective.

Coccidioidomycosis

Disease due to *Coccidioides immitis* occurs in the semiarid regions of the southwestern United States, northern Mexico, and parts of Central and South America.

Infection occurs when wind or construction disturb the surface layer of soil, leading to airborne anthrospores that are then inhaled. The arthrospores develop into spherules in the pulmonary alveoli. These develop multiple endospores that rupture, leading to widespread dissemination. Disease in the HIV-infected host is believed to most commonly represent reactivation from prior exposure.

The clinical manifestations of coccidioidomycosis are very similar to those of histoplasmosis: chronic constitutional symptoms with fevers and wasting predominate, and concomitant respiratory symptoms are common. In one large clinical series, 72% of patients had abnormalities on chest radiograph. Approximately one-half of these were in the form of diffuse infiltrates, and one-third were focal abnormalities. The patterns of focal infiltrates were varied and included alveolar consolidation, discrete nodules, and cavitary lesions. Hilar and mediastinal adenopathy and pleural effusions were also described.

Diagnosis is made by visualization of the giant coccidioidal spherules in respiratory secretions or tissue. In those with respiratory disease, sputum culture, BAL, and transbronchial biopsy are all means of confirming the diagnosis. Coccidioidal serology by either tube precipitin or complement fixation methods was shown to be 83% sensitive in confirmed cases of the disease. False negatives occurred most frequently in the more immunocompromised individuals. Follow-up titers had some value in following the response to therapy.

Therapeutic regimens are similar to those described for histoplasmosis (Table 2). Amphotericin B is given to a total dose of 1.0 to 2.5 g. Chronic maintenance is continued for life with weekly or biweekly amphotericin B or fluconazole 400 mg daily.

Blastomycosis

Blastomyces dermatidis causes systemic fungal disease in the Midwest and southeastern United States. Rates of infection in the HIV-infected host appear to be lower than those seen in the other endemic mycoses. A review of 15 cases of blastomycosis documented advanced immunodeficiency at presentation (CD4 counts less then 200/mm^3 or a prior diagnosis of AIDS) in 13 of 15 cases. Six of these 13 had disseminated disease at presentation; 7 had disease confined to the lungs and pleura. Radiographic patterns varied. As with other endemic mycoses, the diagnosis is made by culture of the organism from body fluid or by direct visualization of the broad-based yeast form in tissue samples. Serologic testing is not helpful. Treatment regimens are similar to those employed with histoplasmosis: an induction course of amphotericin B therapy (1.0–2.5 g) is followed by chronic suppressive therapy with ketoconazole, fluconazole, or itraconazole (Table 2).

Aspergillosis

Although respiratory infections due to *Aspergillus* species are a common cause of morbidity and mortality in other immunocompromised patients, they are relatively infrequent in AIDS patients. Nevertheless, invasive and obstructive pulmonary disease due to *Aspergillus* sp. has been described as a late complication of AIDS. Predisposing conditions cited include neutropenia, corticosteroid use, marijuana use, and recent broad-spectrum antibiotic therapy. Radiographic patterns described are varied and include patchy consolidation, reticulonodular infiltrates, and cavity formation. Diagnosis is made by BAL and transbronchial biopsy. Recommended therapy is amphotericin B at doses of 0.7 to 1.5 mg/kg/day (Table 2). Despite early institution of therapy, disease progression is the rule and early mortality is high, with a median survival of 3 months in one series. Itraconazole as therapy shows some promise, and isolated cases unresponsive to amphotericin B have responded to itraconazole.

VIRUSES

Cytomegalovirus

Cytomegalovirus (CMV) is an important cause of ocular and gastrointestinal disease in advanced HIV infection. It is also a cause of serious pulmonary morbidity in other immunocompromised groups, such as bone marrow transplant patients. Although CMV is a common isolate from pulmonary secretions in patients with HIV-related respiratory disease, its role as a pulmonary pathogen remains uncertain. Patients in whom both CMV and *P. carinii* are isolated from respiratory specimens and are treated for PCP have similar survival to patients with PCP alone.

When CMV does cause pneumonitis, the clinical manifestations are very similar to those of PCP: dry cough, dyspnea, and interstitial infiltrates. To make the diagnosis of CMV pneumonitis, the following criteria should be met: a compatible clinical presentation; positive viral cultures from lung tissue or BAL; lung cytopathology showing the intranuclear inclusion bodies typical of CMV, along with the identification of either specific CMV antigens or of CMV nucleic acid; and the absence of other pathogenic organisms in respiratory specimens.

For those patients who are thought to have CMV pneumonitis, ganciclovir or foscarnet therapy should be given (Table 2). There are few data regarding efficacy of therapy, but response rates appear to be lower than seen with CMV retinitis. Unlike treatment for CMV retinitis, lifelong maintenance therapy is not recommended after the initial episode.

MALIGNANCIES

Malignancies are an important cause of morbidity and mortality in HIV-infected individuals. Kaposi's sarcoma (KS) and non-Hodgkin's lymphoma (NHL) are the most common HIV-related malignancies. Both can present with intrathoracic disease and respiratory symptoms.

Kaposi's Sarcoma

Although KS has occurred in all HIV-risk groups, it is more prevalent among homosexual and bisexual men, leading to the speculation that AIDS-related KS is caused by an additional sexually transmitted pathogen. Pulmonary disease is common, although in the vast majority of cases there is cutaneous involvement at the time that pulmonary KS is diagnosed.

Clinical Presentation

AIDS-related KS can occur in both early and advanced stages of immunosuppression, with CD4 counts in one series ranging from 10 to 540/mm^3 at the time pulmonary KS was documented. Presenting symptoms overlap considerably with those of respiratory infections and include dry cough, dyspnea, and fatigue; constitutional symptoms such as fevers, night sweats, and weight loss may be present as well. Physical examination may reveal lesions compatible with KS on the skin or in the oral cavity. The chest radiograph commonly shows bilateral infiltrates, both interstitial and alveolar in character, as well as poorly demarcated nodules. Pleural effusions may be present in up to 30% of cases; hilar or mediastinal adenopathy are present in approximately 10% of cases, although marked adenopathy due to KS is uncommon. Features that clearly distinguish between KS and AIDS-related infections are difficult to define because concurrent infection occurs in up to 50% of patients undergoing pulmonary evaluation. Images by computed tomography may be useful in staging patients with visceral KS; multiple flame-shaped or nodular lesions are seen radiating out from the hila along bronchovascular bundles. Radionuclide imaging may be useful in the diagnostic workup in very specific cases. Pulmonary KS is thallium-201 avid, but does not take up gallium citrate. Diagnosis is confirmed by bronchoscopic visualization of the characteristic violaceous plaques within the bronchial tree, along with tissue confirmation by biopsy at any other accessible site. Although biopsy of lung tissue has generally been proven safe, the diagnostic yield for KS is variable (0–83%) via this route due to problems with reactive fibrosis, hemorrhage, and crush artifact.

Treatment

Multiple chemotherapeutic agents (vinblastine, vincristine, etoposide, bleomycin, doxorubicin), used either alone or in combination, have been shown to be effective in alleviating symptoms of visceral disease and in shrinking cutaneous lesions. Whole or partial lung irradiation may reduce symptoms as well, although radiation pneumonitis may result. The impact of therapy on survival is not clear. Therapy will be discussed elsewhere in this volume.

Non-Hodgkin's Lymphoma

HIV-associated NHL is usually at an advanced stage at the time of diagnosis, with extensive involvement at extranodal sites. In one early series of AIDS-related NHL, lung involvement was seen in 9% of patients; however, isolated intrathoracic disease was uncommon. Other common sites of involvement are the GI tract, bone marrow, mucocutaneous sites, and the CNS, with presenting symptoms related to the site of disease. Radiographic features include well-delineated pulmonary masses or nodules, and hilar and mediastinal adenopathy may be present. Parenchymal infiltrates and pleural effusions are also described. Diagnosis is made by biopsy of accessible tissue. Combination cytotoxic chemotherapy is effective in reducing tumor bulk but is often poorly tolerated by HIV-infected patients, and durable remissions are difficult to attain. Therapy and prognosis for NHL will be discussed elsewhere in this volume.

SUGGESTED READING

Ampel NM, Dols CL, Galgiani JN. Coccidioidomycosis during human immunodeficiency virus infection: Results of a prospective study in a coccodioidal endemic area. *Amer J Med* 1993;94:234–240.

Chuck SL, Sande MA. Infections with *Crpytococcus neoformans* in the acquired immunodeficiency syndrome. *N Engl J Med* 1989;321:794–799.

Denning DW, Follansbee SE, Scolaro M, et al. Pulmonary aspergillosis in the acquired immunodeficiency syndrome. *N Engl J Med* 1991;324:654–662.

Dropulic LK, Leslie JM, Eldred LJ, et al. Clinical manifestions and risk factors of *Pseudomonas aeruginosa* infections in patients with AIDS. *J Infect Dis* 1995;171:930–937.

Gallant JE, Moore RD, Chaisson RE. Prophylaxis for opportunistic infections in patients with HIV infection. *Ann Intern Med* 1994;120:932–944.

Gill PS, Akil B, Colletti P, et al. Pulmonary Kaposi's sarcoma: clinical findings and results of therapy. *Am J Med* 1989;87:57–61.

Janoff EN, Breiman RF, Daley CL, Hopewell PC. Pneumococcal disease during HIV infection. Epidemiologic, clinical and immunologic perspectives. *Ann Intern Med* 1992;117:314–324.

Kalayjian RC, Toossi Z, Tomashefski JF Jr, et al. Pulmonary disease due to infection by *Mycobacterium avium* complex in patients with AIDS. *Clin Infect Dis* 1995;20:1186–1194.

Levine B, Chaisson RE. *Mycobacterium kansasii*: a cause of treatable pulmonary disease associated with advanced human immunodeficiency virus (HIV) infection. *Ann Intern Med* 1991;114:861–868.

Masur H. Prevention and treatment of *Pneumocystis* pneumonia. *N Engl J Med* 1992;327:1853–1860.

Meduri GU, Stein DS. Pulmonary manifestations of acquired immunodeficiency syndrome. *Clin Infect Dis* 1992;14:98.

Polsky B, Gold JWM, Whimbey E, et al. Bacterial pneumonia in patients with the acquired immunodeficiency syndrome. *Ann Intern Med* 1986;104:38–41.

Small PM, Schecter GF, Goodman PC, et al. Treatment of tuberculosis in patients with advanced immunodeficiency virus infection. *N Engl J Med* 1991;324:289.

Wheat LJ, Conolly-Stringfield PA, Baker RL, et al. Disseminated histoplasmosis in the acquired immune deficiency syndrome: clinical findings, diagnosis and treatment, and review of the literature. *Medicine (Baltimore)* 1990;69:369–374.

A Clinical Guide to AIDS and HIV,
edited by Gary P. Wormser.
Lippincott-Raven Publishers, Philadelphia © 1996.

6

Neurologic Complications of AIDS and HIV Infection: An Overview

Barbara S. Koppel

*Department of Neurology, New York Medical College, Valhalla, New York 10595; and
Metropolitan Hospital, New York, New York 10029*

Neurologic complications are common in HIV infection. At least 10% of cases of AIDS present with neurologic symptoms, and over the course of the illness symptomatic involvement of the central or peripheral nervous system has been found in 30% to 63% of patients. Impressively, one prospective study found that neurologic findings were present in 90% of AIDS patients if they were examined by a neurologist. Postmortem examination of brains from patients dying of AIDS has revealed abnormalities in up to 88% of cases, and more than one disease process was frequently present (Table 1). Some patients develop a mononucleosis-like syndrome with aseptic meningitis or cranial neuropathies as early as 2 weeks after primary HIV infection. Rarely, encephalopathy, brachial plexus neuritis, ganglioneuronitis, myelitis, peripheral neuropathy, stroke, and muscle necrosis with myoglobinuria also occur at, or shortly after, HIV infection and seroconversion.

An asymptomatic period of variable duration follows primary infection, even if early neurologic symptoms had occurred. During this "silent interval" special tests of nervous system function such as EEG and polysomnography, brainstem auditory evoked potentials, long latency evoked potentials, brain magnetic resonance imaging (MRI), cerebrospinal fluid analysis, cerebral blood flow, and neuropsychological assessment may detect subclinical evidence of central nervous system (CNS) involvement or dysfunction by HIV.

Autoimmune disorders with neurologic consequences may occur during the course of HIV infection as the body's immune system becomes dysfunctional. These include polyradiculopathy, peripheral polyneuropathy, mononeuritis multiplex, Bell's palsy, polymyositis, myasthenia gravis, thrombocytopenia leading to brain hemorrhage, and anticardiolipin anitbodies causing cerebral infarction.

The brain may be devastated by a bland encephalitis, so-called AIDS-dementia complex (ADC), caused by HIV itself, even in patients whose immune function is relatively normal. ADC is clinically evident in 30% of cases, although only 2.8% of AIDS cases have ADC as a presenting illness. The incidence of ADC increases with

TABLE 1. *Frequency (%) of neurologic complications in AIDS patients in different series*

Series[a]							
Main risk[b]	HS	HS	HS	IVDU	IVDU	MIX	MIX
Site[c]	SF	NY	LA	NY	NY	BAL	Miami
Patient numbers	390	104	66	28	172	186	83
HIV							
Aseptic meningitis	4	4	—	—	—	7	—
Encephalitis	25	66	85	25	39	16	14
Infection							
Toxoplasma	14	14	9	32	8	8	40
Cryptococcus	17	2	17	25	20	6	14
CMV[d]	3	27	21	—	<1	6	10
PML[e]	2	2	9	4	<1	<1	4
Mycobacteria	<1	3	6	4	6	—	2
Bacteria	<1	—	—	4	2	—	2
Herpes zoster	1	1	—	4	4	<1	—
Candida	<1	2	1	4	—	<1	1
Fungi[f]	<1	—	1	—	—	—	1
Tumor							
1° Lymphoma	6	5	4	11	<1	4	2
2° Lymphoma	<1	5	1	—	—	<1	—
Kaposi sarcoma, plasmacytoma	<1	2	—	—	—	—	—
Cerebrovascular							
Infarction	<1	3	20	—	3	<1	5
Hemorrhage	<1	3	20	—	2	—	—
Metabolic	—	—	9	—	—	3	6
Nerve	6	10	—	—	13	21	11
Muscle	<1	1	—	—	—	—	4

[a]Pathologic series.
[b]HS, homosexual men; IVDU, intravenous drug users; MIX, mixed group.
[c]SF, San Francisco; NY, New York; LA, Los Angeles; BAL, Baltimore.
[d]CMV, cytomegalovirus, including retinitis and encephalitis.
[e]PML, progressive multifocal leukoencephalopathy.
[f]Fungi include *Aspergillus, Coccidioides, Rhizopus,* and *Histoplasma.*

prolonged survival, approaching 75% in patients with end-stage AIDS, and there is pathologic evidence of the encephalitis in many more. In about half the patients with ADC, myelopathy or peripheral neuropathy also develop.

Once the immune system is no longer capable of effective defense, the nervous system also becomes vulnerable to opportunistic infections, neoplasms, and infarction. Standard therapies often fail to control viral, treponemal, fungal, or mycobacterial disease in such immunosuppressed patients, and the course of these infections may be fulminant, although with improved diagnostic and treatment methods as experience with AIDS has evolved, survival times are increasing.

Drugs used to treat patients with AIDS may have neurotoxic side effects. Dideoxycytidine (ddC) causes neuropathy; didanosine (ddI) causes neuropathy and rarely seizures; zidovudine (AZT) causes a mitochondrial myopathy that is related to cumulative dose and is associated with carnitine deficiency, Wernicke's encephalopathy, seizures, headache, and rarely delirium; ganciclovir causes seizures; 2'-fluoro-5-iodo-aracytosine (FIAC) causes myoclonus and delirium; compound Q causes aphasia and coma; trimethoprim-sulfamethoxazole causes aseptic meningitis; and pentamidine causes hypotension and hypoglycemia, which may be associated with abnormal movement. Antiepileptic drugs seem to have an unusually high incidence of adverse effects (26%), such as rash, neurotoxicity, orofacial dyskinesias from phenytoin, and neuroleptic agents often produce severe extrapyramidal effects and sometimes neuroleptic malignant syndrome as well.

This chapter offers an approach to the neurologically impaired patient and provides descriptions of the more commonly encountered syndromes.

DIAGNOSTIC STUDIES

Neuroimaging

Structural lesions of the brain and spinal cord are defined and serially assessed by computerized tomography (CT) or magnetic resonance imaging (MRI). Because of the importance of early detection of opportunistic brain infection and tumor, some investigators have recommended routine CT scans at regular intervals even in asymptomatic patients, although this is generally not standard practice. CT findings of HIV-related conditions are summarized in Table 2.

The most common CT finding in cerebral HIV infection is diffuse atrophy with sulcal and ventricular enlargement (Fig. 1). The white matter changes associated with HIV infection, which are visible with MRI (Fig. 2), are usually not evident with CT. If the amount of ventricular dilation is out of proportion to the degree of cortical atrophy, communicating obstructive hydrocephalus caused by chronic meningitis should be suspected (Fig. 3). Focal atrophy may be the result of infarction, previous trauma, or healed infection. Intracerebral calcification, especially of the basal ganglia, was previously thought to occur only in children with congenital HIV infection. However, as adults with opportunistic infections survive longer, parenchymal calcification may develop, especially in those with cytomegalovirus (CMV) infection (Fig. 4). Thus calcification of lesions generally reflects chronicity, as in immunocompetent hosts, and should never be taken as evidence of inactive disease. Both lymphoma and toxoplasmosis favor periventricular and gray–white matter junction locations (Fig. 5), although they can occur almost anywhere. If a lesion has hemorrhagic elements on the nonenhanced scan, fungal infection, especially aspergillosis, should be considered.

Although parenchymal lesions can often be seen on unenhanced CT as hypodense lesions, with or without evidence of mass effect, contrast infusion greatly facilitates detection of lymphoma and abscesses due to bacterial or toxoplasma infection. Double-dose contrast injection with delayed imaging improves visualization of less intensely enhancing lesions, but use of this technique is often limited by the patient's renal function. When serial studies are performed in the same patient, it is important to use consistent amounts of contrast on each occasion to facilitate meaningful comparisons. Even with optimal use of current CT technology, however, the extent of

TABLE 2. CT scan findings in HIV-infected patients

Pathology	Typical location	Enhancement	Atrophy	Hydrocephalus	Edema or mass effect	Multiple sites
HIV encephalitis	White matter, especially frontal	Rarely	+ + Progressive	+	−	−
Toxoplasma abscesses	Periventricular (basal ganglia, thalamus) corticomedullary	Variable: ring, homogeneous, or none	After treatment	Rare, with meningitis	Usually	Usually
Fungal[a] brain lesion	Cortical or near sinuses	+	−	−	+	Occasionally
Mycobacterial infection	Cortical	+ +	−	+ +, after meningitis	+	Rarely
PML[b]	White matter, 10% posterior fossa	Ring or solid	−	−	−	Occasionally (increased number over time)
Chronic meningitis[c]	−	Meninges, ependyma of ventricles	Generalized and focal	+	−	−
Lymphoma and other tumors	Periventricular, rarely cortical	+ +	−	−	+ +	+

Scale: −, absent; +, present; + +, prominent.
[a]Candida, Asperigillus (may be hemorrhagic), mucormycosis.
[b]Progressive multifocal leukoencephalopathy due to JC papovavirus.
[c]Due to toxoplasma, cryptococcus, mycobacterial species, or tumor. May see infarctions as well.

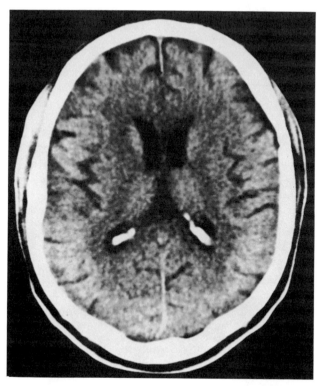

FIG. 1. Brain CT in a 34-year-old woman with ADC showing sulcal and ventricular dilation resulting from diffuse cerebral atrophy. There is hypodensity of the cerebral white matter adjacent to the ventricles, another common finding in patients with HIV infection of the brain.

brain pathology is almost always underrepresented. Ring enhancement correlates with better prognosis, because poor fibroblast recruitment limits capsule formation in many AIDS patients. Thus, in some patients, disappearance of enhancement may represent deterioration rather than response to treatment.

If a presumptive diagnosis of toxoplasmosis is made, an empiric trial of appropriate anti-infective agents can be instituted and the patient rescanned after 10 to 14 days. To assess response to treatment most meaningfully, the size and number of lesions must be carefully determined, as well as the extent to which each enhances, while attempting to control for nonspecific beneficial effects of corticosteroids and technical aspects of the imaging procedure.

MRI is complementary to CT, especially in detecting white matter degeneration caused by HIV, excess water content, or by progressive multifocal leukoencephalopathy. It is more sensitive than CT in detecting lesions and in reflecting the extent of the pathologic process, but findings are generally less specific and margins of lesions are not easily distinguishable from surrounding edema. Unlike iodine-based

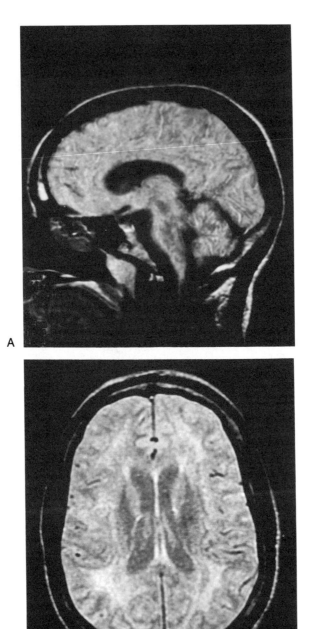

FIG. 2. A: Sagittal T1-weighted MRI of a 32-year-old man with dysarthria, gait ataxia, and dementia showing lucency in the midbrain, pons, and medulla consistent with demyelination. **B:** T1-weighted MRI with gadolinium shows no abnormal enhancement but increased white matter signal.

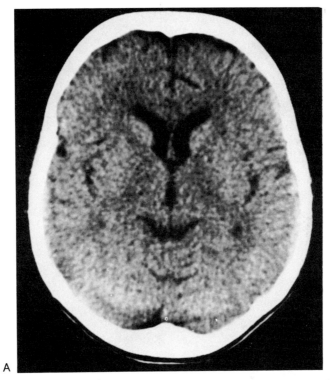

FIG. 3. A: Brain CT in a 30-year-old woman with AIDS and chronic otitis media due to *H. influenzae.* The only finding is mild atrophy.

contrast agents used with CT, gadolinium diethylenetriamine pentaacetic acid (DTPA), the contrast agent used with MRI, almost never evokes an allergic response. Furthermore, the small volume required, about 10 ml, allows gadolinium to be used in patients with renal failure. Like contrast-enhanced CT, gadolinium-enhanced MRI reveals alterations in blood-brain barrier and abnormal perfusion. In general, statements about the effect of contrast enhancement on CT-detected lesions apply to gadolinium and MRI. Patients with claustrophobia need prior conditioning or sedation to tolerate the procedure.

Similar MRI or CT abnormalities may be seen with different infections, or with infections and tumors (Fig. 5). Even viral infections may rarely present as a focally enhancing lesion. Both CT and MRI can facilitate brain biopsy, and immediate postoperative scanning allows early detection of bleeding and confirmation that the lesion was accurately sampled.

MRI or CT accompanied by myelography is necessary to diagnose spinal cord compression from tumor or abscess.

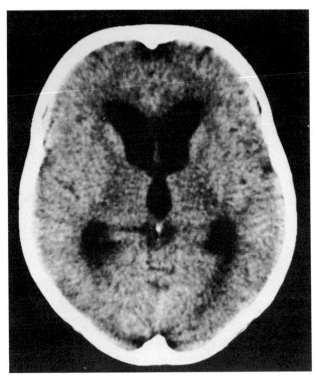

FIG. 3. B: CT of same patient 1 month later during treatment for *H. influenzae* meningitis showing enlargement of third and lateral ventricles with absent cortical sulci, reflecting increased intracranial pressure and hydrocephalus.

Cerebrospinal Fluid (CSF) Examination

CSF examination is required when meningitis is suspected, but findings are frequently atypical in immunocompromised hosts compared with immunocompetent ones. For example, there may be a paucity of white cells in cryptococcal or other infectious meningitides due to the patients' inability to generate an inflammatory response; conversely, pleocytosis can be seen in the Guillain-Barré-like syndrome associated with HIV infection. Low CSF glucose is a reliable indicator of infection, but hypoglycorrhachia can be seen with sarcoid or meningeal tumor as well. A serum glucose level should always be obtained simultaneously for comparison with CSF glucose measurements. Tests for antigen in CSF have been developed for cryptococcus, mycobacteria, and HIV, and for antibody in mycobacterial (tuberculosis), bacterial (syphilis), and viral (HIV, herpes simplex) infections. These are discussed in later sections dealing with specific infections. Amplification by polymerase chain reaction will likely assist in detecting minute quantities of pathogens in the future. Serologic tests that rely on antibody production can be falsely negative. To detect tumor cells

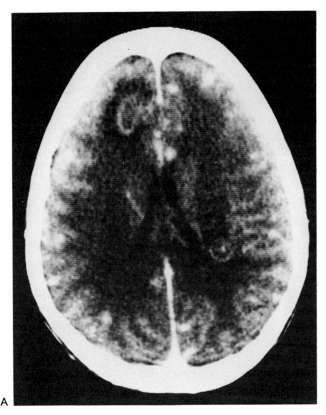

FIG. 4. A: Contrast-enhanced CT and brain scan in a 34-year-old HIV-infected man with seizures, showing right frontal and left parietal ring enhancing lesions surrounded by edema as well as multiple small lesions in the left frontal lobe adjacent to the falx, consistent with toxoplasmosis. (Courtesy of Dr. Michael Daras.)

adequately, at least 3 ml of fluid should be preserved with an equal amount of alcohol and studied by millipore filtration or cytometry. Sometimes cytologic examination must be repeated several times before a positive sample is obtained. Measurement of myelin basic protein may be of interest in quantifying the extent of ongoing demyelination. Atypical oligoclonal band patterns occur as a nonspecific consequence of viral infection or acute destructive processes and thus are usually not helpful. HIV can be cultured from CSF, so appropriate precautions in handling must be observed.

Clinical Neurophysiology

A wide variety of electroencephalographic (EEG) changes have been described in patients with HIV infection or AIDS. EEG is rarely of specific help, but diffuse

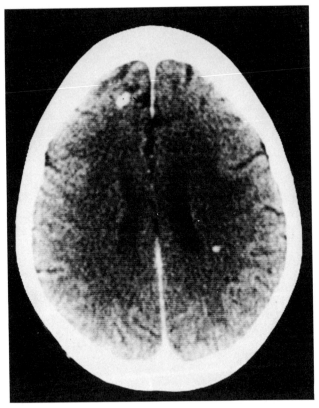

B

FIG. 4. B: Noncontrast scan in the same patient after 8 weeks of empiric antitoxoplasma therapy, showing a decrease in size and number of lesions and increased density of the right frontal and left parietal lesions representing calcification.

abnormalities of background rhythms may assist in documenting organic cerebral dysfunction in patients with equivocal mental or psychological symptoms. Conversely, a normal EEG in an apparently demented patient should raise suspicion of a psychiatric disorder such as severe depression.

Early EEG findings in ADC include slowing of mean alpha rhythm frequency, loss of alpha rhythm, and increased diffuse slow frequency activity. Later, EEG activity becomes low voltage, and there is loss of faster frequency components (Fig. 6). Quantitative computer-assisted methods of EEG analysis may increase the sensitivity for detecting abnormalities in asymptomatic patients with HIV encephalitis and predict progressive dementia. One study has claimed that electrophysiologic tests are the most sensitive indicators of subclinical CNS disease, but another found no abnormal EEGs among nondemented subjects.

Patients with focal lesions usually show focal slowing over the appropriate re-

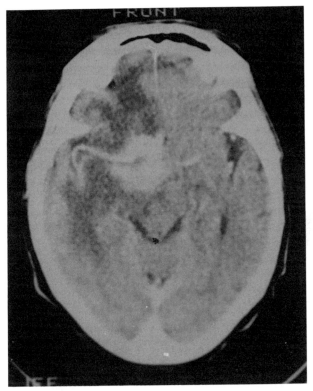

FIG. 5. Contrast-enhanced CT of the brain in a 57-year-old woman with AIDS who presented with headache and left hemiparesis, showing a densely homogeneously enhancing mass with extensive surrounding edema in the right suprasellar region, which proved to be lymphoma on biopsy. (Courtesy of Dr. John Mangiardi.)

gions. Herpes simplex encephalitis may be accompanied by a characteristic periodic sharp-wave pattern. Triphasic waves suggest metabolic encephalopathy. In patients with seizures, epileptiform discharges may be focal, multifocal, or generalized. Nonconvulsive status epilepticus may present as altered mental status and is diagnosable only by EEG.

One group has provided preliminary data that some neurologically asymptomatic HIV-infected individuals, as well as patients with early ADC, have a characteristic attenuation or loss of subcortical components (P14, N18) of the somatosensory evoked potential, and another showed the same for auditory potentials. Polysomnography has demonstrated disruption of stage IV sleep in some patients early in the course of HIV infection. Nerve conduction studies and electromyography are useful in quantifying neuropathy and in detecting myopathy and radiculopathy.

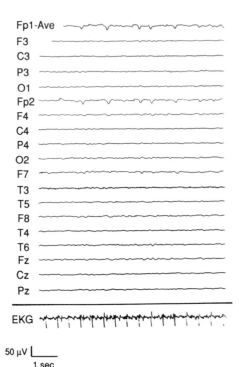

Fp1-Ave
F3
C3
P3
O1
Fp2
F4
C4
P4
O2
F7
T3
T5
F8
T4
T6
Fz
Cz
Pz

EKG

50 µV
1 sec

FIG. 6. Electroencephalogram of a 41-year-old HIV-infected man with dementia showing diffuse low-voltage slowing with reduction in faster frequency activity. (Courtesy of Dr. Cynthia Harden.)

Brain Biopsy

Because of the similarity in clinical and neuroimaging presentations of etiologically different neurologic complications, brain biopsy is often crucial for definitive diagnosis. This is especially important when empiric therapy, based on the most reasonable presumptive diagnosis, fails or new lesions develop. Tissue diagnosis is mandatory in such cases. Brain biopsy is also indicated in patients who are deteriorating too quickly for a therapeutic trial. Having said this, it is important to acknowledge that definitions of treatment failure and timing of biopsy are often disputed.

Brain biopsy has an increased incidence of complications in patients with AIDS, including infection (Fig. 7) and hemorrhage. Although a bleeding diathesis is frequently present that may predispose to hemorrhage, such as thrombocytopenia, liver dysfunction with clotting abnormalities, or disseminated intravascular coagulopathy, AIDS patients seem to have increased bleeding even in the absence of these. Awareness of these problems can reduce their influence on surgical morbidity. Chance of hemorrhage can be minimized by replacing deficient clotting factors and platelets. Stereotactic-guided biopsy using either CT or MRI guidance and only a small burr hole or limited craniotomy allows safer access to deep lesions.

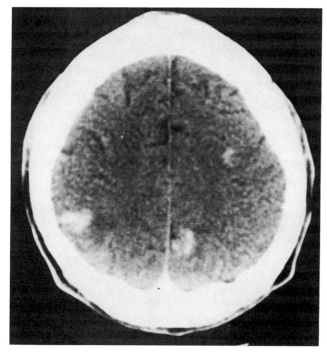

A

FIG. 7. A: Contrast-enhanced CT scan of the brain in a 38-year-old HIV-infected man with fever and seizures, revealing multiple enhancing nodular lesions. Biopsy revealed toxoplasmosis.

The disadvantage of this is that only a small tissue sample is obtained, which is sometimes inadequate for diagnosis (although taking three consecutive samples improves yield). An ultrasound probe, used with a small craniotomy, can help define the perimeter of a lesion, which maximizes detection of organisms in patients with brain abscess (Fig. 8). Ultrasonography is also helpful in detecting hemorrhagic complications.

Even with tissue obtained by biopsy, it is sometimes not possible to make an unambiguous diagnosis. This is usually because the amount of tissue is inadequate or because the sample is obtained from a part of the lesion that does not contain diagnostic pathology. Review of frozen sections is helpful in confirming that an adequate sample has been obtained. An additional problem is that sections stained with hematoxylin and eosin may appear normal even in the presence of infection. Thus special stains and cultures are always necessary and must not be overlooked. It is also important to recognize that multiple infectious agents may be present simultaneously, or that different pathologic processes may coexist, such as toxoplasmosis with lymphoma. Finally, the histopathology may be atypical in the immunodeficient host, causing problems for the unwary. For example, toxoplasma tachyzoites may be round rather than crescentic; microglial nodules may be seen with infections

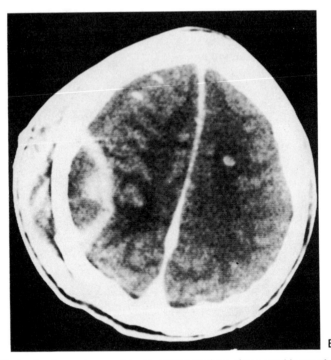

B

FIG. 7. B: Contrast-enhanced scan of same patient 10 days after open biopsy of right frontal lesion, showing dural enhancement and subgaleal swelling due to bacterial empyema.

other than CMV and HIV; and capsules of cryptococcal yeast organisms may appear unusually small (Fig. 9). Polymerase chain reaction may supplement standard techniques to identify organisms.

SYNDROMES DUE TO HIV INFECTION

HIV Encephalitis (AIDS–Dementia Complex)

Clinical and Laboratory Features

Early in the course of HIV infection, in some patients as early as 2 weeks after exposure to the virus, a flu-like syndrome occurs with muscle and joint aches, macular trunk rash, lymphadenopathy, and aseptic meningitis. Symptoms referable to the meningitis include headache, irritability, mild confusion, photophobia, and excessive sleepiness. Seizures are rare. Transient cranial neuropathies, especially facial, may appear. CSF shows a mild lymphocytic pleocytosis with slight elevation in protein content but a normal sugar level. HIV-1 can be detected by polymerase

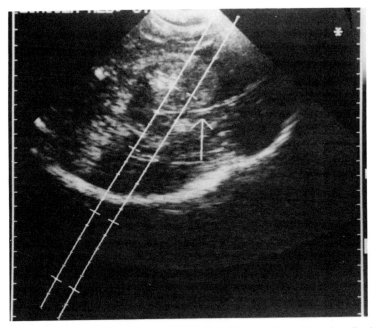

FIG. 8. Real-time ultrasonography performed during the biopsy of the patient described in Fig. 5, showing needle trajectory in center of lesion (lymphoma). (Courtesy of Dr. John Mangiardi.)

chain reaction (PCR) or other techniques. The aseptic meningitis that occurs early is usually symptomatic for only a few days or sometimes weeks, but some patients continue to show a cellular reaction in CSF even after they become asymptomatic. Rarely chronic meningitis develops with persistent headache and confusion. Treatment with corticosteroids has been beneficial, but if required, these should be used only for short periods because of the undesirable immunosuppressive properties.

As brain infection evolves, several nonspecific markers appear in CSF in both patients and experimental animals infected with HIV. Concentrations of quinolinic acid, an excitotoxin, increase proportionally to the degree of neurologic involvement and correlate with the severity of neuropsychological and motor deficits. The ratio of quinolinic acid to kynurenic acid, an antagonist of the excitotoxic effects of quinolinic acid, also increases. CSF levels of neopterin, a putative marker of activated macrophages, also rise in parallel with the severity of neurologic disease and decrease in conjunction with clinical improvement associated with zidovudine therapy. Intrathecal production of α-tumor necrosis factor, one of the cytokines proposed to contribute to neurotoxicity, also occurs with HIV brain infection, and CSF levels may correlate with ongoing active CNS disease. Measurable antibodies to HIV develop, and the virus may be cultured relatively easily.

For the next months to years the patient usually has no neurologic symptoms, although aseptic meningitis can recur. Nonetheless, evidence of latent CNS infec-

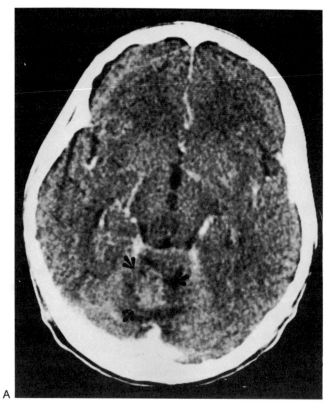

FIG. 9. A: Contrast-enhanced brain CT in a 32-year-old man with cryptococcal meningitis who developed gait ataxia on treatment. The scan shows a round, fairly homogeneously enhancing lesion in the cerebellar vermis. Biopsy revealed a cryptococcoma.

tion can be demonstrated, including the presence of HIV-Ag and β_2-microglobulin in CSF, and intrathecal synthesis of anti-HIV immunoglobulin (IgG), which may precede other serologic markers of infection. The ratio of HIV antibody in CSF to that in serum is highest early in infection, and in acute cases, antibody may be found only in CSF. Although disputed, there is some evidence that careful neuropsychological assessment reveals increased abnormalities in at least a small percentage of neurologically asymptomatic HIV-seropositive individuals compared with controls. However, selection bias may play a role in the controversy regarding psychological findings, because studies other than one in military recruits and a few others in intravenous drug users (IVDUs) have all been of homosexual men. Members of nonhomosexual risk groups, especially IVDUs, tend to seek medical attention only when opportunistic infection occurs. Low education also correlates to poor neuropsychologic performance. It has thus been extremely difficult to correlate neuropsychological findings with HIV encephalitis in this group of patients. Further-

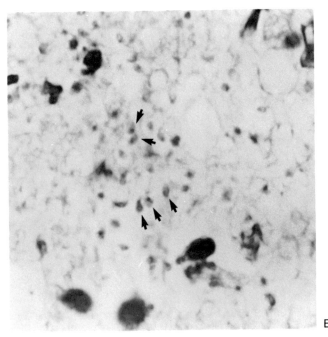

FIG. 9. B: Biopsy specimen of lesion shown in (A), demonstrating cryptococcal yeast forms surrounded by a blank space containing nonstaining capsular material (hematoxylin and eosin stain, ×800). (Courtesy of Dr. Tung Pui Poon.)

more, abnormal neuropsychological findings have been mostly observed in timed trials, which may reflect slowed motor ability rather than impaired cognitive function. Thus the clinical significance of the neuropsychological abnormalities reported to date early in HIV infection is unclear.

Other functional abnormalities in clinically asymptomatic patients have been reported using routine and quantitative electroencephalography, brainstem auditory evoked potentials, somatosensory evoked potentials, long-latency event-related potentials, and oculography. ^{31}P magnetic resonance spectroscopy, positron emission tomography, and single photon emission computed tomography (SPECT) (Fig. 10) have demonstrated *increased* metabolism within the thalamus and basal ganglia in patients with early symptoms and signs of ADC, and *decreasing* cortical metabolism as the disease progresses. Early changes in the central white matter fornices and corpus callosum have been reported using high-resolution MRI, and MRI abnormalities have been correlated with results of neuropsychological testing.

Eventually, clinical symptoms referable to HIV encephalitis emerge in approximately 85% of those with AIDS. The development of dementia correlates with older age at diagnosis of AIDS, low hemoglobin and body mass, and constitutional symptoms. Neurologic abnormalities correlate well with the areas of the brain found

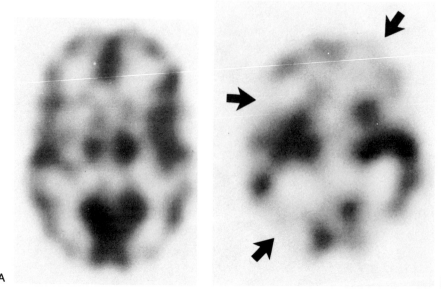

A

B

FIG. 10. A: Normal SPECT brain scan in a healthy control subject in the axial plane at the midthalamic level. **B:** Multifocal perfusion defects (*arrows*) are present in the SPECT scan from a patient with HIV encephalopathy. (Courtesy of Dr. Joseph Masdeu.)

to be most involved pathologically by the virus. Computed tomography and MRI show atrophy, the degree of which parallels the stage of disease.

Children who are infected with HIV *in utero* or perinatally may be developmentally delayed and then, at about 2 to 3 years of age, develop a progressive syndrome characterized by loss of milestones, pyramidal tract signs, acquired microcephaly, seizures, and a behavioral and cognitive decline. Computed tomography (CT) in these children reveals diffuse brain atrophy with calcifications in the basal ganglia that correspond to mineral deposits in blood vessels. MRI also demonstrates atrophy, delayed myelination, and calcification.

Adults with HIV encephalitis develop apathy and depression and have trouble concentrating and organizing tasks, difficulties that are probably due to neuron loss within frontal lobes. Memory loss, language impairment, difficulty with other higher cortical functions, and occasional hallucinations can be attributed to involvement of the limbic system and temporal lobe. Bradykinesia, impaired eye movements, and involuntary movements such as myoclonus, tremor, asterixis, and posturing result from abnormalities of basal ganglia and other subcortical nuclei. Ataxia is often noted first in walking, with patients taking cautious steps to maintain balance; this reflects brainstem or basal ganglia involvement. Loss of myelin within fiber tracts leads to delayed information processing, slow responses, impaired fine motor skills, and loss of bladder control. Pathologic reflexes such as grasp, snout, and root responses appear as the disease progresses. Terminally, patients are mute, incontinent, quadriplegic and contracted, but awake.

Demyelination precedes inflammatory changes and frank atrophy. The rate of desease progression varies but onset is usually abrupt. Asymptomatic subjects of neuropsychologic studies usually do not show minor deficits prior to the development of ADC. Once dementia is evident, the patient's average life span is less than 6 months, although survival length is increasing recently, especially among homosexuals. Sporadic generalized seizures occur in 25% to 30% of patients, possibly reflecting increased levels of excitotoxins such as quinolinic acid, and the incidence goes up with disease progression.

Pathophysiology

Pathologic evidence of HIV encephalitis, including microglial nodules and multinucleated giant cells, are found in up to 90% of patients with AIDS but do not correlate well with the presence or severity of dementia. Viral entry into brain is by HIV-infected monocytes and macrophages or directly across capillary endothelium and occurs as early as 15 days after exposure.

Monocytes and macrophages, together with endothelial cells of blood vessels, provide a repository for HIV within the brain. HIV has been identified in cortical and subcortical tissue using polymerase chain reaction methodology. Even when gross pathologic signs of encephalitis are absent, viral antigens such as gp41 and p24 have been demonstrated in neocortex using immunocytochemistry. The degree of neocortical damage, including gliosis and loss of dendritic arborization, correlates with these antigen levels. Although neurons can be infected with difficulty in tissue culture, they probably are not infected *in vivo*. Defective viral infection of astrocytes is possible.

Cytokines include interleukins 1 and 6 (IL-1,IL-6), tumor necrosis factor-α (TNF-α), granulocyte-macrophage colony-stimulating factor (GM-CSF), and transforming growth factor-β (TGF-β), all of which are normally present in the brain to regulate inflammatory and immune responses. Elevated CSF levels of inflammatory markers such as TNF, GM-CSF, IL-1, ferritin, and prostaglandin correlate with dementia and implicate macrophage stimulation in pathogenesis. Experimentally, high levels of TNF-α and IL-1 cause nonspecific necrosis in astrocytes and neurons that adhere to HIV-infected monocytes, but the exact mechanism is not known. In the presence of HIV, normal regulation of immune activity is altered so that persistent infection results in continuous cytokine production. Therefore, although the inflammatory reaction triggered by the release of IL-1 may be mild, it is never shut off and cumulative damage accrues over time. Other mediators such as interferon-γ further activate macrophages, which release quinolinate. For instance, astrocytes are stimulated to proliferate leading to gliosis and disruption of normal neuronal circuitry. Once it was understood that most cytokines are cell bound and, therefore, their levels in CSF and blood may not reflect intraparenchymal activity, postmortem brain analysis was able to correlate local amounts of HIV viral particles, cytokines, and other markers of inflammation such as neopterin and β-microglobulin with local pathology. In addition, cytokine secretion allows cell death to go on in areas remote from HIV itself.

Quinolinate, a cytokine and weak *N*-methyl-D-aspartate (NMDA) agonist, can contribute to death directly or by causing nearby neurons to release glutamate which stimulates NMDA receptors. This overstimulation may eventually cause cell death. In addition, the cytokines TNF-α and -β destroy oligodendrocytes, the cells responsible for normal myelin maintenance, leading to white matter disease in the brain and spinal cord. Cofactors such as nitric oxide and free radicals may be required for tissue damage to occur with cytokines. In addition to their effects on cortex and white matter, cytokines amplify the infectious process itself by upregulating the synthesis of HIV. The absence of CD4 cells allows polyclonal B-cell stimulation, resulting in production of brain autoantibodies whose role in AIDS dementia is not yet determined.

Trophic factors are required for normal neuronal and myelin maintenance and cell survival; a section of the HIV envelope shares some amino acid sequences with neuroleukin and vasoactive intestinal peptide and may interfere with their trophic action on normal cortex. Cytokines may likewise block delivery of trophic factors to their site of action by causing astrocytes to proliferate.

HIV or gp120, an envelope protein of HIV, can contribute to cell death through excessive release of glutamate or by opening calcium channels. Conversely, blocking calcium influx and glutamate receptors protects cells in experimental situations. Similarly, fetal neurons that have not yet developed NMDA receptors are not vulnerable to the cytotoxic effects of HIV. The sequential effect on cell populations depending on the number of NMDA receptors they contain may explain the degenerative sequence seen in children and adults (i.e., subcortical before cortical cell loss).

Eventually, the loss of synaptic connections, the reduction in numbers of dendritic spines, and the decrease in neuron density must lead to dysfunction in the neocortex. In addition, the Tat protein made by HIV causes depolarization of cell membranes, further contributing to neuronal dysfunction and, in high concentrations, leads to pore formations in the membrane with resulting cell death.

The blood-brain barrier, which normally protects the brain from toxins circulating in the rest of the body, is leaky in about half of all HIV-infected patients' brains, even in the absence of encephalitis. This may be the cause of the frequently found chronic white matter edema, which is often described as demyelination, even though pathologic studies have failed to demonstrate loss of myelin. The dysfunctional white matter probably contributes to delayed reactions and overall slowing of thought and motor processes, which can be measured and followed using event-related evoked potentials and electroencephalography. In addition, impairment of the blood-brain barrier allows destruction to take place in the absence of direct viral invasion because circulating toxins, such as tumor necrosis factor, cross over from the systemic circulation. This may account for the increased incidence of dementia late in the course of AIDS, when signs of cachexia or wasting suggest the presence of systemic cytokines.

Studies now indicate that HIV strains associated with prominent neurologic disease differ biologically from those linked to immune deficiency. Although the presence of opportunistic infection or tumor may obscure signs of ADC in nonhomosexual patients, differences in neurotropism of viral strains may explain the occasional occurrence of neurologic symptoms due to HIV encephalitis without major changes in immune status and may partially account for the disparate frequency of ADC among the different risk behavior groups. Alcohol or other drug abuse has synergistic deleterious effects on the nervous system.

Prospective studies have not yet linked early episodes of aseptic meningitis or facial nerve palsy to the development of HIV encephalitis, but the ability of the virus to mutate may explain the high incidence of encephalitis in patients with prolonged (>3 years) infection. That is, even if the virus were not neurotropic at the time infection occurred, it may become so over time.

Therapy

Therapy of ADC consists, first, of reducing the viral burden using antiretroviral agents, even though direct infection of neurons has not been documented and therapy with zidovudine (ZDV) does not necessarily clear the virus from the CSF.

ZDV can reverse some signs of dementia in adults and children, with CSF levels correlating with the dose. The optimal dose and duration of treatment are not yet established. The motor dysfunction of ADC is especially reversible. Epidemiologic data provide circumstantial evidence for the efficacy of ZDV; the incidence of dementia has declined since its introduction. Radiologic and CSF abnormalities have also improved in patients receiving ZDV. SPECT studies show reversal of abnormal uptake, and pathologic studies have demonstrated decreased numbers of multinucleated giant cells and less overall neuropathology in ZDV-treated patients.

Antiviral therapy may limit the secretion of cytokines such as quinolinic acid, and inflammatory stimulants such as neopterin, interferon-γ, IL-1, IL-6, and TNF. ZDV and other reverse transcriptase inhibitors successfully cross the blood-brain barrier, with measurements in the CSF approximately 50% of those in the blood.

Resistance to ZDV is a growing problem. However, the clinical response to ZDV can continue despite *in vitro* resistance of the viral strain grown from blood, which may be due to distinct viral isolates in brain, CSF, and blood. Conversely, immunologic or cognitive function may decline despite continued viral sensitivity in peripheral blood to ZDV. In these cases, the virus may have undergone neurotropic (or macrophage tropic) mutation within the brain, or patient noncompliance may have led to inadequate cellular levels of ZDV. The convergent or sequential use of antiretroviral drugs such as didanosine (2',3'-dideoxyinosine, ddI) or 2',3'-dideoxycytidine (zalcitabine, ddC) may limit the emergence of resistance, but further studies are necessary to prove this. Attempts to reduce HIV binding to CD4 cells or specific brain receptors are being made, but so far they have been unsuccessful in preventing neuropathy or dementia.

Neuroprotective agents act nonspecifically to prevent cell damage in the presence of HIV infection. Calcium channel blockers such as nimodipine and flunarizine have prevented cell death in *in vitro* models of HIV including rat hippocampal and retinal ganglion cell cultures; both cross the blood-brain barrier and have few side effects. Clinical trials with nimodipine in ADC are ongoing. A separate mechanism leading to cell death is regulated by NMDA receptors, which can be blocked by antagonists such as memantine and dextromethorphan. Cofactors such as nitric oxide are probably required to sensitize or open these receptors, but there is as yet no mechanism to interfere with them without affecting normal cognitive function. Antibodies to the gp120 section of the viral envelope can also block neurotoxicity *in vitro*.

If patients are to be selected for prophylactic neuroprotection, more longitudinal studies are necessary to predict who will eventually develop dementia. The neurotropic quality of a viral strain is not easily apparent before clinical deterioration. So far, testing of asymptomatic patients using available diagnostic tools has led to conflicting results that are therefore not suitable to guide the choice of patients for prophylaxis. Although a disproportionate risk of dementia might be expected in patients with aseptic meningitis or persistent headache, longitudinal studies to confirm this association are lacking. If such an association is confirmed, early aseptic meningitis could serve as a marker for infected patients in whom neuroprotection is warranted. Alternatively, as with current guidelines for opportunistic infection prophylaxis, all patients reaching a stage of immunosuppression usually associated with dementia (e.g., T4<400) or increased level of HIV p24 antigen in serum could be candidates for nimodipine, memantine, dextromethorphan, or other agents.

Antiinflammatory drugs such as pentoxifylline and interferon-α and -γ are also being studied.

Symptomatic treatment for ADC is based on the individual's complaints. Dopamine deficiency has been documented in CSF of HIV-infected patients, and Parkinsonian features respond to L-dopa supplementation. Conversely, neuroleptics are particularly likely to produce extrapyramidal side effects or even neuroleptic malignant syndrome in patients with AIDS, and they should be avoided except when necessary to treat psychosis. Even patients with psychosis or dyskinetic movement disorders such as hemichorea prefer benzodiazepines or no treatment to neuroleptics, which may induce or worsen depression. Depression can contribute to slowed mentation and is somewhat responsive to the stimulant methylphenidate. Metabolic disorders such as hyponatremia, hypoxia, sepsis, and kidney and liver failure can exacerbate ADC and are potentially treatable, although rarely are they completely reversible. Cobalamin (vitamin B_{12}) deficiency is present in up to 20% of patients, especially those with malabsorption or nutritional deficiency; treatment with B_{12} supplementation only rarely improves symptoms of dementia.

HIV Myelopathy

Up to 40% of patients with ADC develop progressive spastic paraparesis that is usually accompanied by loss of bladder and bowel control. Eventually the arms may become weak as well, but a sensory level is rarely found.

Myelopathy is associated with a characteristic pathologic picture mainly involving the lateral and posterior columns of the thoracic spinal cord which resembles subacute combined degeneration seen in vitamin B_{12} deficiency (Fig. 11). Although B_{12} levels are low in some of these patients, supplementation with B_{12} has not led to neurologic improvement. No other primary nutritional or metabolic abnormality has been identified. Furthermore, unlike the brain in which there is evidence of inflammation and where HIV can readily be demonstrated by appropriate probes, HIV-associated myelopathy is not associated with pronounced inflammatory changes and HIV has been directly demonstrated only in regions of vacuolar change. However, activated macrophages that secrete cytokines such as tumor necrosis factor and IL-1 are present in the posterior and lateral columns of thoracic spinal cord and may precede vacuolar degeneration but cause myelin damage. Some investigators have

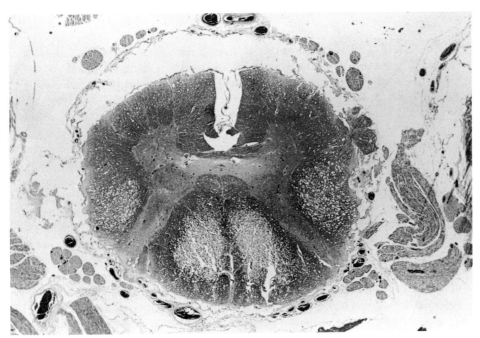

FIG. 11. Cross section of spinal cord stained with hematoxylin and eosin and luxol fast blue for myelin showing vacuolar changes in the posterior and lateral columns. (Courtesy of Dr. Seymour Levine.)

proposed that these spinal cord changes may be secondary to Wallerian degeneration resulting from a primary process in the brain or dorsal root ganglia. In children, the spinal cord may fail to myelinate fully. Other possible but unlikely causes for the vacuolar myelopathy include toxic effects from chemicals used in wound cleaning; nutritional deficiency or toxicity from therapeutic drugs such as isoniazid; and coinfection with other agents, most often the related retroviruses human T-lymphotropic virus type I (HTLV-I) and HTLV-II. In most cases, however, HTLV-I, the causative agent of tropical spastic paraparesis, cannot be demonstrated. Whether other agents, acting alone or in synergy with HIV, cause myelopathy in AIDS patients is unknown.

There is no proven treatment for HIV myelopathy. Steroids may have helped in one case in which an inflammatory component attributed to coinfection with HTLV-I may have played a pathogenic role. Spasticity may be relieved by baclofen (although often at the expense of loss of strength), and urinary urgency is improved by oxybutynin or imipramine.

At least two cases of amyotrophic lateral sclerosis (ALS) have occurred in a patient with AIDS, but another patient with a syndrome resembling motor neuron disease actually had severe, extensive peripheral neuropathy and myopathy.

HIV Peripheral Neuropathy

In up to 35% of AIDS patients a clinical sensory neuropathy occurs manifested by stocking/glove numbness, painful dysesthesias (mainly burning feet), and uncommonly, weakness or autonomic dysfunction. Electrophysiologic studies are consistent with axonal degeneration or, rarely, segmental demyelination; these findings have been confirmed by nerve biopsy. Unlike the chronic inflammatory demyelinating polyneuropathy that resembles Guillain-Barré syndrome, inflammatory changes are generally absent in HIV sensory neuropathy, and the virus has not been demonstrated directly. However, virus has been grown from sural nerve, gp120 binding to the sensory ganglion has been shown by immunoflorescence, PCR has demonstrated HIV in the dorsal root ganglion, viral antigen has been found within monocytes infiltrating the vasa nervorum of peripheral nerves, and viral-like particles have been seen with electron microscopy in the axoplasm of peripheral nerve. Although the pathologic changes are consistent with direct viral invasion of the nerve or "dying back" consequent to dorsal root ganglia infection, circulating immune complexes, toxins, cytokines, or nutritional deficiency such as B_{12} may be contributing factors in some patients. This sensory neuropathy must be distinguished from the inflammatory polyneuritis which occurs as a manifestation of immune dysregulation (see below). A self-limited polyradiculopathy associated with mononuclear CSF pleocytosis may be due to HIV, and is responsive to steroids. Symptoms and signs of peripheral neuropathy usually stabilize but may improve with zidovudine. Tricyclic antidepressants (amitriptyline, imipramine) or antiepileptic drugs (carbamazepine, phenytoin, gabapetin) can alleviate neuritic pain in some patients. Substance P releasing creams, such as capsaicin, can also be useful in suppressing neuralgic pain. Plasmapheresis and peptide T have not proven effective.

Muscle Disease

Most patients, especially depressed patients and injecting drug users, suffer from myalgias and weakness preterminally, and some patients have an inflammatory syndrome mimicking polymyositis. Affected patients have had myalgias, especially of the thighs, slowly worsening proximal weakness, and mild elevations of creatine phosphokinase (>500 IU/L). The electromyogram shows fibrillations, positive sharp waves, and polyphasic motor units. Muscle biopsy has revealed lymphocyte and macrophage infiltrates that stain for HIV gp41 antigen, but generally shows myofiber degeneration and rare signs of inflammation. Myoglobinuria not accompanied by inflammatory changes on muscle biopsy was reported in one HIV-infected patient before other symptoms of muscle disease, and myoglobinuria has also been reported rarely at the time of HIV seroconversion. Treatment with steroids, antiretroviral drugs, nonsteroidal antiinflammatory drugs, or, rarely, plasmapheresis leads to improvement in the majority of patients. Fatigue, although a common complaint, is not associated with altered metabolism.

HIV wasting syndrome, which accounts for 15% of new cases of AIDS reported to the CDC, may rarely be due to a steroid-responsive myopathy in patients without signs of malabsorption.

Syndromes of Immune Dysregulation

In intermediate stages of HIV infection, autoimmune diseases can appear, probably because the virus has adversely affected lymphocyte function without yet causing complete immunosuppression. The most common of these is a subacute or chronic inflammatory demyelinating polyneuropathy (CIDP) or polyradiculopathy. Acute forms more typical of Guillain-Barré syndrome have been described, which may occur even at the time of HIV seroconversion. Clinical features include symmetric weakness of the arms and legs, which is most marked distally, and relatively milder sensory abnormalities, mainly of the hands and feet, with the ability to sense vibration being especially affected. Involvement of the autonomic nervous system is rare. Occasionally the disease is severe enough that respiratory insufficiency develops. Although this is mainly a disorder of adults, at least one child has been affected. Isolated facial palsy may be a restricted variant of the more widespread disorder. Nerve biopsies reveal inflammatory segmental demyelination with a variable amount of axonal degeneration. CSF protein is generally elevated to two to three times normal, and there may be a slight pleocytosis (<50 WBCs/mm^3). Cytomegalovirus has been seen in the Schwann cells of two patients.

Polymyositis, vasculitis, mononeuritis multiplex, myasthenia gravis, and multiple sclerosis also probably represent autoimmune phenomena, as does thrombocytopenia. Thrombocytopenia may lead to cerebral hermorrhage. Anticardiolipin antibodies or lupus anticoagulant are found in some AIDS patients with cerebral infarction, as is vasculitis.

Despite the concern about accelerating immunosuppression, corticosteroids and plasmapheresis have been used with apparent benefit in some patients with immune dysregulation disorders, including a multiple sclerosis-like syndrome. However, it is also clear that symptoms subside spontaneously in some patients. In one of three refractory patients with HIV-related CIDP, intravenous immunoglobulin therapy was associated with improvement, but this failed in two patients with acute poly-radiculoneuropathy.

NEUROLOGIC SYNDROMES DUE TO OPPORTUNISTIC INFECTION, TUMOR, AND VASCULAR DISEASE

The clinical manifestations of opportunistic infections, tumors, and vascular disease affecting the nervous system in patients with AIDS can be conveniently grouped into syndromes that reflect predominantly focal cerebral, meningeal, spinal cord, or neuromuscular involvement.

Focal Cerebral Syndromes

A neurologic picture marked by headache and focal signs is most often due to opportunistic infection or tumor affecting the brain parenchyma. Other causes of focal brain disease such as infarction or hemorrhage are much less common. The particular manifestations of a cerebral lesion are a function of its location, acuity, and size. Focal hemispheric lesions commonly cause aphasia, spatial neglect or denial, lateralized changes in tone or strength, hemisensory loss, gaze preference, visual field defect, reflex assymmetry, and unilateral extensor plantar response. Hiccups, though nonlocalizing, are an early sign of brain pathology. Focal or secondarily generalized seizures are common. Sometimes the focal signature must be carefully looked for, because the clinical picture may be dominated by evidence of more global cerebral dysfunction due to multiple lesions, increased intracranial pressure, or involvement of the reticular activating system in the brainstem. Although hemispheric lesions frequently'involve the basal ganglia (e.g., as in toxoplasmosis), classical signs of extrapyramidal disease such as hemiballismus, tremor, bradykinesia, rigidity, and other involuntary movements are uncommon. Brainstem and cerebellar lesions cause nystagmus, diplopia, gaze palsy, dysphagia, ataxia, and "crossed" syndromes in which some signs occur ipsilateral to the lesion while others are contralateral. Fever may occur with either tumor or infection and is therefore not helpful diagnostically.

It is usually impossible to definitively determine clinically the nature of the specific pathogen or even whether a focal lesion is due to infection or tumor. Although it is often said that deterioration caused by tumor occurs more rapidly than that caused by infection, this dictum is completely unreliable in the immunodeficient patient.

Meningitis

Meningitis manifests in both acute and chronic forms. Acute manifestations include headache, photophobia, confusion, lethargy, and seizures. Papilledema may be present. In chronic meningitis, headache is often less prominent, and encephalopathic features (lethargy, impaired mentation) are correspondingly more common. Communicating hydrocephalus with increased intracranial pressure occurs frequently, and infarction may result from inflammatory arteritis. Chronic meningitis may lead to abscess formation, usually near a meningeal surface, with accompanying focal signs. Meningitis or ependymitis inconsistently results in diffuse enhancement of the meninges or ventricular lining (Fig. 3).

Metabolic disturbances sometimes mimic the encephalopathy of chronic meningitis. When asterixis or multifocal myoclonus is present, it should strongly suggest a metabolic disorder. Common causes of metabolic encephalopathy in AIDS patients include chronic hypoxia, liver and kidney failure, and hyponatremia. Wernicke's encephalopathy has been reported in association with zidovudine therapy, and the pathologic features of thiamine deficiency were incidentally noted at autopsy in another patient.

Spinal Cord

The most common cause of spinal cord dysfunction in HIV infection is the vacuolar myelopathy associated with ADC. Myelopathy can also result from compression due to epidural infection or tumor (Fig. 12), viral myelitis, or, rarely bacterial or parasitic (Fig. 13) infection of the cord itself. Some cases of severe peripheral neuropathy have been associated with sufficient retrograde degeneration to produce myelopathic signs and symptoms.

Clinical features of myelopathy include bilateral symptoms and signs with the legs more affected than the arms. A transverse sensory level is often present, usually on the trunk, and sensory loss below this is usually greater for pin and light touch than for other modalities. Leg weakness is usually worse proximally, and if the disease process is sufficiently chronic, muscle tone is likely to be increased and spontaneous flexor spasms of the legs can be observed. Stretch reflexes are hyperactive below the level of the lesion, and the plantar reflexes are typically extensor. Patients with spinal cord disease complain early of urinary urgency and increased frequency and, as the myelopathy worsens, they develop complete loss of bladder and bowel function. Occasionally, patients note a change in sweat pattern, or they report radicular pain or a belt-like tightness around the chest at the involved level. When spinal cord compression occurs from epidural tumor or infection, there is usually localized pain or tenderness at the involved level. In patients with infection

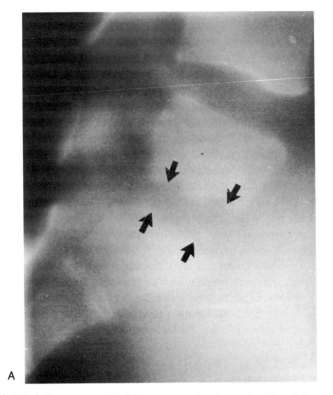

FIG. 12. A: Tomogram of L5-S1 interspace showing destruction of disc space.

of the bone or epidural space, careful examination of the back may reveal an area of warmth or tenderness when the vertebral processes are percussed.

In cases of neoplastic meningitis, spinal nerve roots are commonly involved by tumor deposits, usually at multiple levels, and this results in radicular pain, segmental sensory loss, and areflexia. Some cases of CMV radiculitis simulate a conus lesion with radiating sacral pain followed by sacral numbness and then loss of bladder and bowel control with urinary retention.

Neuromuscular Syndromes

Distinguishing features of the various disorders affecting the peripheral nervous system are summarized in Table 3. Disorders of peripheral nerves cause both sensory and motor symptoms, but strength and sensation are often affected unequally. In peripheral polyneuropathy, there is symmetric, distal loss of cutaneous sensation in a "glove-and-stocking" distribution. The sensory loss may affect only one modality (e.g., pin or light touch). When individual nerves are damaged ("mono-

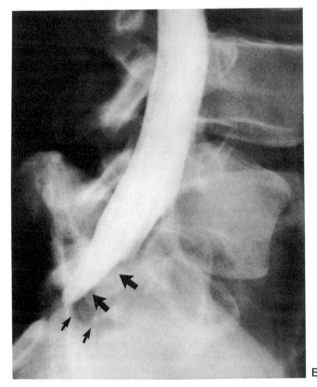

FIG. 12. B: Myelogram shows indentation of dye column from a mass that was proved to be *M. tuberculosis* infection in a 31-year-old HIV-infected man, who had radicular pain and a positive PPD. (From Koppel B, et al. *Arch Neurol*, with permission.)

neuritis"), there is weakness and sensory loss limited to the distribution of the affected nerve(s). Muscle disease causes limb weakness without sensory symptoms or signs. Stretch reflexes can be diminished or lost whenever the lower motor neuron or muscle is affected and are not helpful in specifying the site of the pathologic process in the absence of other data.

Mononeuritis can result from localized vasculitis or cryoglobulinemia. A severe polyneuropathy of unknown cause has produced a clinical picture simulating progressive muscular atrophy with widespread weakness and atrophy. Some patients taking zidovudine have developed weakness without cramps from a mitochondrial myopathy, which probably results from competition by zidovudine with thymidine for the polymerase required in mitochondrial DNA replication. Symptoms of zidovudine myopathy resolve 1 to 8 weeks following drug withdrawal, although CPK levels may remain elevated longer. ddI (didanosine) and ddC (zalcitabine) cause a peripheral neuropathy in some but not all patients. In affected individuals, severity of the neuropathy is proportional to both the daily dose and cumulative

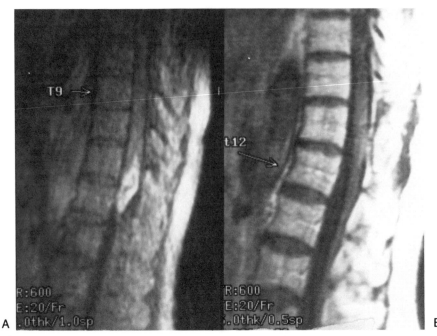

FIG. 13. A: Sagittal T1-weighted MRI with gadolinium of the thoracic spine of a 29-year-old man with urinary retention and minimal leg weakness showing an enhancing mass at T11 within the conus medullaris. Biopsy revealed toxoplasmosis. **B:** After 4 weeks of sulfadiazine and pyrimethamine therapy, gadolinium MRI scan shows resolution of mass.

dose. Most patients recover when the drug is stopped, although there may be temporary intensification of symptoms following drug withdrawal. ddI and ddC should be used cautiously in patients with preexisting neuropathy, although alternation with zidovudine may improve tolerance. Cramps on exertion may be nonspecific symptoms of anemia and hypoxia.

SEIZURES

Seizures are always symptoms of brain dysfunction and may be caused by focal cerebral lesions, meningitis or encephalitis, or metabolic derangements (especially hypoglycemia and hyponatremia). A reversible cause of acute confusion and mental status change is nonconvulsive status epilepticus, diagnosable by EEG. AIDS dementia complex alone is found in about half of the patients. Sleep deprivation and alcohol use may lower seizure threshold in susceptible individuals. If a correctable cause is not found (e.g., metabolic abnormality), antiepileptic drug therapy should be started. Because most seizures in AIDS patients have a focal origin, drugs of choice are phenytoin or carbamazepine. In acute situations, therapeutic phenytoin

TABLE 3. *Localization of neurologic symptoms*

Symptom		Features		Cause
Weakness	Proximal	←	Reflexes, Babinski	Myelopathy
	Isolated	←	Reflexes	Myopathy
		←	Reflexes	Mononeuritis multiplex
	Distal		Proximal or distal	
			May be asymmetric	Neuropathy (inflammatory) (HIV related)
		→	NCV slowed	
		→	Amplitude, NCV normal or slow	
Pain	Bandlike		Usually thoracic	Myelopathy (compressive mass)
	Patchy		Radicular, can involve cranial nerves	Carcinomatous meningitis
	Cramps		Exertional	Myopathy
		←	CPK	
	Distal feet > hands ——		Burning, numb, tingling	Neuropathy (HIV related)
	Distal (stocking/glove) —	→	All modalities	Neuropathy (HIV related)
		→	Amplitude	
		→	Velocity on NCV	
Numbness	Spinal level		Usually thoracic	Myelopathy (cord compression)
		→	Pin, touch	
Urination change	Urgency, frequency		Culture negative, constipation	Myelopathy, rarely hydrocephalous
	Incontinence, dribbling		Flaccid bladder	CMV sacral radiculitis or cauda equina mass
	Bilateral Babinski			Myeolopathy
Pathologic reflexes	Unilateral Babinski			Brain (mass or PML)
	Bilateral Babinski with snout, grasp, glabellar			Brain (dementia, usually HIV)

CMV, cytomegalovirus; NCV, nerve conduction velocity.

levels can be achieved rapidly by loading with 1 to 1.5 g orally or, if necessary, intravenously. When given intravenously, phenytoin should not be administered at rates faster than 40 to 50 mg/min, and ECG and blood pressure should be monitored continuously during the infusion. Blood levels should be determined frequently if the patient is systemically ill or taking other medications. About 15% to 20% of patients taking carbamazepine develop a benign leukopenia that is not clinically significant, even in immunosuppressed patients.

SPECIFIC OPPORTUNISTIC INFECTIONS

Protozoan Infections

Toxoplasmosis

Toxoplasmosis is the most frequent CNS opportunistic infection among adult patients with AIDS. Up to 30% of Americans have asymptomatic infection with *Toxoplasma gondii* as determined by serologic testing. Encephalitis develops in up to 30% of patients with AIDS who have toxoplasma antibodies, and this is usually not accompanied by a rise in serum antibody titer. In fact, antibodies may be undetectable in 20% of patients, although more sensitive assays may still allow detection. The incidence of toxoplasma encephalitis or meningitis is higher in Haitians, Europeans, and intravenous drug users (IVDUs) than in other HIV-infected groups, and it is rare in children.

The clinical presentation of brain involvement may be that of a mass lesion (60%), confusion, personality change or lethargy, nonspecific symptoms of increased intracranial pressure, or, less frequently, meningitis or panhypopituitarism. The predilection for localization in the basal ganglia makes movement disorders a common finding. Ataxia and tremor result from brainstem sites. Combinations of symptoms and signs are common. Fever is inconsistently present, and seizures occur in 30%. Rapid deterioration may be due to hemorrhage into lesions.

Presumptive clinical diagnosis is made by finding multiple nodular lesions on CT or MRI of the brain combined with a positive serum serology. Using special cell cultures, toxoplasma can be grown from blood. CSF examination is rarely helpful, although PCR may increase the sensitivity of CSF studies. Lesions are typically found in the cortex, especially at the gray–white matter junction, or in the basal ganglia. Computed tomography consistently underestimates the number of lesions compared with MRI or postmortem examination. Contrast infusion typically results in enhancement, although this may be absent (a poor prognostic sign) in patients not capable of reactive vascular proliferation or mounting more than a minimal inflammatory response. Scans done immediately after contrast infusion show peripheral ring enhancement, but delayed scans may result in more homogeneous enhancement of the lesion. The amount of surrounding edema varies, and CT is more accurate than MRI in delineating the lesion's boundaries.

Neuropathologic findings include necrotizing abscesses with vascular proliferation. Occasionally, thrombosed blood vessels and petechial hemorrhages are seen. Disseminated cases are associated with little inflammatory reaction.

Once suspected, the diagnosis of CNS toxoplasmosis is confirmed empirically by observing the response to appropriate treatment. Clinical and radiographic improvement, as judged by resolution of neurologic abnormalities and a measurable decrease in the size and number of lesions and in the associated edema, occurs within 2 or 3 weeks (Fig. 14) and often even earlier. If new lesions emerge on treatment, or if there is no change in existing ones, the diagnosis must be regarded as suspect, and brain biopsy becomes necessary. Special techniques for processing brain biopsy specimens are often required. Differentiating lymphoma from toxoplasmosis may be especially difficult when the organism is not visualized.

Standard treatment is pyrimethamine (50–100 mg/day following a loading dose of 100–200 mg) and sulfadiazine. Lifelong therapy is recommended, although lower doses may be used for maintenance. In patients allergic to sulfa, desensitiza-

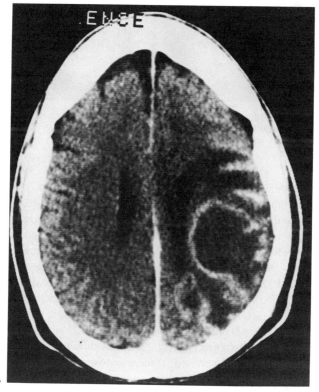

A

FIG. 14. A: Contrast-enhanced brain CT scan showing large left parietal ring-enhancing lesion with surrounding edema and gyral enhancement of the adjacent cortex.

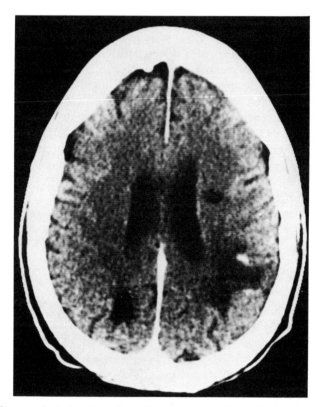

FIG. 14. B: Same patient after 6 weeks of therapy for toxoplasmosis showing small area of calcification and an irregular low-density lesion in the same region as well as in the right occipital lobe and the left basal ganglia.

tion can be attempted, or clindamycin can be effectively substituted. Pyrimethamine alone, even at high doses, may be inadequate to prevent relapse. Folinic acid is given concomitantly with pyrimethamine to prevent hematologic toxicity. Other efficacious, well-tolerated alternatives include azithromycin and atavaquone.

Use of corticosteroids should be avoided unless required to prevent herniation. Therapeutic trials can be misleading if specific anti-infective agents are combined with corticosteroids, because apparent improvement may be due only to nonspecific beneficial effects of corticosteroids on edema and the blood-brain barrier.

Toxoplasmosis is uncommon in children with HIV infection, probably because its occurrence usually depends on reactivation of latent infection, and children may not yet have been exposed. Toxoplasma serologic status should be determined in adults at the time HIV infection is diagnosed. If there is no evidence of toxoplasma infection, patients should be warned of the usual routes of transmission through accidental ingestion of cat feces or by consuming undercooked infected meat. Primary prophylaxis has been an adjunctive benefit of oral preventive therapy of *P. carinii* using trimethoprim-sulfamethoxazole, dapsone, and cotrimoxazole. Pyrimethamine alone may be effective. In patients with serologic evidence of toxoplasma exposure, periodic radiographic screening may be used to guide institution of prophylactic therapy.

Atypical sites of infection include muscle and spinal cord (Fig. 13).

Other Parasitic Infections

Parasitic disease other than toxoplasmosis has only rarely involved the nervous system. Two cases of cysticercosis were discovered on autopsy in a series reported from Miami. Acanthamoeba memingoencephalitis has been reported, which may resemble toxoplasmosis on CT. Trypanosomiasis (Chagas' disease) presenting as a cerebral tumor was diagnosed at surgery and successfully treated with nifurtimox. Reactivation of infection can lead to meningoencephalitis as well as mass lesions in patients from South America.

Fungal Infections

Which fungal infection a patient acquires reflects, in part, environmental exposure, thereby explaining why children have proportionally fewer fungal infections, although they are at increased risk for candida meningitis. Unusual organisms, such as blastomycosis, are being described as pathogenic in AIDS patients.

Cryptococcus

Cryptococcus neoformans is an encapsulated yeast found worldwide, especially in the soil of areas that support large pigeon populations. In patients with impaired T-cell immunity, *C. neoformans* causes a chronic meningitis that accounts for the majority of CNS fungal infections. Among AIDS patients, the prevalence of cryptococcal meningitis ranges from 4% to 25%. Although the organism gains entry through the lungs, pulmonary infection is usually asymptomatic. Dissemination to other organs, including the brain, occurs via the bloodstream. Meningitis is the most common manifestation, occurring in 67% to 84% of patients with cryptococcosis, and it is frequently the presenting illness that leads to a diagnosis of AIDS. Although the Centers for Disease Control (CDC) has reported that intravenous drug users have an incidence of cryptococcal meningitis almost three times higher than that of other HIV-infected groups, this was not confirmed in the series by Malouf et al.

Cryptococcal meningitis usually begins insidiously, and signs or symptoms typical of meningeal irritation are minimal. Stiff neck and photophobia occur in a minority of patients. Usually, there is a history of malaise, lethargy, low-grade fever, altered mentation, or behavioral changes for several weeks or even months before the diagnosis is made. Rarely, nausea, vomiting, and seizures occur, but these signs of increased intracranial pressure due to blockage of CSF outflow by yeast cells are associated with a worse outcome. Lumbar punctures and acetazolamide may be used therapeutically in patients with impaired consciousness and normal scans, as ventriculoperitoneal shunts are associated with further infection risk. Infarction due to infective arteritis is not seen, although transient ischemic attacks occurred in one patient. Occasionally, cryptococcal brain involvement is associated with the formation of cryptococcal abscesses or cryptococcal granulomas (torulomas), which can act as mass lesions to produce symptoms and signs that reflect their location. These probably arise by direct extension from infected meninges or the ependymal lining of ventricles (Fig. 5).

Diagnosis of cryptococcal meningitis depends on a high index of clinical suspicion, demonstrating cryptococcal antigen in the CSF using latex agglutination and, ultimately, by culture. Routine CSF markers for meningitis are unreliable in AIDS patients. Pleocytosis is variable. In one series, lymphocytosis of more than 20 cells/mm^3 was a predictor of good outcome. The protein content is usually moderately elevated, but it can be normal in about one-third of cases. Similarly, the CSF glucose level is low in only 30% of patients. India ink preparations of CSF provide a rapid means of making a presumptive diagnosis, as yeast forms can be identified in centrifuged samples in 75% of patients. However, false positives due to artifacts misinterpreted as yeast are common, and in some AIDS patients the organism may be difficult to recognize because of an atypical appearance resulting from incomplete capsule formation (Fig. 9).

Rarely, CSF cultures have been positive despite absence of detectable antigen. Very high titers of cryptococcal antigen (>1:10,000) are associated with increased mortality. Hyponatremia and symptomatic systemic disease are also poor prognostic features.

Treatment of choice is intravenous amphotericin B unless precluded by renal failure. Salt loading and calcium channel blockers protect the kidneys, allowing more consistent treatment. Initially, 1.5 g is given over 6 weeks. Liposomal delivery reduces toxicity and facilitates CNS entry; in one trial 74% of 23 patients responded clinically. Flucytosine has been used as adjunctive therapy, but it contributes to bone marrow suppression and does not seem to improve outcome. Relapses occur in 50% of cases, and these are especially likely if end-of-treatment CSF antigen titers are greater than 1:8. Extrameningeal sites, such as the prostate, can cause reseeding after treatment, as relapse strains are genetically related to initial strains. Accordingly, maintenance suppression with fluconazole has been recommended. Fluconazole has a high degree of CSF penetration following oral administration. Doses of 400 mg, followed by 200 mg/day, with adjustment for renal failure, may be given orally or intravenously. Relapses have occurred in patients receiving amphotericin B, even when given intrathecally or ketoconazole. Despite its inability to cross the blood-brain barrier, ketoconazole has reduced mortality from recurrent cryptococcal meningitis, possibly by preventing blood-borne dissemination of the organism from extracranial foci. Similarly, intraconazole, which is highly lipophilic, may be able to penetrate the blood-brain barrier when meningitis induces inflammation, as it has been successful in treatment and maintenance suppression.

Improvement is slow in patients treated with amphotericin or fluconazole, and clear indications of beneficial effect may not be evident for up to 3 weeks. Declining antigen titers in serum and CSF usually indicate successful treatment, although this is not invariable.

Primary prophylaxis in endemic areas is being studied.

Candidiasis

Overall, *Candida* species are the most common cause of fungal infection in humans. They are part of the normal body flora but become pathogenic in the presence of depressed cellular immunity. Nearly 60% of AIDS patients have oral candidiasis or candida esophagitis. Despite this ubiquity, candida is only rarely responsible for brain infection. Meningitis has been reported in children who seem particularly predisposed to this complication, and brain microabscesses have been found at autopsy in adults who have other cerebral infections, including toxoplasmosis. Subdural empyema secondary to sinusitis has been described.

Diagnosis of candida brain abscess can be made in life only from biopsy specimens, which allow the organisms to be demonstrated microscopically, using PAS, methanamine, or silver stains, and cultured.

Amphotericin is the preferred treatment, but its effectiveness is hard to evaluate. Fluconazole may prove useful, especially because it allows discontinuing the intravenous catheters required for amphotericin, which are often a source of continuing candida infection.

Coccidioidomycosis

Coccidioides immitis is a fungus found mainly in the deserts of the southwestern United States and Mexico. Infection is usually asymptomatic, but the organism can cause both self-limited and chronic respiratory disease. Up to 95% of the population in Arizona and southern California have positive skin tests to *C. immitis*; with advancing immunosuppression, 25% of a group of patients developed active disease. Disseminated coccidioidomycosis is rare but manifests as chronic meningitis in 30% to 50% of cases. Jarvik et al. have described the MRI findings in an HIV-infected patient with a brain abscess due to *C. immitis*. Intrathecal amphotericin has been the mainstay of treatment, although oral fluconazole is also successful, and itraconazole is being studied. Ketoconazole does not prevent dissemination.

Histoplasmosis

Histoplasmosis is the most common endemic mycosis in the United States, occurring mainly in the Caribbean and in the Mississippi, Missouri, and Ohio River valleys. It usually causes a self-limited pulmonary infection, but disseminated cases occur, especially in persons whose immune systems are suppressed. The most fulminant examples of dissemination have been reported in AIDS patients. The brain has been involved only rarely, but both chronic meningitis and focal cerebritis have been described. More often, metabolic encephalopathy from pulmonary or liver failure is encountered. Disseminated infection has been controlled in some patients with amphotericin B. Failures sometimes respond to itraconazole.

Mucormycosis

Mucormycosis accounts for about 15% of fungal infections in immunocompromised patients. It generally presents in a rhinocerebral form, with brain infection occurring by direct extension from infected nasal mucosa, orbits, and sinuses. Common neurologic findings include ophthalmoplegia, corneal, and upper face hypoesthesia, blindness, and mental changes due to frontal lobe involvement. Invasion of blood vessels can lead to thrombosis and cerebral infarction. Chronic meningitis may occur once intracranial integrity is breached. Isolated brain abscess is rare, but a predilection for the basal ganglia has been alleged.

Once cerebral manifestations are evident, the course is usually one of rapid progression; successful therapy is rare. Hyperbaric oxygen may improve response to treatment, but this has not yet been tried in AIDS patients.

Aspergillosis

Unlike in transplant recipients, *Aspergillus fumigatus* is a rare cerebral pathogen in AIDS patients. As of mid-1990, only six cases had been reported. Brain infection occurs by hematogenous spread from pulmonary aspergillosis. CNS aspergillosis results in necrotizing, suppurative abscesses, which may be single or multiple. One case involved spinal cord compression by an epidural abscess that formed by direct extension from infected lungs. Because the organism invades blood vessel walls, abscesses are often accompanied by hemorrhage or hemorrhagic infarction. In addition to abscesses, chronic meningitis can occur.

Antemortem diagnosis of CNS aspergillosis is difficult without biopsy. It can be suspected in a patient with known or probable pulmonary aspergillosis who develops a brain abscess or meningitis. CSF studies, including culture and precipitin titers, are not helpful. By the time CNS disease is recognized, it is almost invariably fatal. The usefulness of itraconazole is presently under evaluation, as amphotericin B does not usually work.

Viral Infections

Cytomegalovirus (CMV) Infection

CMV was originally believed to be the causative agent for the subacute encephalitis that occurred in AIDS patients. It is now recognized that most of the pathologic findings considered "typical" for CMV encephalitis are equally characteristic of HIV infection. Furthermore, CMV may potentiate the spread and destructive effects of HIV. Nonetheless, CMV has likely been the primary cause for subacute encephalopathy in some patients, especially those with prominent brainstem involvement. More often, CMV causes demyelination and vasculitis of the spinal cord and nerve roots, particularly the cauda equina. Individual peripheral nerves, cranial nerves, or their branches (e.g., the laryngeal nerve) and muscles can also be symptomatically infected. CMV retinitis probably accounts for most cases of visual loss in patients with AIDS. Finally, CMV can also infect the adrenal glands and rarely cause adrenal insufficiency. Unless infection is disseminated, CMV is often undetected clinically. Progressive polyradiculopathy should be suspected in patients with rapidly evolving flaccid paraparesis and bladder retention with pain in sacral dermatomes; it is confirmed by CSF examination showing many polymorphonuclear leukocytes and low glucose. MRI shows clumping of deposits on lumbosacral nerve roots.

Evidence for CMV infection in these cases includes positive CSF cultures for CMV, characteristic findings on routine and electron microscopic examination of affected tissue, and positive results from various molecular probes and immunohistochemical techniques for CMV. CMV has also been isolated from blood, urine, and CSF from individual patients with myelitis, chorioretinitis, and an illness resembling Guillain-Barré syndrome. Routine serum serology is not helpful; rises in viral titer with CMV infection are only rarely documented. CT or MRI show periventricular enhancement.

Treatment with ganciclovir helps in controlling viremia and stabilizing retinitis or colitis. One patient with biopsy proved CMV encephalitis also improved, and another with culture-proven meningoencephalitis responded transiently to high doses of ganciclovir and foscarnet. Its use is limited by neutropenia, and it cannot be given concurrently with zidovudine. Relapses are common when the drug is stopped or the dose lowered. Alternate day therapy with foscarnet limits toxicity of both. Alpha-interferon was not beneficial. Granulocyte-macrophage colony stimulating factor (GM-CSF) combined with ganciclovir has helped reduce bone marrow toxicity. Polyradiculopathy responds well to ganciclovir, although a 2-week delay in response is common. Addition of plasmapheresis may help. Foscarnet is an effective alternative for retinitis and systemic disease and in one case of nerve root involvement. Hyperimmune globulin fails to enter the CNS and is associated with development of myelitis.

Herpes Simplex Virus

Like syphilis, genital ulcers due to herpes simplex virus (HSV) may predispose to easier acquisition of HIV. Furthermore, the incidence of HSV infection seems to be increasing in HIV-infected populations. Both HSV-1 and HSV-2 can cause encephalitis, meningitis, or myelitis, although HSV-1 is more often the cause of encephalitis, and HSV-2 of meningitis and myelitis.

The presentation and course of HSV encephalitis in HIV-infected individuals are much more variable than in immunocompetent hosts. Although many patients present with the familiar acute features of fever, headache, seizures, and abrupt deterioration in behavior and mental status accompanied by CSF pleocytosis and focal changes on EEG and CT or MRI, others have a more indolent course extending over weeks. Patients with this subacute variant of HSV encephalitis present with a slowly progressive neurologic syndrome in which lethargy, behavioral changes, weakness, and seizures predominate. Diabetes insipidus was the presenting symptom in one case. Fever may be absent, the spinal fluid unremarkable, and EEG changes nonspecific. In other patients, clinically asymptomatic, autopsy examination has demonstrated HSV in the brain.

These differences in the clinical spectrum of disease must reflect a modified pathogenesis caused by immunodeficiency. Severely immunocompromised patients are incapable of mounting a massive inflammatory response, and as a result, the disease can be much more protracted and the evidence of inflammation less marked. The encephalitis may also be more diffuse and less localized to frontal and temporal lobes in AIDS patients, and this possibly reflects a different route of entry into the brain. CSF analysis using experimental techniques to assay viral antigen, or PCR to amplify viral DNA from lymphocytes, may be helpful in diagnosis. When necessary, brain biopsy remains the definitive procedure for establishing a diagnosis. Cultures can determine the viral strain and exclude other infections or neoplasms that may produce a similar clinical picture. Rapid diagnosis is possible using *in situ* hybridization and electron microscopy.

Treatment of choice is acyclovir. Relapses occur, even in patients with reasonable immune function. Fear of developing acyclovir-resistant HSV strains from long-term maintenance therapy appears well founded: 7% of AIDS patients treated chronically for herpetic anogenital lesions demonstrated resistance using a rapid nucleic acid hybridization method and one patient developed fatal HSV-2 encephalitis while being treated with acyclovir. Because there are presently no guidelines for maintenance therapy of patients treated for encephalitis with acyclovir, it is probably advisable to treat for 10 to 20 days and then observe patients carefully for new neurologic symptoms. If a relapse occurs, acyclovir should be resumed. In acyclovir-resistant cases, foscarnet has been effective for skin lesions, but it has not been evaluated in patients with encephalitis.

Progressive Multifocal Leukoencephalopathy (PML)

PML is a progressive demyelinating disease of the brain due to reactivation of latent papovavirus infection, usually of JC type. Latent virus has been demonstrated in bone marrow and spleen and presumably spreads through the circulation to brain, where it infects oligodendroglia. However, antibodies to JC virus were present in 64% of a series of 94 patients. PML occurs in patients with T-cell dysfunction due to a variety of causes; it was first described in a patient with AIDS in 1982. In one series of 79 AIDS patients, PML occurred in 3.8% over a 4-year period, although only 0.8% of AIDS cases present with PML.

Signs and symptoms of PML infection develop gradually and reflect progressive white matter disease. Initial symptoms are usually mental changes, weakness, visual loss, or ataxia. Hemiparesis or weakness of an arm or leg was the initial presentation in 12 of 25 patients reviewed by Berger et al. There are never signs of meningitis or raised intracranial pressure. Although a disease of white matter, seizures have been reported. As suggested by the name, white matter lesions are classically multifocal, but only one area of demyelination can be demonstrated in about 10% of cases. Children are rarely infected.

The mean survival of AIDS patients with PML has averaged approximately 4 months. There have been rare cases of survival longer than 3 years, and stable disease or partial recovery has been demonstrated, especially when inflammation is present. Prognosis is worse when demyelination affects mainly the brainstem or cerebellum. In one case, infection with JC papovavirus seemed to induce an accelerated form of HIV encephalitis, possibly by recruiting HIV-infected macrophages.

MR or CT brain imaging characteristically shows nonenhancing lesions with irregular borders that are confined to white matter and not associated with edema or

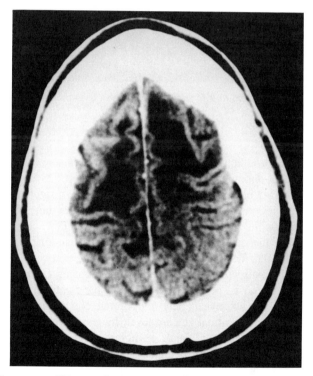

A

FIG. 15. A: Noncontrast CT scan of a 38-year-old HIV-infected man with mild dementia and progressive right hemiparesis, showing a hypodense lesion in the left frontal lobe. Enhanced scan did not show contrast in area. Presumed diagnosis was progressive multifocal leukoencephalopathy.

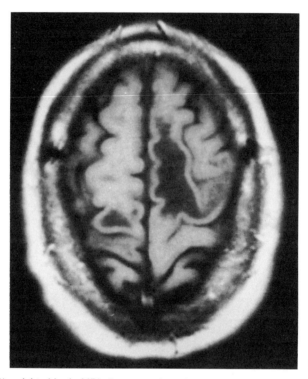

B

FIG. 15. B: T1-weighted brain MRI of same patient shows bilateral lesions without edema or mass effect.

mass effect (Fig. 15), although exceptions showing a thin rim of contrast enhancement have been reported and gray matter may be involved. On T2-weighted MRI, additional lesions may be detected as irregular areas of high signal intensity within white matter. The lesions of PML as visualized by MRI are more discrete than the diffuse subcortical white matter changes that occur with HIV encephalitis. Early in the illness, it is not unusual for patients to appear sicker than imaging abnormalities would seem to indicate. The EEG demonstrates moderate to severe focal or multifocal slow wave abnormalities, with nonspecific diffuse changes later. Serologic tests are not helpful in diagnosis, because 90% of adults have antibody titers to JC papovavirus. CSF examination reveals only mild protein elevation (<100 mg/dl) with no cellular response and a normal glucose level. Increased myelin basic protein can be demonstrated, and oligoclonal bands or increased IgG are found occasionally. Polymerase chain reaction of CSF is highly specific but has sensitivity of 43% to 75%. If lymphocytic pleocytosis is present, it usually reflects HIV encephalitis or meningitis, or another separate process.

Neuropathologic features include areas of demyelination of various ages and sizes that microscopically contain enlarged, bizarre multinucleated astrocytes, especially at the periphery, and hypertrophied oligodendroglia that contain characteristic intranuclear basophilic or eosinophilic inclusions. Sparing of axons is only relative, and in large lesions, there may be frank necrosis at the center with a phagocytic reaction. Immunofluorescent techniques usually demonstrate papovavirus antigen in the intranuclear inclusions. Electron microscopy reveals the typical virus particles within the intranuclear inclusions of oligodendrocytes and in neurons.

So far, antiviral treatment using cytosine arabinoside, vidarabine, or acyclovir, and immunostimulation methods such as platelet transfusions have been unsuccessful. Interferon-α worked in one patient with sarcoid and PML. Zidovudine has also been used, but results have not yet been reported. With all therapies, interpretation of results is complicated by the rare occurrence of spontaneous remission.

Herpes Zoster

The most common form of disease due to the varicella-zoster virus is shingles, which occurs in 5% to 10% of patients with HIV infection. Indeed, shingles often precedes development of severe immunodeficiency and may be the symptom that calls attention to the underlying disorder. Both spinal and cranial nerve roots can be involved. Zoster encephalitis can develop following resolution of the rash, even in patients who completed a course of treatment with acyclovir and has been demonstrated in a patient who never had a rash. Myelitis can cause either segmental myoclonus or isolated leg weakness when the infection is limited to cervical or lumbar dermatomes, or a more complete myelopathy with a level corresponding to the dermatome exhibiting shingles.

Although acyclovir may attenuate pain and limit spread from radicular involvement, resistance has emerged with chronic oral treatment. Furthermore, as already noted, encephalitis has developed following "appropriate" treatment. Patients with herpes zoster should be placed in strict isolation to avoid nosocomial transmission.

Mycobacterial Infection

Mycobacterial infection in AIDS patients is most often due to *M. avium-intracellulare* or *M. tuberculosis* but other atypical pathogens, such as *M. kansasii*, *M. fortuitum*, and *M. leprae*, have been seen as well. Extrapulmonary involvement is common, although meningitis is found more often in HIV-infected (10%) than normal hosts (2%). *M. tuberculosis* is more frequent in Haitians and parenteral drug users than in other AIDS patients in the United States. All AIDS patients are at increased risk for atypical mycobacterial infection. Culture, which takes up to 4 to 6 weeks, has been required to determine which mycobacterium is present, but recently special blood culture techniques, genetic probes, anti-P32 antibody, and selective skin testing have shown promise in making a specific diagnosis more rapidly.

Mycobacterial infection typically causes meningitis or brain abscess (Fig. 16).

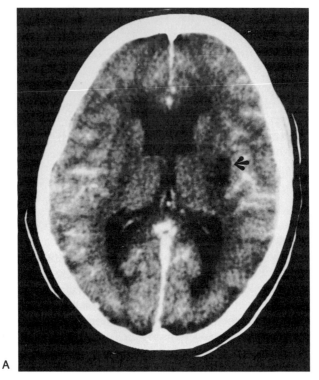

FIG. 16. A: Contrast-enhanced CT scan of the brain in a 30-year-old HIV-infected woman with headache, obtundation, and acute onset of right hemiplegia due to tuberculous meningitis. *Arrow* points to lacunar infarction of the left internal capsule. Meninges diffusely enhance with contrast.

Intervertebral disc space infection and spinal epidural abscess have also been reported. Meningitis has been followed by tuberculoma formation (Fig. 16). Conversely, rupture of an abscess into the subarachnoid space or ventricle may lead to meningitis. Mycobacterial infection can also cause polymyositis, meningomyelitis, and peripheral neuropathy. Abscesses due to *M. avium-intracellulare* are more apt to occur in previously damaged brain or in conjunction with other organisms such as toxoplasma.

Mycobacterial meningitis tends to be less fulminant and more subacute in AIDS patients than in non–HIV-infected groups and is more often associated with concurrent brain abscess. Thus patients often present with signs indicating both focal and diffuse neurologic disease, and CT or MRI may demonstrate single or multiple mass lesions even in patients whose clinical course suggests a diffuse encephalopathy. Another cause for focal neurologic abnormalities in patients with mycobacterial meningitis is cerebral infarction, a common complication that results from an associated infective arteritis of the major cerebral blood vessels. The infarctions are

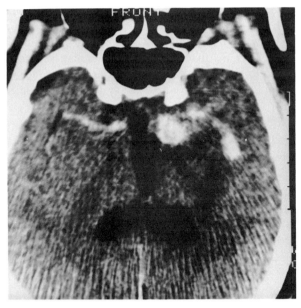

B

FIG. 16. B: Contrast-enhanced scan of same patient after she developed decreased vision and impaired extraocular movements of the left eye despite 10 weeks of triple drug antituberculous therapy. The scan reveals a small densely enhancing round lesion adjacent to the middle cerebral artery. This eventually disappeared after several months of treatment with streptomycin in addition to isoniazid, ethambutol, and rifampin.

often in the basal ganglia. Inflammatory debris in the basilar cisterns and arachnoid granulations obstructs normal CSF circulation and leads to hydrocephalus.

CSF examination reveals increased protein content, variable lymphocytosis, and depressed sugar content, although protein and glucose may be normal in cases of atypical mycobacteria meningitis, and even in cases of tubercular meningitis fluid may be acellular. Acid-fast organisms can be found on stained smears of CSF in only 10% of cases, and CSF cultures are positive in less than 50% of cases. Special tests of CSF for the presence of anti-BCG cells, antibody to tuberculous antigens, or PCR may increase the diagnostic yield but are not readily available or completely reliable. Organisms are recovered most often from tissue obtained by brain biopsy. In HIV-infected patients with tuberculosis of the central nervous system, tuberculin skin testing may or may not be positive, depending on the degree of immunosuppression.

Treatment of infection due to *M. tuberculosis* is usually successful, even in immunocompromised patients. The organism is typically sensitive to isoniazid, rifampin, and pyrazinamide, all of which cross the blood-brain barrier in effective concentrations. However, multiple drug-resistant strains are increasing, especially in patients with AIDS who have been hospitalized; hospital workers are also at risk.

Treatment failures occur most often when abscesses are present or when patients are noncompliant with long-term therapy. Malabsorption of medication can also cause failure. Standard treatment regimens are of at least 9 to 12 months duration. Ventricular drainage or other CSF diversionary techniques may be necessary in patients with hydrocephalus. In non-AIDS patients, corticosteroids reduce morbidity from tuberculous meningitis, but they have not been systematically studied in AIDS patients.

In contrast, atypical mycobacterial infections in AIDS patients are notoriously resistant to most therapies. Combined drug regimens are almost always necessary, but results are almost invariably poor. Newer agents such as clofazimine, rifabutin, amikacin, and ciprofloxacin may prove more successful than have conventional anti-tuberculous drugs, and prophylactic use has improved well-being in patients.

Spirochetal Infection

Syphilis

Syphilis and HIV infection are intimately related, and serologic tests for syphilis are positive in up to 30% to 50% of HIV-infected patients. A syphilitic chancre increases the risk of acquiring HIV, and syphilitic meningitis or syphilis-induced depression of cell-mediated immunity enhances the likelihood of HIV penetrating the brain. Other important issues related to coinfection with HIV and *Treponema pallidum* include the following:

1. HIV-immunocompromised patients may have falsely negative serologic tests for syphilis, which hinders identification of infection. Titers may decline due to immunosuppression of advanced AIDS instead of successful treatment. The PCR test for *T. pallidum* (which is not yet generally available) should aid in more accurate detection.
2. Standard treatment to prevent progression may be ineffective, and relapses may occur in previously treated patients.
3. Neurologic manifestations of syphilis in AIDS patients may occur early and may be unusual and include Bell's palsy, polyradiculopathy, transverse myelitis, stroke, or seizures with a mass lesion.

Although there is general agreement that *Treponema pallidum* invades the CNS early in the course of syphilitic infection, it is not clear that the actual incidence of neurologic manifestations is higher in HIV-infected patients. On the other hand, there is growing evidence that the course of syphilis in AIDS patients is more fulminant and atypical than in non–HIV-infected persons. CSF findings, especially early, do not always permit distinction between syphilitic and HIV brain infection. A positive CSF VDRL test, however, indicates neurosyphilis except when blood contaminates CSF, a well-recognized cause of false-positive CSF serology.

Recommendations for treating primary syphilis and neurosyphilis in HIV-infected patients are still evolving, but penicillin continues to be the mainstay of therapy; resistance has not yet been documented. It is possible that high-dose penicillin regimens, such as 24 million units of penicillin IV daily for 10 days, are required for all AIDS patients with syphilis regardless of clinical stage or interval since infection, but this is unclear and not standard practice for disease outside the CNS. Maintenance treatment regimens or use of a penicillin carrier combination that allows better passage across the blood-brain barrier are additional areas for future study. Improved methods for detecting and monitoring active infection are also needed.

Borreliosis

There is one reported case of Lyme disease in an HIV-infected patient. This 39-year-old man had a typical annular rash, followed several weeks later by bilateral facial palsy and numbness. Specific antibody titers to *Borrelia burgdorferi* were present, and there was a good response to a standard treatment regimen. Potential clinical issues include false-negative serology in patients with coinfection; cross reactivity of *B. burgdorferi* with other spirochetes including *T. pallidum*; a possible need for more intensive antibiotic treatment; and confusion between neurologic manifestations of Lyme disease with other, more common, causes of nervous system dysfunction in AIDS patients.

Bacterial Infections

Compared with the prevalence of infections caused by opportunistic organisms, bacterial infections are relatively uncommon in AIDS patients. Children, who have limited exposure to opportunistic organisms, are an exception in that they are more likely to develop bacterial infections, especially gram-negative meningitis. However, HIV may indirectly impair B-cell function in all patients, and drugs such as zidovudine or ganciclovir may lead to bone marrow suppression and neutropenia, all factors that may predispose to bacterial infection. Infections due to encapsulated bacteria occur with increased frequency, more acute presentations, and with greater tendency to relapse. Cerebral abscesses caused by *Listeria*, *Nocardia*, *Salmonella*, *Staphylococcus epidermidis*, *Streptococcus mitis*, and *Streptococcus pneumoniae* have been recognized (Fig. 17). Many of these were diagnosed only at autopsy. Spinal epidural abscess due to *S. aureus* or *S. epidermidis* fails to respond to antibiotic treatment alone and mandates surgery. Intramedullary spinal cord abscess due to *Pseudomonas cepacia* has been observed in one HIV-seropositive patient.

Listeria, *E. coli*, *S. pneumoniae*, and *H. influenzae* have caused meningitis in HIV-infected patients (Fig. 3). Standard doses of penicillin or ampicillin have been successful in treating *Listeria* meningitis. Nath et al. have described CNS Whipple's disease, presumably due to a bacilliform bacterium, in an AIDS patient. With

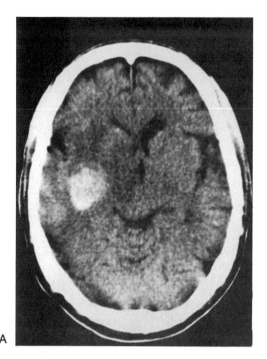

A

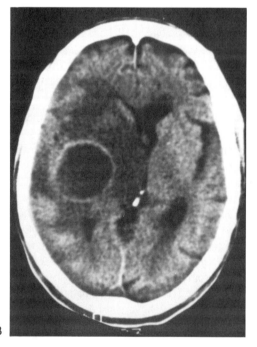

B

FIG. 17. A: Noncontrast head CT scan of a 40-year-old hypertensive man with acute right hemiplegia and streptococcal sepsis shows hyperdense mass in the right basal ganglia consistent with a cerebral hemorrhage. **B:** Six weeks later, after recovery from the hemorrhage, the patient was readmitted with fever, obtundation, and increased left-sided weakness. CT with contrast shows a round mass with rim enhancement in the region of the previous hematoma. The abnormality is now consistent with a brain abscess.

the development of more sophisticated techniques to detect and culture fastidious organisms, recognition of unusual bacterial CNS infections may increase.

Intravenous drug users are at higher risk for bacterial infections than other HIV-infected groups, especially before severe immunosuppression develops. Risk factors include skin ulcers, endocarditis, and contaminated needles. Trauma often precedes cases of epidural spinal abscess. The incidence of infection following surgical procedures is higher in AIDS patients than in non-HIV-infected individuals (Fig. 7B).

Diagnosis of meningitis requires lumbar puncture to obtain fluid for culture. CSF cultures can be positive even when gram stains on centrifuged samples are negative. CT or MRI scans may suggest meningitis if they demonstrate meningeal enhancement. Suspicion of spinal epidural abscess necessitates either myelography followed by CT or spine MRI.

NEOPLASMS

Primary Brain Lymphoma

Primary brain lymphoma is a rare CNS tumor in the general population, but its increased frequency in patients with acquired immune suppression, including transplant recipients and HIV-infected individuals, is now well established. In AIDS, the risk for developing primary brain lymphoma is nearly 100 times that in the general population. Lymphoma accounts now for 2% to 7% of the CNS complications in AIDS and is secondary only to toxoplasmosis as a cause of mass lesion. Its incidence rises with prolonged survival after AIDS is diagnosed, even with zidovudine treatment.

Reasons for the increased risk of lymphoma in this population are not fully understood, but most likely relate to defective internal surveillance mechanisms, oncogenic viruses, or dysfunction of immune regulation. Depression of T-cell numbers increases the likelihood that the immune system no longer effectively recognizes or destroys mutant, potentially neoplastic cells. The Epstein-Barr virus has been increasingly implicated in the development of CNS lymphoma. AIDS patients have impaired ability to suppress the growth of lymphocytes infected by Epstein-Barr virus. Other DNA viruses, including CMV, herpes simplex, and human papillomaviruses, may play a causative role in some patients, as may RNA viruses, including human T-cell leukemia virus-type I and even possibly HIV itself. It is perhaps most reasonable to speculate that with sufficient derangement of the immune system, several viruses may play etiologic roles in the development of cancer.

Primary brain lymphoma presents mainly as a parenchymal mass lesion with signs reflecting its particular location and, often, increased intracranial pressure. Aphasia, hemiparesis, ataxia, and altered mentation are common early findings, and isolated oculomotor palsy has been described. Seizures occur in about one-third of patients, but they are more apt to occur as the illness evolves than at its presentation. Although meningeal involvement is common with metastatic spread from systemic lymphoma, it is infrequent with primary brain lymphoma. Skull involvement may cause constant headaches.

The CSF is almost always abnormal but usually nonspecifically. The protein content is usually elevated, and some patients show mild pleocytosis (<50 cells/mm^3) and depressed glucose concentration. Because extensive meningeal infiltration does not usually occur with primary brain lymphoma, CSF cytology is almost always unhelpful.

Although the MRI or CT appearance of primary brain lymphoma is generally similar in AIDS and non-AIDS patients, some differences have been described. In AIDS the role of Epstein-Barr virus is prominent. However, there are no pathognomonic features that reliably distinguish this mass lesion from that caused by toxoplasmosis. Increased metabolic activity is seen in malignant CNS lesions using fluorodeoxyglucose PET scanning, but this is not widely available. Lesions are usually deep with periventricular and cerebellar sites especially common (Fig. 5). Multifocal tumors are not rare. Primary brain lymphoma almost always shows enhancement after intravenous contrast administration, although the pattern is quite variable and may be nodular, patchy, or ringlike. However, in a recent series of non-AIDS-related lymphoma, 10% of patients failed to show enhancement in CT or MRI. Enhancement results from both local alterations in the blood-brain barrier and neoplastic angiogenesis. Surrounding edema and some element of mass effect are the rule, and, rarely, there may be diffuse gyral enhancement.

Primary brain lymphoma is exquisitely sensitive to corticosteroids, and their use may be associated with a rapid and sometimes dramatic reduction in lesion size. However, because diagnosis can only be made with certainty by biopsy, preoperative steroid administration may actually hinder attempts to locate the lesion. Biopsy is facilitated by using a CT-guided stereotactic approach. Attempts at complete resection have been disappointing and resulted in a high incidence of severe neurologic sequelae.

Although radiation and corticosteroids almost always result in initial improvement and probably prolong survival, prognosis remains depressingly poor, and death usually occurs within a few months. Intensive chemotherapy is increasingly used after radiation, but neurologic and systemic toxicities are significant. One group reported a 52% response rate and a median survival of 7 months using a MACOP-B regimen (methotrexate, adriamycin, cyclophosphamide, vincristine, prednisone, and bleomycin). Patients without previous or concurrent opportunistic infection survived longer. Other investigators had a similar response rate (54%) using M-BACOD (dexamethasone substituted for prednisone), but only a 33% response rate using high-dose cytosine arabinoside and methotrexate. Lower dose combination therapy has been effective in systemic lymphoma, with fewer complications.

Metastatic Lymphoma and Other Tumors

Systemic non-Hodgkin's lymphomas also occur with increased frequency in AIDS patients, and the CNS is commonly involved, probably more often than in non–HIV-infected populations. The pattern of CNS involvement with metastatic lymphoma is usually leptomeningeal or epidural. Seventeen percent of a recent series had CSF involvement on routine screening. Thus the presentation of intracranial metastatic lymphoma is usually that of subacute meningitis with headache, lethargy, and cranial nerve palsies. Tumor deposits on spinal nerve roots cause radicular pain and segmental symptoms or signs. Epidural metastases, most often to the midthoracic spine, are common and frequently lead to spinal cord compression. Back pain is almost invariable. Other common findings are sensory loss, sphincter dysfunction, and paraparesis.

Diagnosis of meningeal lymphoma is made by cytological examination of CSF. Intrathecal chemotherapy using methotrexate and cytosine arabinoside is the mainstay of treatment. With spinal cord compression, decompressive surgery and radiotherapy may also be required. Prophylactic treatment with intrathecal cytosine arabinoside has been successful.

Kaposi's sarcoma and other tumors only rarely affect the nervous system, and always in the setting of metastatic spread from systemic involvement. The neurologic complications of metastatic Kaposi's sarcoma have been described, and brain parenchyma, dura, spinal cord, and nerve roots have all been sites of involvement. Immunoblastic sarcoma has also metastasized to brain, and we and others have seen patients with nasopharyngeal tumors that involve the brain by direct extension (Fig.

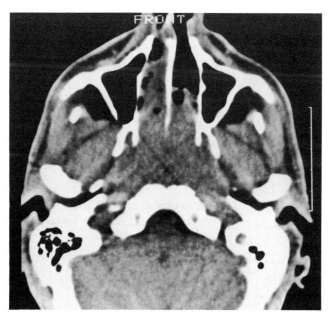

FIG. 18. Noncontrast CT scan of a 36-year-old HIV-infected man who presented with bilateral extraocular muscle palsies. Tumor mass fills the nasal passages and adjacent sinuses and, at higher levels, invaded the orbits (not shown). Biopsy revealed Burkitt's lymphoma.

18). Children have developed leiomyosarcoma, which is rare in the absence of AIDS. Rhabdomyosarcoma, plasmacytoma, and immunoblastic sarcoma have metastasized to the epidural space and produced spinal cord compression. Solid tumors are especially common among injecting drug users with AIDS and are more virulent than in non-HIV patients (Fig. 19). Two HIV-seropositive patients developed rapidly progressive astrocytomas. As patients survive longer with AIDS, more malignancies are diagnosed.

CEREBROVASCULAR DISEASE

Cerebral Infarction

Cerebral infarction and hemorrhage are not unusual in autopsy series of AIDS patients, with prevalence estimates ranging from 24% to 34%. Nonetheless, cerebrovascular complications associated with AIDS have been diagnosed clinically in only 1.6% of adults and 6% of children. Annual incidence rates of 0.75% and 1.3% have been estimated. Several reasons may account for the discrepancy between clinical and autopsy series. First, many cerebrovascular events probably occur late in the course of a patient's illness when new neurologic symptoms or signs may be missed altogether, attributed to other, previously diagnosed neurologic disease, or assumed to reflect preterminal hypoxia or hypotension. Second, cerebrovascular complications seem to be especially common in children with AIDS, an age group where they are not ordinarily suspected. Third, lesions may be "silent" because they are small or occur in areas of the brain that do not result in easily detectable clinical abnormalities. Finally, in our experience transient neurologic disturbances occurring in patients with focal cerebral lesions are commonly attributed to seizures or postictal Todd's phenomena, often without adequate justification.

Cerebral infarction probably results from several mechanisms, although in half the cases, no presumptive cause can be identified. It is well established that mycobacteria, varicella zoster virus, *T. pallidum*, and *Candida* cause an infective arteritis that may lead to stroke (Fig. 16), and that cryptococcal infection may be associated with transient ischemic attacks. In addition, occlusion of both small and medium to large vessels occurs from arteriopathies marked by endothelial prominence, fibrinoid deposits, intimal fibrodysplasia, and thickening of the vessel wall with variable inflammatory response. In some of these patients, the presence of intranuclear inclusions within endothelial or inflammatory cells, as well as more direct immunocytochemical evidence, has suggested an association with infective organisms, including CMV, the virus of PML (JC virus), aspergillus, and, most convincingly, HIV. Vasculitis has been described in several patients with HIV infection, including one patient with simultaneous primary HIV and CMV infection, and another patient who developed a necrotizing vasculitis of the nervous system. Although it is tempting to speculate that some of the cerebrovascular complications seen in AIDS patients result from viral infection of vascular cells that either directly

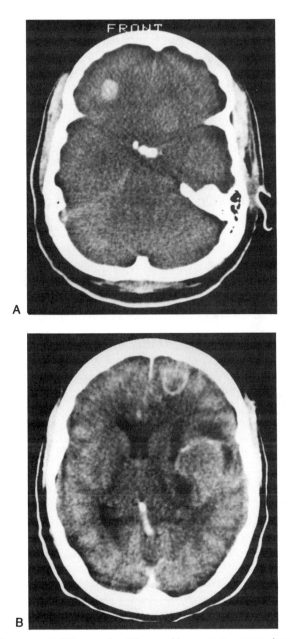

FIG. 19. A: Noncontrast CT scan of a 34-year-old pregnant woman showing a right frontal hyperdense lesion and possible left temporal and frontal lesions as well, attributed to toxoplasmosis. **B:** A scan with contrast one week later showing an enhancing lesion in the left basal ganglia causing ventricular effacement, and left frontal lobe lesions.

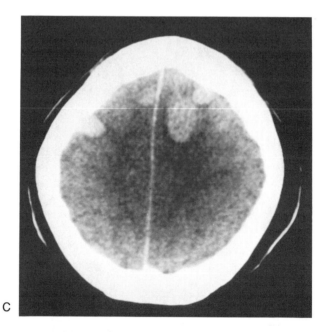

C

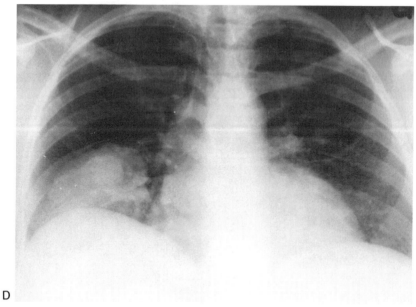

D

FIG. 19. C: One month later, despite treatment for toxoplasmosis, lesions are increased in size and number. **D:** Chest radiograph shows lesion in the right lower lobe, which bronchoscopic biopsy proved to be an undifferentiated bronchogenic adenocarcinoma. Postmortem brain examination showed several mucinous brain metastases.

causes thrombotic occlusion or indirectly mediates vascular injury through immune complex deposition, this mechanism remains hypothetical at the present time. Lymphoma has been associated with vasculopathy in one patient.

Cardiogenic emboli are another important cause of stroke in this group of patients. In addition to cardiomyopathy, both infective and nonbacterial thrombotic endocarditis may occur. Bacterial or fungal endocarditis is especially common in active intravenous drug users. Anticardiolipin antibodies or lupus anticoagulant have been detected in up to half the AIDS patients surveyed, but the role of these "hypercoagulant" serum factors in producing cerebral infarction is unclear.

Cerebral Hemorrhage

Cerebral hemorrhage is easily diagnosed by CT scan (Fig. 20), and additional cases are discovered at autopsy. Like cerebral infarction, there are several reasons for the increased frequency of hemorrhage in AIDS patients. Both adults and children with AIDS develop idiopathic thrombocytopenic purpura (ITP) on an autoim-

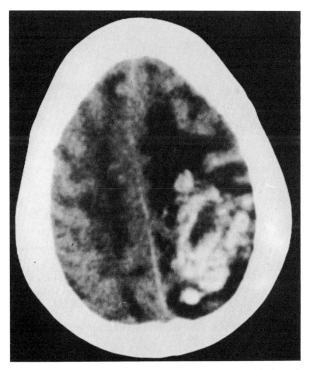

FIG. 20. Noncontrast scan of a 28-year-old HIV-infected woman with thrombocytopenia who collapsed with sudden onset of right hemiplegia and the rapid development of coma. There is a large, multilobulated hyperdense area with surrounding edema and mass effect consistent with intraparenchymal hemorrhage.

mune basis or from decreased platelet production. ITP may appear early or late in the course of HIV infection and is often asymptomatic. However, some investigators have rated the thrombocytopenia as severe in 5.3% of a group of HIV-seropositive drug users. Others found platelet counts less than $100,000/mm^3$ in 9% of intravenous drug users and in 3% of homosexual men who were HIV seropositive. Development of thrombocytopenia correlated with falling CD4 cell counts.

Hemophilia, aneurysmal dilatation, mycotic aneurysms (usually in intravenous drug users), and CNS aspergillosis predispose to cerebral hemorrhage. Bleeding into metastatic Kaposi's sarcoma has been described.

CONCLUSION

Although HIV infection has devastating consequences for the central and peripheral nervous systems, some specific therapies and preventive measures are being developed. In addition, mass lesions, meningitis, and spinal cord disease caused by opportunistic infections or lymphoma are now well characterized, clinically diagnosable, and often treatable. It is important that all clinicians be aware of how HIV infection affects the nervous system and have an organized approach to diagnosis and treatment whenever possible. All patients can, at the least, be offered symptomatic relief and meaningful supportive care.

ACKNOWLEDGMENTS

I thank my husband, Dr. Timothy A. Pedley, for editing the manuscript and watching our children. I am grateful to Ken Bailey for excellent photography; to Shirley Susarchick and Amelia Gulston for expert typing; and to the patients and staff of Metropolitan Hospital, especially Dr. Ted Lenox, for teaching me about AIDS and the nervous system.

SUGGESTED READING

Balfour HH Jr, Benson C, Braun J, et al. Management of acyclovir-resistant herpes simplex and varicella-zoster infections. *J Acquir Immun Def* 1994;7:254–260.

Barohn RJ, Gronseth GS, LeForce BR, McVey AL, McGuire SA, Butzin CA, King RB. Peripheral nervous system involvement in a large cohort of human immunodeficiency virus-infected individuals. *Arch Neurol* 1993;50:167–171.

Berenguer J, Moreno S, Laguna F, et al. Tuberculous meningitis in patients with the human immunodeficiency virus. *N Engl J Med* 1992;326:668–672.

Dickson DW, Llena JF, Nelson SJ, Weidenheim KM. Central nervous system pathology in pediatric AIDS. *Ann NY Acad Sci* 1993;693:93–106.

Feiden W, Bise K, Steude U, Pfister H-W, Moller AA. The stereotactic biopsy diagnosis of focal intracerebral lesions in AIDS patients. *Acta Neurol Scand* 1993;87:228–233.

Forsyth PA, Yahalom J, DeAngelis LM. Combined-modality therapy in the treatment of primary central nervous system lymphoma in AIDS. *Neurology* 1994;44:1473–1479.

Gordon SM, Eaton ME, George R, et al. The response of symptomatic neurosyphilis to high-dose intravenous penicillin G in patients with human immunodeficiency virus infection. *N Engl J Med* 1994;331:1469–1473.

Gozlan J, El Amrani M, Baudrimont M, et al. A prospective evaluation of clinical criteria and polymerase chain reaction assay of cerebrospinal fluid for the diagnosis of cytomegalovirus-related neurological disease during AIDS. *AIDS* 1995;9:253–260.

Johnston MI, Hoth DF. Present and future prospects for HIV therapies. *Science* 1993;260:1286–1293.

Labar DR. Seizures and HIV infection. In: Pedley, TA, Meldrum B, eds. *Recent advances in epilepsy.* London: Churchill Livingstone, 1991;Ch. 8.

Lipton SA, Gendelman HE. Dementia associated with the acquired immunodeficiency syndrome. *N Engl J Med* 1995;332:934–940.

O'Connor PG, Selwyn PA, Schottenfeld RS. Medical care for injection-drug users with human immunodeficiency virus infection. *N Engl J Med* 1994;331:450–459.

Porter SB, Sande MA. Toxoplasmosis of the central nervous system in the acquired immunodeficiency syndrome. *N Engl J Med* 1992;327:1643–1648.

Price RW, Perry SW, eds. *HIV, AIDS and the brain* (ARNMD vol. 72), New York: Raven Press, 1994.

Saag MS, Powderly WG, Cloud GA, et al. Comparison of amphotericin B with fluconazole in the treatment of acute AIDS-associated cryptococcal meningitis. *N Engl J Med* 1992;326:83–89.

So YT, Olney RK. Acute lumbosacral polyradiculopathy in acquired immunodeficiency syndrome: experience in 23 patients. *Ann Neurol* 1994;35:53–58.

Steiger MJ, Tarnesby G, Gabe S, McLaughlin J, Schapira AHV. Successful outcome of progressive multifocal leukoencephalopathy with cytarabine and interferon. *Ann Neurol* 1993;33:407–411.

Tirelli U, Franceschi S, Carbone A. Malignant tumors in patients with HIV infection. *Br Med J* 1994; 308:1148–1153.

A Clinical Guide to AIDS and HIV,
edited by Gary P. Wormser.
Lippincott-Raven Publishers, Philadelphia © 1996.

7

The Gastrointestinal and Hepatobiliary Systems in HIV Infection

Donald P. Kotler

*Department of Medicine, Division of Gastroenterology,
College of Physicians and Surgeons, Columbia University,
Saint Luke's Roosevelt Hospital Center,
New York, New York 10025*

Gastrointestinal (GI) dysfunction is common in HIV-infected individuals, with or without AIDS, as it is in other immune deficiency disorders. The specialized functions of mucous membranes, such as nutrient absorption by enterocytes or gas exchange by pulmonary epithelium, require intimate contact with the external environment and thereby render them vulnerable to pathogens. This vulnerability has promoted the evolution of complex immunologic and nonimmunologic defenses.

Gastrointestinal involvement in HIV infection and AIDS has serious consequences. Chronic enteropathy has been associated with increased mortality. Progressive malnutrition, which may be associated with intestinal disease, has been shown to be an independent predictor of death in patients with AIDS. Chronic diarrhea has been associated with diminished quality of life.

In this chapter the effects of HIV and AIDS on the GI tract and liver are discussed. Diagnosis and management are organized into a series of clinical syndromes.

HIV AND MUCOSAL IMMUNITY

Immune defenses of the mucous membranes are linked as a common mucosal immune system. Gut-associated lymphoid tissue (GALT) is composed of lymphoid aggregates in the tonsils, Peyer's patches, and mucosal lymphoid follicles, plus diverse immunologically active cells in the lamina propria. Different subpopulations of mononuclear cells are found in the lamina propria than in the epithelium. The mucosa contains elements of both humoral (secretory) and cell-mediated immunity. The nonimmunologic defense system includes gastric acid, salivary, pancreatic and biliary secretions, secreted mucus, and intestinal motility. A stable luminal flora also contributes to homeostasis.

Mucosal immunity in HIV infection has received relatively little study. Immunohistochemical studies as well as studies of cells isolated from mucosal biopsies have demonstrated reductions in the helper T cell population (CD4$^+$) in intestinal mucosa and an increase in suppressor T cells (CD8$^+$), similar to that seen in peripheral blood. The lamina to propria CD4 lymphocyte population is disproportionately depleted early in the disease course. CD4$^+$ lymphoid cells in lymphoid aggregates are relatively preserved, compared with cells in lamina propria. Immunohistochemical and flow cytometric studies have also found evidence of altered expression of cell surface markers of lamina propria lymphocytes. Electron microscopic studies have demonstrated ultrastructural evidence of cell activation of intraepithelial lymphocytes in AIDS patients, while flow cytometry studies of isolated mucosal mononuclear cells have revealed increased cell membrane expression of DR antigen, implying cell activation. Immunohistologic studies have demonstrated depletion of plasma cells containing immunoglobulin A (IgA) in mucosal biopsies from AIDS patients, possibly accounting for the observed reduction in salivary IgA secretion. In contrast to evidence of decreased secretory immunity, serum IgA concentrations are often elevated in HIV-infected individuals.

Few studies have examined the functional status of the immune system in the GI tract of HIV-infected persons. Ericksson demonstrated normal responses to oral vaccination with cholera toxin B subunit in HIV-infected subjects, which contrasts with studies demonstrating poor systemic antibody responses to tetanus toxoid vaccination. Evidence of specific anti-HIV activity of lamina propria lymphocytes has been reported.

HIV AND THE GI TRACT

Investigators have detected cellular reservoirs for HIV in the GI tract by a variety of techniques, including the polymerase chain reaction. In situ hybridization studies demonstrated HIV-1 RNA and DNA in lamina propria mononuclear cells, and some studies have also shown HIV DNA in crypt epithelial and enterochromaffin cells. Cells containing HIV RNA were found both in mucosal lymphoid follicles and lamina propria. Dendritic cells in germinal centers of follicles in the GI tract exhibit a pattern of diffuse staining identical to that seen in peripheral lymph nodes, thought to be due to trapping of immune complexes containing HIV virions.

HIV P24 antigen has been detected in GI mucosa. Primary intestinal cell lines and colonic tumor epithelial cell lines have been productively infected with HIV. Additional *in vitro* studies have demonstrated apparent endocytosis of HIV by an epithelial cell line. The possible role HIV may play in intestinal disease is discussed below.

CLINICAL SYNDROMES

General Principles of Evaluation and Treatment

Proper clinical management of an HIV-infected patient requires appreciation of differences in disease presentation. More than one enteric complication may coexist in AIDS patients. In one study, multiple infections were found in almost one-third of such patients. One organism may produce several different clinical syndromes, while many organisms can produce identical clinical syndromes. Disease complications of AIDS are notable for their susceptibility to suppression but resistance to cure, so that treatments must often be given indefinitely. The specific pathogens producing disease in AIDS patients may be the same but are often different from those that typically cause illness in immunocompetent individuals. In either case, the pathologic features usually match the clinical symptoms and physical findings.

Pathologic processes may affect the GI tract with either a focal or diffuse pattern. For example, focal ulcers may be found anywhere in the GI tract. They may be infectious, noninfectious, or neoplastic. Certain viral infections, such as cytomegalovirus (CMV) infection, and fungal infections, such as histoplasmosis, produce multifocal disease. The GI tract can also be involved diffusely. The most common diffuse lesion is candidiasis of the oral cavity and/or to the esophagus. The epithelial cell layer of the small intestine is a target for certain protozoal infections including *Cryptosporidium parvum, Isospora belli*, and the microsporidia, *Enterocytozoon bieneusi* and *Septata intestinalis*. The lamina propria and submucosa may be involved by chronic infections caused by *Mycobacterium avium* complex (MAC). Bacteria such as salmonella, shigella, and campylobacter may cause a diffuse colitis or enterocolitis.

The pathologic processes described above may lead to several types of clinical syndromes: disorders of food intake, dyspepsia, diarrhea, anorectal diseases, tumors, hepatobiliary diseases, pancreatic diseases, gastrointestinal bleeding, and the acute abdomen.

Which patients require extensive evaluation is an important question. Virtually all patients develop GI symptoms at some point during the course of HIV infection, but many of these episodes are self-limited. Extensive evaluation for all cases would be expensive and burdensome. Evaluation is mandated for patients whose symptoms are persistent, increasing in severity, or associated with fever and/or weight loss. When such symptoms have been present for more than one month, it is likely that they will continue indefinitely unless diagnosed and treated.

The diagnostic evaluation should be streamlined and yet thorough enough to detect multiple infections, should they exist. Proper GI diagnosis after careful history, physical examination, and stool tests may require biopsy with histopathologic examination. If evaluation is negative and symptoms persist, workup should be repeated after several weeks, since a second evaluation may yield a diagnosis missed initially.

Disorders of Food Intake

Etiology and Pathogenesis

Oral candidiasis is the most common infectious complication of HIV infection, developing in more than three-quarters of patients at some time during the disease course. Candidiasis decreases taste sensation and affects swallowing, in addition to causing oral or substernal discomfort. Most cases are due to *Candida albicans*.

Three types of candidiasis are recognized: pseudomembranous such as thrush (Fig. 1A), erythematous, and angular stomatitis. Thrush is most florid in the soft palate and posterior pharynx. Candidiasis is quite distinct from oral hairy leuko-plakia, which is found along the sides of the tongue and occasionally on the adjacent

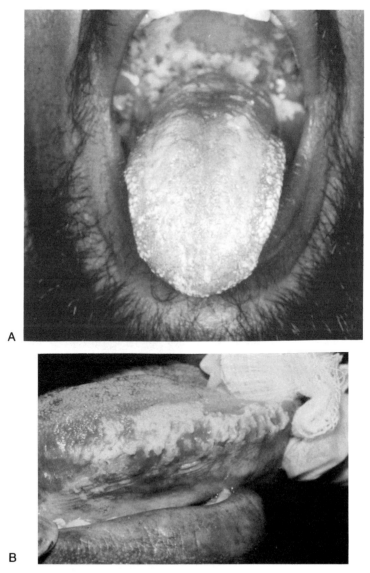

A

B

FIG. 1. A: Oral candidiasis. **B:** Hairy leukoplakia (courtesy of J. S. Greenspan).

buccal mucosa. Oral hairy leukoplakia has a fissured or serrated border and cannot be scraped off (Fig. 1B). Evidence for Epstein-Barr virus in the affected tissue has been demonstrated by molecular techniques as well as by electron microscopy. In contrast to candidiasis, hairy leukoplakia is asymptomatic and does not affect food intake. Severe gingivitis or periodontitis may also affect eating. Ulcerations due to herpes simplex or CMV and aphthous ulcers may cause pain and interfere with eating. Mass lesions such as those caused by Kaposi's sarcoma or lymphoma occur in the oral cavity and can interfere with chewing or swallowing. The esophagus is affected by the same lesions as the oral cavity. A particularly striking lesion is the idiopathic esophageal ulcer, which may be large and produce debilitating symptoms. In contrast to herpetic ulcers, no etiologic agent is found even with biopsy of the lesion. Studies have documented the presence of HIV RNA in these ulcers, although HIV may also be detected in ulcers due to known etiologies, such as CMV-associated ulcers. HIV has also been detected in the ulcers that have occurred transiently during primary HIV infection.

Patients may also experience diminished food intake in the absence of oral or esophageal disease. Focal or diffuse neurologic lesions can affect food intake. Patients with malabsorption do not increase food intake sufficiently to compensate for the lost calories, due to inhibitory factors related to the presence of unabsorbed nutrients in the distal intestine. Anorexia is often a prominent feature of systemic

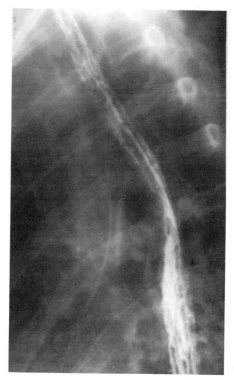

FIG. 1. continued. **C:** Barium esophagram demonstrating diffuse mucosal involvement as a result of candida esophagitis.

C

opportunistic infections, and appears to be related to altered cytokine release. Diminished food intake may also occur as a result of an adverse effect of a specific medication.

Diagnosis

Determining the etiology of disorders of food intake can be approached using a diagnostic algorithm (Table 1). Local disease can be diagnosed by the careful history and physical examination, assisted by ENT or dental consultation. The presence of malabsorption is usually suggested by history (see below) and can be confirmed with biopsy or an absorption study. Systemic disease is suggested by fever or other localizing signs and symptoms. The clinician should not conclude that anorexia is due to a medication until other possibilities are ruled out or the patient responds favorably to a supervised trial of medication withdrawal.

Candidiasis is a diffuse lesion in the esophagus and may occur independently of thrush. The diagnosis may be suggested by barium studies (Fig. 1C) and confirmed by biopsy or brushings. In an AIDS patient with suspected esophageal candidiasis, it is advisable to treat empirically with an antifungal agent such as fluconazole and further evaluate only those patients with persisting symptoms. A transnasal cytology brush has been developed for nonendoscopic diagnosis of candidiasis.

All esophageal ulcerations should be investigated by direct examination and biopsy. Herpetic esophagitis presents as groups of small, shallow ulcers; on histopathologic examination typical inclusions are found in the epithelial layer. CMV may produce esophageal ulcers with characteristics CMV inclusions seen histo-

TABLE 1. *Diagnostic algorithm for disorders of food intake*

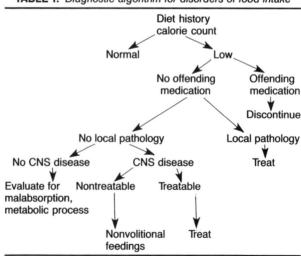

logically in the ulcer base. No etiologic diagnosis can be reached in a significant proportion of patients with esophageal ulcers. These ulcers may be large and deep, with undermined edges.

Treatment

The management of eating disorders is based upon the precise cause of the problem. Oral candidiasis responds to a variety of antifungal therapies including topical, nystatin, and clotrimazole, or the systemically active azole drugs. Esophageal candidiasis is best treated using systemically active compounds, since the organism is invasive. Fluconazole was shown to be superior to ketoconazole in one study. The presence of achlorhydria may decrease the bioavailability of ketoconazole, which requires gastric acidity for dissolution. Candida infection may develop resistance to azole therapy in some cases, and some strains of this fungus may be inherently resistant. In these patients intravenous amphotericin B therapy may be required. Anecdotal reports suggest that amphotericin B may also be effective when given orally. The most important unresolved management issue is the benefit of prophylactic therapy. While most clinicians provide maintenance suppressive therapy in the event of recurrent disease, the use of primary prophylaxis is unsettled.

Herpes simplex virus infection responds to oral treatment with acyclovir. Hairy leukoplakia responds to acyclovir or ganciclovir. Ganciclovir or foscarnet are effective treatments for CMV esophageal disease. Deep painful aphthous ulcers not due to an identifiable pathogen may respond to locally injected or systemic corticosteroids, although the danger of worsening immune suppression in patients with AIDS should be kept in mind. Corticosteroid therapy was associated with an increased risk of developing CMV infection in one study. Prolonged treatment may be required for complete healing to occur. The ulcer also may recur after steroid therapy is discontinued.

A major complication of oral and esophageal diseases is decreased food intake. Dietary consultation with creative diet planning and choice may be quite beneficial in milder cases. Caloric supplementation with formula diets also may be helpful. In patients with local lesions that cannot be treated successfully or in refractory cases of anorexia, some form of nonvolitional feeding is required (see section Nutritional Interventions, below).

Dyspepsia

Etiology and Pathogenesis

Nausea and dyspepsia are very common symptoms in AIDS patients but rarely dominate the clinical picture. The stomach may be involved by disseminated infections due to CMV, MAC, or fungi, or by tumors. Gastritis due to *Helicobacter pylori* has been seen, but its incidence appears to be lower in HIV-infected than in noninfected patients. Some medications, such as nonsteroidal antiinflammatory agents, promote gastric ulceration and produce dyspepsia. Studies have shown a high incidence of achlorhydria in AIDS patients. Achlorhydria may alter the absorption of drugs, such as a ketoconazole, and may promote an increase in bacterial colony counts in the stomach and upper smaller intestine, with potential adverse affects upon nutrient absorption. Intrinsic factor secretion might also be decreased, and promote decreased vitamin B_{12} absorption.

Clinical symptoms are nonspecific. The presence of weight loss or fever implies a serious complication such as a systemic infection or ulcerating tumor. Dyspepsia is due to a low-grade pancreatitis in some patients and may precede the diagnosis of biliary tract disease in others (see below). As in the non–HIV-infected person, gastric pathology may be detected even in the absence of gastric symptoms.

Diagnosis

Diagnosis of gastric diseases can be made by imaging or endoscopic procedures. Radiologic examinations are sensitive in detecting mass lesions, pose little risk, involve a low risk of contamination by patient secretions, and cost less than endoscopic examinations. However, radiologic imaging has a variable sensitivity for detection of mucosal lesions and has poor specificity for the etiologic diagnosis of mass lesions or ulcers. The need for subsequent endoscopy and/or the use of sophisticated examination such as computed tomography (CT) scans also decreases the cost advantage.

Treatment

Symptomatic *H. pylori* infection in an AIDS patient is treated in a similar manner to other patients. A diagnosis of CMV or MAC infection is an indication for systemic antiinfective therapy. Widespread or ulcerating Kaposi's sarcoma is an indication for systemic chemotherapy, as is the presence of lymphoma. Associated eating disorders should be evaluated and sufficient caloric intake assured.

Diarrhea and Wasting

Etiology and Pathogenesis

Alterations in bowel habits occur in more than one-half of HIV-infected patients at some point during the disease course. The spectrum of enteric pathogens continues to increase, although a substantial proportion of symptomatic patients have no identifiable etiology for their problems. Unexplained intestinal dysfunction and injury was an early observation, and the term *AIDS enteropathy* has been applied to this group of patients.

Prevalence

The prevalence of enteric pathogens varies greatly in reported series, from 15% to 75%. The most likely explanations are differences in diagnostic evaluations and varying experience with certain infections. Prevalence rates for enteric pathogens also differs in patients seen by primary care physicians compared with GI consultants due to selection of the most severe and protracted cases for referral. We prospectively evaluated 250 HIV-infected individuals referred for GI symptoms, using stool analyses plus light and transmission electron microscopic examination of intestinal biopsies. Enteric pathogens were identified in 83% of 141 AIDS patients with diarrhea, compared with 2% of 53 AIDS patients without diarrhea and 3% of 56 HIV-infected patients who had not progressed to AIDS. Two or more coexisting infections were found in 28% of AIDS patients with diarrhea. Thus, AIDS patients with chronic diarrhea are very likely to have one or more enteric pathogens. In contrast, only a small minority of HIV-infected individuals without advancing immune deficiency have enteric pathogens, with the possible exception of HIV itself (see below).

Small Intestinal Pathogens

Pathophysiology

Histopathologic studies have shown that small intestinal pathogens produce partial villus atrophy and crypt hyperplasia, while most patients without pathogens have normal or mild-moderate hyporegenerative atrophy. Studies of small intestinal function using D-xylose as a measure of effective surface area also demonstrate a bimodal distribution of function, with both normal and grossly abnormal results. In some studies, function abnormalities were disproportionate to the extent of structural changes. In different studies, brush border enzyme-specific activities were found to be normal or low in patients without enteric pathogens. Epithelial cell proliferation is affected by alterations in the expression of cytokines and other inflammatory mediators in the lamina propria. Such changes were noted in a fetal explant model after infection with HIV.

Other evidence of intestinal disease has been reported. Ileal dysfunction may occur, as documented by malabsorption of vitamin B_{12}/intrinsic factor complex (Schilling test, part 2), abnormal bile salt breath tests, and decreased retention of a synthetic bile salt (SeHCAT). Studies of intestinal permeability show frequent alterations that are unassociated with enteric pathogens. The contribution of bacterial overgrowth is unsettled.

Cryptosporidiosis

Cryptosporidiosis has received the most attention of enteric infections in AIDS. Cryptosporidiosis is generally believed to account for about 10% of cases of chronic diarrhea in AIDS patients. The illness is self-limited in most immune-competent patients. The clinical course in AIDS patients is variable, but is usually protracted. Only a small percentage of patients undergo spontaneous remission. On occasion the infection may be fulminant and involve extraintestinal structures. A histopathologic study demonstrated variability in the intestinal location of cryptosporidiosis in AIDS (Fig. 2). Most patients (65%) had diffuse small intestinal involvement with or without mild colonic involvement. A smaller percentage of patients have cryptosporidial ileocolitis, without evidence of jejunal disease. Patients with small intestinal localization have more severe villus alterations and malabsorption. Patients with diffuse small intestinal disease also had significantly shorter survivals, and more often received parenteral hydration or nutritional support. The factors underlying this variability are unknown.

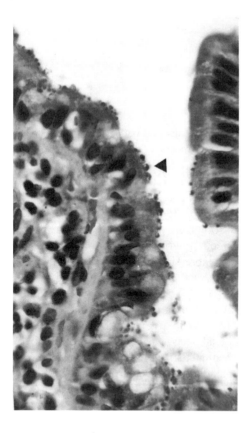

FIG. 2. Cryptosporidial infection of the small intestine. Organisms are seen at the level of the epithelial cell brush border (*arrow*) (H&E 480×).

Microsporidiosis

Microsporidia are primitive protozoa only recently recognized to infect man, although they have long been known as pathogens in animals. Microsporidia are characterized by the presence of a coiled polar tubule with an intracellular extrusion apparatus. Cellular infection occurs through extrusion of the polar filament, followed by ejection of the sporoplasm through the hollow tube.

Two species have been identified in intestinal biopsies from AIDS patients: *Enterocytozoan bieneusi* and *Septata intestinalis*. While *E. bieneusi* infection is limited to enterocytes, *S. intestinalis* has been shown to produce disseminated disease. Spores of *S. intestinalis* can be found in epithelial cells in the urinary sediment. Autopsy studies have demonstrated this organism in the kidney as well as the liver.

Microsporidiosis is being recognized with increasing frequency. The diagnosis was often missed in the past due to the small size and poor staining of the organism (Fig. 3). Prevalence rates in different population groups range from 2% to 50%. The prevalence rate in our laboratory has remained constant since 1988, at about one-third of cases of chronic diarrhea with weight loss. A recent report identified *E. bieneusi* in an immunocompetent individual with a self-limited diarrheal illness. This observation implies that human infection may be widespread and could be a significant cause of community-acquired or traveler's diarrhea. One prospective study found prevalence rates for microsporidiosis by electron microscopy of over 20% for HIV-infected patients with and without diarrhea. If confirmed by other investigators, the results suggest that *E. bieneusi* is a common infection in man, and that infection may not necessarily be associated with diarrhea.

The mode of transmission of *E. bieneusi* infection has not been defined, although it is likely to be by the oral route. Little is known about immunity to *E. bieneusi* infection. Several studies have examined the development of symptomatic microsporidiosis as a function of the level of immune deficiency and found that patients typically have severe depletion of CD4 lymphocyte counts (<50 cells/mm^3). The one study finding similar prevalence rates in patients with and without diarrhea also found infection in patients with much higher CD4 lymphocyte counts.

Isospora belli has been reported frequently in AIDS patients from Haiti and West Africa, although fewer cases have been seen in the continental United States. The symptoms are similar to those of cryptosporidiosis. Organisms may be rare in stool specimens and in biopsies, so the diagnosis may be missed (Fig. 4).

Giardia lamblia is not a common cause of acute diarrhea in AIDS. Drug therapy with metronidazole is indicated if cysts or trophozoites are found, although suspicion of other etiologies should be high. Like giardiasis, amebiasis is not a common cause of severe illness in HIV-infected patients in the United States. In the majority of cases, *Entameba histolytica* appears to act as a commensal organism. While therapy should be given, the possibility of coexisting pathogens should be considered. Other parasites have been reported in AIDS patients, including *Strongyloides stercoralis*, which may produce a hyperinfection syndrome. *Blastocystis hominis*,

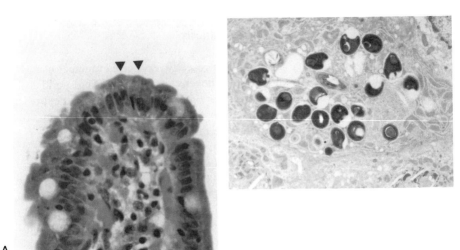

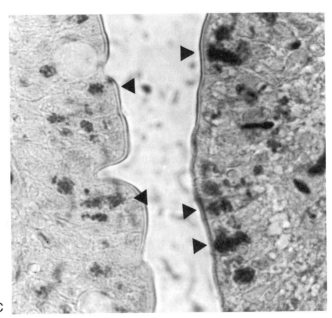

FIG. 3. Microsporidial infection of the small intestine. **A:** Cytoplasmic inclusions are noted in the apical cytoplasm of villus tip epithelial cells (*arrows*) (H&E 250×). **B:** Transmission electron micrograph of *E. bieneusi* spores in an epithelial cell (90000×). **C:** Chromotrope 2R modified trichrome stain demonstrating spores of *S. intestinalis* in epithelial cells (*arrows*) (880×).

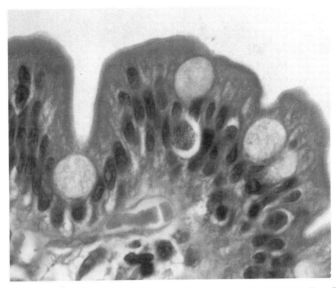

FIG. 4. Isoporiasis of the small intestine. A microgametocyte is located in the epithelium (H&E 480 ×).

which is felt by some authors to be an enteric pathogen, has been found in HIV-infected people with diarrhea.

Enteropathogenic Bacterial Infection

A syndrome of chronic diarrhea and malabsorption associated with bacterial-epithelial cell adherence and damage has been recognized. Infection is localized to the terminal ileum, cecum, and colon. The histopathologic findings are similar to those seen in infants with enteropathogenic *Escherichia coli* infection. It is unclear if the same mechanism applies in AIDS patients, or if the immune deficiency renders the mucosa vulnerable to "non-pathogens." Alternatively, the problem might result from community-acquired, low-grade intestinal infection that cannot be cleared due to the severity of the immune deficit.

Enterocolitis

Cytomegalovirus

Disseminated CMV infection is a frequent and serious complication in AIDS and can present as a variety of gastrointestinal syndromes including oral and esophageal ulcers, esophagitis, gastritis, isolated intestinal ulcers, terminal ileitis, spontaneous intestinal perforation, and focal or diffuse colitis. Colitis is the most common GI

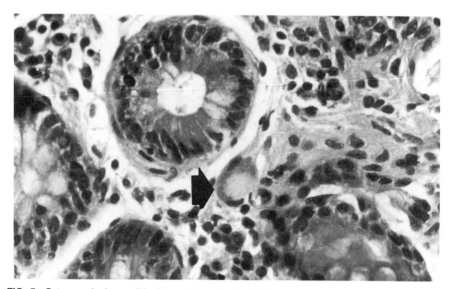

FIG. 5. Cytomegalovirus colitis. Large intracytoplasmic inclusion and small intranuclear inclusion are seen in an endothelial cell (*arrow*) (H&E 480 ×).

problem produced by CMV. The cecum and ileocecal valve are usually involved earliest in the disease. The major cell affected is the vascular endothelial cell (Fig. 5). Clinical disease occurs as a result of vasculitis and presents as focal or multifocal ulcerations that become progressively diffuse. Colonic perforation, "toxic megacolon," and progressive wasting with refractory diarrhea are possible clinical outcomes in untreated cases.

Mycobacterium Avium Complex

Infection with *Mycobacterium avium* complex (MAC) is a common cause of intestinal disease in AIDS patients with severe immune suppression. Infection is probably acquired through the ingestion of contaminated water. Clinical disease results from infiltration of infected macrophages into tissue compartments, similar to Whipple's disease, and from the effects of cytokines released by the macrophages. The luminal gastrointestinal tract is involved by MAC. Massive thickening of the proximal intestine may occur. Small intestinal biopsy reveals infiltration of the lamina propria by macrophages containing large numbers of acid-fast bacilli (Fig. 6).

Bacterial Enteritides

Bacterial enteritides in AIDS have distinctive features. Salmonella, shigella, or campylobacter infections occur in HIV-infected patients with or without AIDS. In

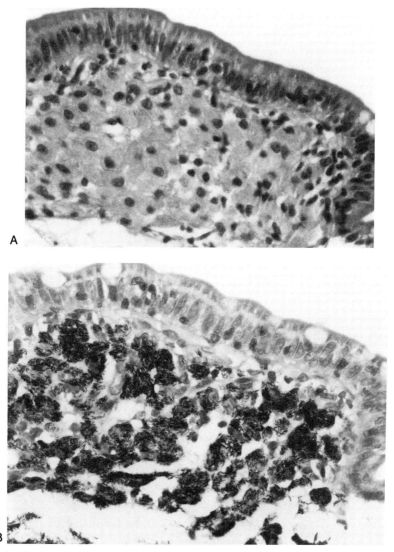

FIG. 6. Mycobacterium avium complex infection of the small intestine. **A:** Foamy macrophages located in the superficial lamina propria (H&E 480 ×). **B:** Acid-fast bacilli located predominantly in cells corresponding to the foamy macrophages (Ziehl Nielson 480 ×).

one study, shigella infections tended to occur early in the disease course, while salmonella and campylobacter infections were more common in AIDS patients. It is unclear if the incidence is increased over the surrounding population, although enhanced susceptibility could be related to decreased gastric acid secretion, as noted above. The clinical presentation of salmonella infection may be reminiscent of the classical descriptions of typhoid fever.

Antibiotic-Associated Colitis

Antibotic-associated colitis, related to elaboration of *Clostridium difficile* toxin, has been reported in AIDS patients. AIDS patients may be particularly vulnerable to this complication, as they often receive broad-spectrum antibotics. Clindamycin use and prolonged hospitalization are risk factors for its development. The clinical syndrome is similar in AIDS and non-AIDS patients.

Adenovirus

Adenoviruses are occasionally isolated from rectal swabs or biopsies from AIDS patients with diarrhea and a stable or deteriorating course. Electron microscopic studies have demonstrated cytoplasmic inclusion bodies containing adenovirus in superficial epithelial cells, including goblet cells.

Newly Described Pathogens

Several novel microbes have been described in immunodeficient patients, including AIDS patients. In one study, stool specimens from HIV-infected individuals were shown to contain enteric viruses, such as astrovirus and picobirnavirus, each in about 10% of cases. Infection with a cyclospora, a large coccidian parasite, has been detected in AIDS patients. Infection with a facultative anaerobic gram-negative coccobacillus, dysgonic fermenter-3, has been reported. This fastidious organism requires special culture conditions.

Role of HIV in Intestinal Disease

Several authors have suggested that HIV itself may play a role in intestinal disease. Most AIDS patients with diarrhea but very few HIV-infected individuals without AIDS have identifiable enteric pathogens. In one study, expression of p24 in GI mucosa correlated both with altered bowel habits and with histopathologic alterations, including lymphoid cellularity. The lymphoid composition of intestinal mucosa varies during disease progression and cell numbers are increased in many HIV-infected patients without AIDS. Expression of HIV p24 in the GI tract is determined by enzyme-linked immunosorbent assay (ELISA) and by immunohistochemical staining, and is highest during the phase of peak mucosal cellularity. In the study cited above, tissue contents of the cytokines, tumor necrosis factor-α (TNF-α) and interleukin-1β, and the inflammatory mediators, prostaglandin E_2 and leukotriene B_4, were higher in HIV-infected than in control subjects, adding biochemical evidence of mucosal inflammation. In another study, generalized cytokine expression in such patients was detected using the technique of *in situ* RNA hybridization. Furthermore, cells expressing HIV RNA and TNF mRNA colocalized in the lamina propria immediately beneath the epithelium. Studies from other laboratories have also correlated tissue HIV expression with chronic colitis. Since several cytokines and other inflammatory mediators are known to modulation HIV replication *in vitro*, it is possible that tissue cytokine expression affects HIV production *in vivo*.

Clinical Symptoms

The ability to localize a pathologic process to the small intestine or colon presumptively is valuable in directing and streamlining the diagnostic evaluation. Important information can often be obtained from the clinical history. Symptoms related to small intestinal infection are typical of malabsorption. Patients complain of 3 to 10 nonbloody bowel movements per day, with urgency but no tenesmus. When severe, the diarrhea is associated with dehydration and electrolyte abnormalities, typically hypokalemia and hypomagnesemia. A mild hyperchloremic acidosis may be seen. Stool volume is variable but often large. Patients may have little diarrhea or even formed stools at times, yet suffer from episodes of profuse diarrhea at other times. Diarrhea does not occur consistently throughout the day and is often worst at night or early in the morning. There may be no *specific* food intolerances, as diarrhea is worsened by any significant food intake. However, stool volumes are decreased by fasting. In some patients, stool volumes are very high (up to 10 L/day) and not affected by food intake, implying a secretory process. Infections that cause malabsorption are usually not associated with fever or anorexia, although food intake may be decreased voluntarily to avoid diarrhea. A notable exception to this rule is MAC. Weight loss is typically slow and progressive, or patients may stabilize at a lower weight.

Enterocolitic diseases produce symptoms typical of colitis. There are numerous (up to 30) small volume bowel movements that occur at regular intervals throughout the day and night. Cramped and tenesmus may occur but are usually not severe. The clinical course is often associated with fever, anorexia, rapid and progressive weight loss, and extreme debilitation.

Diagnosis

Stool examinations are an integral part of the diagnostic evaluation of an HIV-infected individual with diarrhea. Many organisms can be detected in stool. Special diagnostic techniques are available for cryptosporidia and microsporidia, although there is still relatively little clinical experience with the recently introduced techniques for detection of microsporidia in stool. A substantial proportion of patients have enteric pathogens that can be detected only by intestinal biopsy (Figs. 2–6), so that negative stool examinations are not the end of the evaluation. An algorithmic approach may be used to evaluate AIDS patients with diarrheal illnesses (Tables 2 and 3).

TABLE 2. *Evaluation of acute diarrhea*
(less than 7 days)

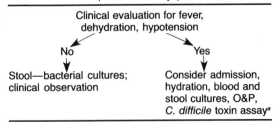

Clinical evaluation for fever,
dehydration, hypotension

No → Stool—bacterial cultures;
clinical observation

Yes → Consider admission,
hydration, blood and
stool cultures, O&P,
C. difficile toxin assay[a]

[a]Recent or concurrent antibiotic use.
O&P, ova and parasites.

TABLE 3. *Evaluation of chronic diarrhea (greater than 14 days)*

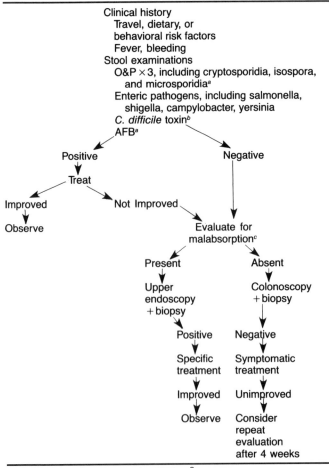

Clinical history
   Travel, dietary, or
   behavioral risk factors
   Fever, bleeding
Stool examinations
   O&P × 3, including cryptosporidia, isospora,
      and microsporidia[a]
   Enteric pathogens, including salmonella,
      shigella, campylobacter, yersinia
   C. difficile toxin[b]
   AFB[a]

Positive → Treat

Negative

Improved → Observe

Not Improved

Evaluate for
malabsorption[c]

Present → Upper
endoscopy
+ biopsy

Absent → Colonoscopy
+ biopsy

Positive → Specific
treatment → Improved → Observe

Negative → Symptomatic
treatment → Unimproved → Consider
repeat
evaluation
after 4 weeks

[a]If CD4[+] lymphocyte count <100/mm^3.
[b]Concurrent or recent antibiotic use.
[c]For example, D-xylose absorption test, fecal fat.
AFB, acid-fast bacillus.

The ability to diagnose *E. bieneusi* on tissue biopsy has improved greatly (Fig. 3). Initially, there was complete reliance upon transmission electron microscopy. Recognition of the characteristic patterns of cytopathy by light microscopy, coupled with confirmatory special stains, has contributed to a marked increase in the number of diagnoses made. Several stains have been employed, including tissue Gram, Giemsa, acid fast, Warthin-Starry, a modified tissue trichrome Chromotrope 2R stain, as described for examination of fecal specimens, and Giemsa-stained touch preparations of fresh mucosal biopsies. In one study, the specificity and positive predictive value of light microscopic stains ranged from 94% to 100%. Other studies have shown that luminal aspirates, luminal lavages, or mucosal cytobrush preparations are sufficient to detect microsporidia. Ongoing development of molecular techniques for the identification of *E. bieneusi* carries the promise of even higher rates of diagnosis.

Microsporidial infection is associated with variable degrees of villus atrophy and crypt hyperplasia. There is increased parasite burden in the proximal jejunum and distal duodenum, compared with the proximal duodenum. In some cases, villus heights are almost normal and there is marked crypt hyperplasia. In other cases, there is significant villus atrophy, usually with less marked crypt hyperplasia. *E. bieneusi* causes a typical pattern of cellular injury, which is concentrated in the upper third of the villus. The histopathology and ultrastructural characteristics have been reviewed in detail.

The spectrum of endoscopic lesions in CMV colitis varies from essentially normal-appearing mucosa, to scattered groups of vesicles or erosions, to broad shallow ulcerations that may coalesce. CMV usually causes a pancolitis, although the cecum and right colon may be affected earlier then elsewhere. Histopathologic examination demonstrates characteristic intracellular inclusions (Fig. 5). Specialized immunohistochemical or *in situ* hybridization techniques are available and can increase the sensitivity of diagnosis, but these techniques showed no improvement over routine histology in the diagnosis of CMV colitis.

Diagnosis of mycobacterial infection is made by culture or histology. Stool smears may demonstrate acid-fast bacilli, but specific correlation with tissue localization has not been made. However, such patients should be considered at high risk for disseminated infection, and should be evaluated and treated accordingly. Blood culture, using a special transport medium (Dupont isolator), is sensitive and often can detect bacteremia prior to the development of clinical symptoms. Mucosal thickening on barium x-rays and thickening of the intestinal wall, plus enlargement of mesenteric and retroperitoneal nodes on CT scan, are characteristic of MAC, although lymphoma or fungal infections may have similar appearances. Histologic demonstration of acid-fast bacilli in intestinal tissue is straightforward (Fig. 6). Diagnosis by biopsy can often be made in one day, as compared with cultures, which may take up to six weeks to become positive. Molecular hybridization techniques are being developed to allow species identification on tissue sections.

Diagnosis of antibiotic-associated colitis is the same in AIDS and non-AIDS patients. Diagnosis of bacterial enterocolitis should be straightforward with routine stool cultures. Blood cultures should be included in the evaluation of diarrhea in the febrile HIV-infected patient, as salmonella may be cultured from blood but not from stool. An unusual feature of salmonella infections in AIDS patients is the tendency for clinical and/or microbiologic relapse after antibiotics are discontinued.

Treatment

Treatment for the patients with diarrheal diseases can be divided into antimicrobial therapies, and treatment for the associated diarrhea, dehydration, and malnutrition. There is no known effective therapy for cryptosporidiosis. Many agents have been tried, but results have been disappointing. Some patients have improved greatly during treatment with paromomycin, while others have no response. The report of successful therapy with hyperimmune bovine colostrum in an agammaglobulinemic child sparked interest in the use of passive immunotherapy to treat cryptosporidiosis in patients with AIDS.

Few studies of drug therapy of *E. bieneusi* infection have been published. Albendazole (Smith-Kline Beecham) has been used experimentally with mildly favorable results. However, follow-up studies continue to show evidence of infection. It is unclear if the drug has a specific beneficial effect, or if concurrent therapies such as dietary alterations and antidiarrheal medications are responsible for any observed improvement. A number of other antimicrobials have been used anecdotally, including metronidazole, paromomycin, and trimethoprim-sulfamethoxazole. As with Albendazole, therapy may be associated with symptomatic improvement, but evidence of continued infection, intestinal injury, and malabsorption persists after therapy. On the other hand, Albendazole (Smith-Kline Beecham) appears to be effective therapy for *S. intestinalis* infection, and results in a complete clinical response.

Isosporiasis may be treated with trimethoprim sulfamethoxazole. Due to a high rate of recurrence, repeated courses or chronic maintenance therapy with this drug may be needed.

Two agents are clinically effective in the treatment of CMV colitis. The most widely used is ganciclovir. A double-blind, placebo-controlled trial demonstrated a beneficial effect of ganciclovir therapy both clinically and virologically. Ganciclovir therapy also has been associated with nutritional repletion and with prolonged survival. Foscarnet is another antiviral drug with activity against CMV. Evidence of clinical benefit with this agent has been reported.

There are several unresolved issues in the treatment of CMV colitis. The need for maintenance therapy has never been addressed formally. The relationship between drug sensitivity and disease progression has not been studied in the intestine. In some patients, colitis has recurred during antiviral therapy, and is well known to occur in cases of CMV retinitis. Emerging data from studies of retinitis have shown that cross-resistance to both ganciclovir and foscarnet does not occur, and that combination therapy may be effective when clinical resistance to a single agent is present. The effect of oral ganciclovir for induction and maintenance therapy is unknown. If proved effective, prophylaxis and therapy of CMV infection could be greatly simplified.

The precise indications for anti-CMV therapy are unsettled. Histopathologic evidence of CMV infection, i.e., tissue injury associated with viral inclusions, is felt to represent a high risk of serious local disease or widespread reactivation with wasting, which justifies therapy. Recommendations for treatment based upon results of viral cultures are less absolute, since intermittent viral shedding without tissue injury can occur. Serologic evidence of viral infection is extremely common and is not an indication for beginning antiviral therapy.

Current therapy of MAC is evolving. Recent studies have shown that a substantial proportion of patients may respond clinically and microbiologically, with a reduction in bacterial colony counts in peripheral blood. Several drugs have in vitro efficacy against MAC including the macrolide clarithromycin, as well as ethambutal, rifabutin, and clofazamine. Other drugs with *in vivo* or *in vitro* efficacy include amikacin, ciprofloxacin, cycloserine, and ethionamide. Two drugs, rifabutin and clarithromycin, have been shown to be effective as prophylactic agents.

Treatment of enterocolitis due to *Salmonella, Shigella*, or *Campylobacter* sp. is modified in that intravenous therapy with antibiotics is more commonly used, due to the frequent occurrence of bacteremia. In addition, repeated or chronic courses of antibiotics such as trimethoprim-sulfamethoxazole or ciprofloxacin are often needed because of disease recurrence. Since many enteric bacterial pathogens are intracellular pathogens, it is possible that disease recurrence is a function of impaired intracellular macrophage killing due to deficient T cell help. Furthermore, an intracellular location may protect the organisms from the antimicrobial effects of certain antibiotics. Ciprofloxacin can penetrate into macrophages and is bactericidal for intracellular organisms. Further studies are needed to determine if complete eradication of enteric bacterial pathogens in AIDS is possible, or if chronic suppressive therapy will be needed.

Treatment of chronic bacterial enteropathy with broad-spectrum antibiotics has brought clinical improvement in several patients. There is difficulty in choosing an antibiotic due to the inability to determine which bacteria in stool are the offending organisms. In addition, widespread use of antibiotics could lead to the development of multidrug resistance strains.

Other Therapies

Maintenance of adequate nutritional status and fluid balance are important clinical tasks, especially in patients with malabsorption syndromes. Oral rehydration solutions may help maintain hydration status, but are hypocaloric and may promote wasting if used excessively. A low-fat, lactose-free diet may be beneficial and medium-chain triglycerides are useful adjuncts in the treatment of patients with significant fat malabsorption (Table 4). On the other hand, polymeric formula diets are

TABLE 4. *Choice of formula diets*

Diet	Indication
Standard polymeric diets	Oral supplement
With added fiber	Diarrhea with oral supplement
Lactose-free	Lactose intolerance
Chemically defined diets	Standard polymeric diet not well tolerated
Lactose-free	Lactose intolerance
Fat substituted (MCT)	Fat malabsorption
Micronutrient fortified	Immune enhancement[a]
Semielemental/elemental	Severe small intestinal disease with malabsorption

[a]Benefits of micronutrient supplementation have not been proven.
MCT, medium-chain triglycerides.

generally tolerated poorly and lead to substantial diarrhea. A variety of antidiarrheal therapies may be used (Table 5). Some patients with nonspecific diarrhea or ileal dysfunction respond well to the bile salt binding resin cholestyramine. The most commonly used antidiarrheal agents are loperamide and opiates, although escalating doses often are required. Octreotide has been used in the treatment of diarrhea of several etiologies, with mixed results. Excess fluid losses from the small intestine due to malabsorption or abnormal secretion will overcome any pharmacologically produced inhibition of motility and lead to diarrhea.

Nutritional therapy of AIDS patients with diarrhea depends entirely upon the pathogenic mechanism underlying the diarrhea. Different approaches are required in patients with and without malabsorption. It is unclear if nutritional repletion can be accomplished by the enteral route in patients with severe small intestinal disease and malabsorption. In severe cases, total parenteral nutrition (TPN) has been employed with success. However, ongoing observations suggest that use of elemental diets, which contain simple sugars, amino acids, and medium-chain triglycerides, may give similar results to TPN in some cases. The topic is of great interest, given the relatively large numbers of AIDS patients with malabsorption plus the great expense, resource utilization, and morbidity associated with the use of TPN.

TABLE 5. *Usefulness of different agents for the management of diarrhea*

	Malabsorption	Enterocolitis
Dietary alterations	+ +	0
Oral rehydration solutions	+ +	+
Formula diets		
Polymeric formulae	0	0
Lactose/fat reduced	+	0
Elemental	+ +	0
Bulk forming agents	0	0
Opiates	+ +	+ +
Octreotide	+	0
Bile salt binding agents	+ +	0

0, ineffective; +, mildly effective; + +, moderately to very effective.

Nutritional support is less effective in patients with enterocolitis associated with systemic infections. The metabolic rate is elevated and metabolic derangements promote protein wasting. Alterations in lipid metabolism often result in the development of fatty liver when nutritional support is attempted. In one study, total parenteral nutrition resulted in weight gain, but the increase was due entirely to an in increase in body fat content, while body cell mass did not change. While nutritional support might help prevent progressive protein depletion, the key to successful therapy is proper diagnosis and treatment of the specific disease complication. Ganciclovir treatment of CMV colitis was shown to lead to body mass repletion in the absence of formal nutritional support.

NUTRITIONAL INTERVENTIONS

As in other diseases, a prudent course is to apply nutritional interventions on a progressive basis, starting with the least intrusive measures, unless the clinical situation dictates otherwise (Table 6). Initially, oral, pharyngeal, or esophageal conditions that impair food intake should be diagnosed and treated and food-based dietary regimens should be tried, including food delivery for the homebound, in the case of weakness and debilitation. If caloric intake is sufficient but improvement is slow, anabolic agents might be tried to maximize the gain of lean body mass. If intake remains inadequate, appetite stimulants can be employed.

If the patient is unable to maintain an adequate intake by oral means despite appetite stimulants, and there is no evidence of malabsorption, obstruction or severe vomiting, the enteral route should be used for alimentation. The route of administration, i.e., transnasal vs. transabdominal, should be based upon the expected duration of therapy and upon the risks of recurrent sinus infections, aspiration pneumonia, or esophageal ulceration associated with long-term nasogastric tube placement (Table 7). If parenteral nutrition becomes necessary, partial parenteral nutrition via a peripheral IV may be used for short periods of time (<2 weeks) in patients likely to resume normal intake. TPN is needed in patients with irreversible gut

TABLE 6. *Feeding options in AIDS patients*

Pathogenesis	Treatment
Offending medication	Discontinue and observe
Obstruction/pain	Dietary alteration[a], tube feeding
CNS disease	Tube feeding
Malabsorption	Dietary alteration[b], TPN[c]
Systemic infection	Appetite stimulants[d], oral supplements
Unexplained anorexia	Oral supplements, appetite stimulants

[a]Pureed or liquid diet for incomplete obstruction, percutaneous gastrostomy for intractable odynophagia or complete obstruction.
[b]Lactose and fat-reduced diet or formula, elemental diet in severe cases.
[c]Total parenteral nutrition.
[d]For example, megestral acetate (megace), 800 mg in one dose per day of oral suspension.

TABLE 7. *Decision tree for tube feeding*

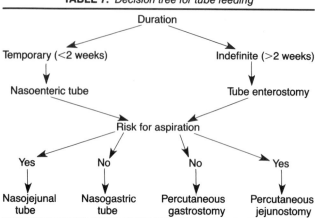

failure, characterized by severe, intractable malabsorption, frequent and persistent vomiting, irreversible obstruction, or other conditions precluding adequate absorption (Table 8). The choice of tube used is often based on personal preferences. For patients with aesthetic concerns a subcutaneous reservoir, which is accessed by a removable needle, may be preferred, rather than an external catheter. Success has been achieved using peripherally inserted central venous catheters for TPN (PICC line).

TABLE 8. *Decision tree for parenteral nutrition*

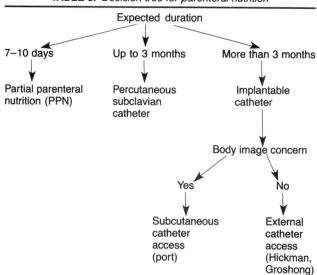

ANORECTAL DISEASE

Etiology and Pathogenesis

Anorectal diseases seen in AIDS patients include both infections and tumors. Herpes simplex virus is the most common infectious agent found. The primary lesion occurs at the pectinate line. Vesicles in the anal canal may be missed as they rupture during defecation or examination. Herpes simplex infection in AIDS patients most often presents as a painful, shallow spreading perineal ulcer. A smaller group of patients present with idiopathic ulcers originating at the anorectal junction. Perianal and intraanal condylomata occur in AIDS patients as well as non-AIDS patients and are related to infection with human papilloma virus. Lesions may be enlarged and flat (leukoplakia) and may show dysplasia on histologic examination. The lesions are likely precursors to squamous cell cancers. Tumors in the anorectal region include Kaposi's sarcoma, lymphoma, and squamous cell carcinoma for its variants.

Hemorrhoidal disease is also seen frequently. Factors predisposing to hemorrhoids may have predated HIV infection. Severe diarrhea or proctitis may promote local thrombosis, ulceration, and secondary infection. Fleshy skin tags, resembling those seen in Crohn's disease, are also seen. Thrombosed hemorrhoids are common, but it is unclear if the incidence is higher in AIDS patients than in a comparable non–HIV-infected population.

A variety of classic venereal diseases can produce anorectal ulcerations. Diagnosis and therapy of *Neisseria gonorrhoeae* proctitis is similar in AIDS and non-AIDS patients. Syphilis may have an atypical presentation in HIV-infected subjects, and serologic diagnosis may be affected by the presence of immune deficiency. Chlamydia are prevalent in sexually active groups. The frequency of chancroid, caused by *Haemophilus ducreyi*, in HIV-infected patients is unknown. Rectal spirochetosis has been recognized in homosexual men with or without HIV infection. This infection usually is asymptomatic and an incidental finding on evaluation.

Diagnosis

In many cases the correct diagnosis can be made by inspection. If necessary, the diagnosis can be confirmed by culture or biopsy. Specialized techniques, such as *in situ* hybridization are available for the diagnosis of papilloma virus infection but are rarely needed clinically.

Treatment

Resolution of herpetic lesions occurs after treatment with oral or intravenous acyclovir. Herpes simplex virus resistant to acyclovir has been demonstrated in patients with refractory ulcerations. These patients will usually respond to foscarnet. Anorectal ulcers containing CMV respond to antiviral therapy. Symptomatic idiopathic ulcers may respond to intralesional corticosteroid therapy and healing may occur after repeated treatments. Areas of leukoplakia can be followed clinically, while large or enlarging lesions should be excised. Some caution should be noted regarding surgical therapy. Poor wound healing may occur, especially in severely malnourished patients, patients with serious, untreated diseases such as CMV, and patients with continued diarrhea due to nutrient malabsorption.

Epidermoid cancers, including squamous cell and cloacogenic cancer, occur in anal skin in rectal glands, respectively. While these cancers rarely metasitize in immunocompetent persons, they may do so in patients with AIDS. For these lesions, management after diagnostic biopsy includes excision, chemotherapy, or laser photocoagulation. Laser therapy of rectal Kaposi's sarcoma also is effective and may cause dramatic regression of bulky disease.

TUMORS

Kaposi's sarcoma in AIDS is indistinguishable histopathologically from classic Kaposi's sarcoma, endemic forms of Kaposi's sarcoma found in Africa, or the form that occurs during immunosuppressive therapy. Visceral involvement in AIDS patients with Kaposi's sarcoma is more common than in non–HIV-infected individuals with Kaposi's sarcoma. Visceral involvement may be asymptomatic. Diagnosis is made by visual inspection and confirmed by biopsy, although endoscopic biopsy may be falsely negative if the tumor is in the submucosa. No treatment is needed in most cases. Chemotherapy may be tried in symptomatic patients or in those with rapidly progressive disease. Obstructive lesions can be treated effectively by laser ablation.

A high prevalence of extranodal, high-grade non-Hodgkin's B cell lymphomas has been noted in AIDS patients. Gastrointestinal lymphomas in AIDS are biologically aggressive, especially the Burkitt's subtype. Lesions may respond to chemotherapy, using combination therapies. There are few long-term survivors, however, because of the underlying immune deficiency.

Sporadic reports of AIDS patients with carcinomas in the gastrointestinal tract have been published, but a higher incidence has not been convincingly documented.

HEPATOBILIARY DISEASES

Etiology and Pathogenesis

Liver dysfunction is common in AIDS patients. There are three distinct clinical syndromes of AIDS-related hepatobiliary disease: diffuse hepatocellular injury, granulomatous hepatitis, and sclerosing cholangitis.

Many HIV-infected patients have had prior exposure to hepatitis B. A relatively high proportion of HIV-infected individuals have circulating hepatitis B surface antigen and e antigen. However, there is no evidence that immune deficiency will cause a reactivation of prior hepatitis B. On the other hand, hepatocyte injury as a direct result of viral or drug toxicity is unaffected by the immune deficiency so that delta hepatitis and drug-induced hepatitis are as severe in HIV-infected as in non-HIV-infected individuals. Chronic hepatitis C infection also occurs in HIV-infected patients, and there is evidence for a more rapid progression to liver failure.

Granulomatous hepatitis in AIDS patients occurs in the setting of disseminated systemic infection. The causative organisms include mycobacteria and fungi, such as *Histoplasma capsulatum, Coccidioides imitis*, and *Cryptococcus neoformans*. Viral diseases such as CMV also may cause hepatic granulomas. Other causes of granulomatous hepatitis include rare cases of disseminated protozoal infection including pneumocystosis.

A syndrome of sclerosing cholangitis has been recognized to occur in AIDS patients. This disease in AIDS bears a striking resemblance to the non-AIDS variety, although it may be more rapidly progressive in AIDS. The etiology and pathogenesis of sclerosing cholangitis are as obscure in AIDS patients as in non-AIDS patients. Some AIDS patients have biliary involvement with protozoa, namely cryptosporidia and microsporidia. Other patients have CMV infection of the liver and biliary tree. In others no etiologic agent has been identified.

Some patients with abnormal liver chemistries have macrovesicular or microvesicular fatty infiltration, or other nonspecific changes. Peliosis hepatis has been described in AIDS patients and is associated with infection by a rickettsia-like organism.

Clinical

There are few specific clinical signs to indicate liver involvement except in cases of diffuse hepatocellular injury or obstruction with jaundice. Liver disease is usually suggested because of abnormal liver function tests in serum samples. Mild abnormalities in liver function tests are commonly seen and are often of no clinical importance. When part of an obvious systemic process with chronic fevers and wasting, the presence of a progressively rising serum alkaline phosphatase level and an enlarged liver point to specific hepatic involvement in the infection. Patients with sclerosing cholangitis present with nonspecific abdominal complaints, sometimes associated with pruritis. Severe liver dysfunction with liver failure is rare but can occur in patients with hepatitis C or delta hepatitis virus infections, and has been seen in a few patients with sclerosing cholangitis.

Diagnosis

Evaluation of liver disease can be approached with the assistance of an algorithm (Table 9). Indication for biopsy is a progressive rise in liver function tests, not the absolute level of these enzymes. The techniques used to diagnose liver and other

TABLE 9. *Algorithm for hepatobiliary disease in AIDS*

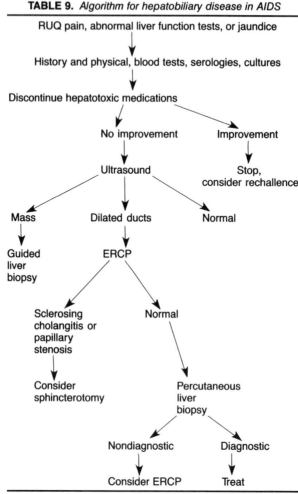

ERCP, endoscopic retrograde cholangiopancreatography; RUQ, right upper quadrant.

visceral diseases are the same in AIDS and non-AIDS patients. Focal lesions may be detected with ultrasound or CT scans and approached by directed biopsy. Percutaneous liver biopsy has been used to diagnosis MAC, tuberculosis, and fungal infections (Fig. 7). In these entities infectious liver biopsy reveals focal collections of histiocytes, which may be organized into poorly formed granulomas, scattered throughout the parenchyma. Giant cells are seen only rarely. In MAC infection, acid-fast stains usually disclose large numbers of organisms. This finding differs from the usual paucity of acid-fast bacilli in non–AIDS-related tuberculosis. Since tuberculosis cannot be differentiated from MAC by biopsy alone, culture of a por-

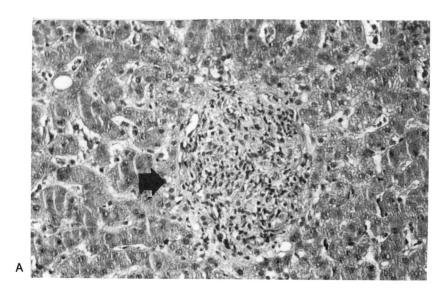

A

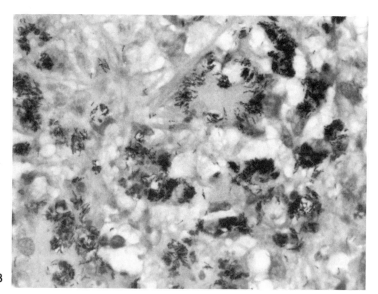

B

FIG. 7. Granulomatous hepatitis. **A:** Granuloma located in the hepatic parenchyma (H&E 400 ×). **B:** Acid-fast bacilli located in macrophages (Ziehl Nielson 640 ×).

tion of the liver sample should be done, and therapy should be based upon clinical judgment until results are known. Histoplasmosis and coccidioidomycosis can be diagnosed with great certainty on biopsy using specific histologic stains. However, a sample of liver should also be submitted for fungal culture. In addition to percutaneous liver biopsy, percutaneous needle aspiration of retroperitoneal nodes

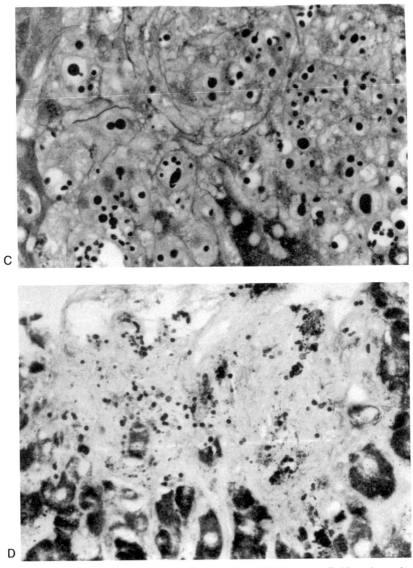

FIG. 7. continued. **C:** Cryptococci located in a granuloma (GMS 480 ×). **D:** Histoplasma located in a granuloma (GMS 480 ×).

using sonographic or CT guidance is an effective means of making a diagnosis of infection or tumor.

The diagnosis of sclerosing cholangitis (AIDS cholangiopathy) can be made by endoscopic retrograde cholangic pancreatography (ERCP) (Fig. 8), although sonographic or CT studies also may support the diagnosis. Endoscopic retrograde

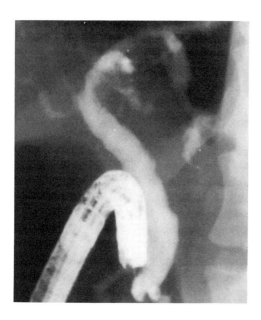

FIG. 8. Sclerosing cholangitis. Dilatation of the common bile duct with ulcerations and plaques, plus beading of the intracellular hepatic ducts are noted.

cholangiography demonstrates multiple areas of narrowing and dilatation of the intrahepatic and/or extrahepatic ducts, sometimes with ulceration and plaque formation. Examination of bile and pancreatic juice may reveal bacterial overgrowth, CMV, and/or cryptosporidia. Absence of ductal dilatation on imaging studies does not exclude sclerosing cholangitis.

Treatment

A diagnosis of mycobacterial or fungal infection is an indication for antimicrobial therapy. Likewise, a diagnosis of lymphoma or widespread Kaposi's sarcoma is an indication for systemic antineoplastic therapy. Attempts have been made to treat sclerosing cholangitis, especially if associated with papillary stenosis, by sphincterotomy, either during ERCP or at laparotomy. The short-term results are variable and the long-term results are poor. Attempts at operative decompression are not indicated unless there exists a very strong suspicion that a single stricture is responsible for the obstruction. Other patients have been treated for CMV infection with ganciclovir, without any effect upon the cause of the biliary disease.

There are no currently accepted therapies for viral hepatitis in AIDS, although treatment regimens using α-interferon are being evaluated. Several small studies of α-interferon therapy of chronic hepatitis C infection in HIV-infected individuals have been done. Treatment responses are seen but at a lower frequency than in HIV-seronegative patients. The probability of responding to treatment falls as immune function wanes.

PANCREATIC DISEASES

Pancreatic disease in AIDS has received little attention and may not be recognized premortem. The pancreas may be affected by systemic diseases, such as CMV, MAC, fungi, Kaposi's sarcoma, or lymphoma. Drug-induced pancreatitis is the most commonly recognized form. Hyperlipidemic pancreatitis has been observed. There are no reports of chronic pancreatitis occurring as a specific complication of HIV infection. Pancreatic insufficiency is an uncommon cause of fat malabsorption in AIDS patients.

GASTROINTESTINAL HEMORRHAGE

Etiology and Pathogenesis

Gastrointestinal hemorrhage is not a common consequence of AIDS, but serious or life-threatening bleeding does occur. Hemorrhage may result from the same conditions that cause bleeding in the non–HIV-infected patient, plus the tumors and ulcers seen in AIDS. Many causes of GI bleeding associated with complications of AIDS have been reported, including localized solitary ulcers in the esophagus or bowel, bleeding duodenal or gastric ulcers with or without associated use of nonsteroidal antiinflammatory agents, and extensive mucosal Kaposi's sarcoma. Extremely debilitated patients may develop deep anal fissures that bleed.

The clinical presentation of gastrointestinal hemorrhage in the AIDS patient is identical to a non-AIDS patient and the basic concepts of resuscitation are also the same.

Diagnosis

The endoscopic and radiologic techniques available for evaluation of GI hemorrhage should be used. Bleeding lesions often can be visualized by endoscopy and controlled locally, while diagnostic material is obtained.

Treatment

The basic approach to GI hemorrhage is the same in AIDS and non-AIDS patients. Proper management of GI bleeding depends upon the precise cause. An attempt to determine the cause should be made in every case of hemodynamically significant bleeding. If bleeding is related to a solitary ulcer, surgical excision should be performed, if possible. Proper management of bleeding neoplasms involves effective local control followed by systemic chemotherapy. Techniques that have been utilized successfully include injection sclerotherapy of bleeding lesions of Kaposi's sarcoma, and angiography embolization of a bleeding ulcer in the terminal ileum. Thus, proper management of GI bleeding in an AIDS patient is probably not different from in an immunocompetent patient.

THE ACUTE ABDOMEN

Etiology and Pathogenesis

Abdominal pain is an important symptom in AIDS patients. The major enteric pathogens such as cryptosporidium, CMV, salmonella, and shigella cause abdominal *cramps* and not *pain*. Severe acute abdominal pain often is a sign of a significant pathologic process, such as a perforated viscus. The clinical signs of abdominal tenderness, guarding, and rebound have the same significance in AIDS patients as in immunocompetent patients. Widespread intestinal MAC infection may present with chronic abdominal pain. It is important to remember that AIDS patients may develop peritonitis for the same reasons as patients without AIDS, plus reasons specific for AIDS itself. Cholecystitis may occur but usually is acalculous. Perforated viscus occurs in AIDS, but the cause may be a solitary intestinal ulcer rather than peptic ulcer disease or diverticulitis. Malignant intestinal obstruction is usually due to Kaposi's sarcoma or lymphoma rather than adenocarcinoma. Kaposi's sarcoma and lymphoma also may be responsible for perforation or be the leading edge in an intussusception. Some patients have developed an acute abdomen, but have had only a mild fibrinous peritonitis at laparotomy.

Clinical

The clinical presentation of appendicitis, cholecystitis, or generalized peritonitis are the same in AIDS and non-AIDS patients and the correct diagnosis can be made using similar criteria. It is important to recognize that extensive MAC infection in the retroperitoneum may lead to liquefaction necrosis of retroperitoneal nodes and production of peritonitis similar to that seen in tuberculosis peritonitis. In this circumstance, surgery is not helpful and should be avoided.

Diagnosis

While physical findings in a patient with an acute abdomen may be unaffected by the presence of AIDS, laboratory findings may differ. This is particularly true of the white blood count. Elevations of the leukocyte count with a left shift count may be absent, especially if there is preexisting leukopenia or prior treatment with myelosuppressive drugs such as zidovudine. Imaging studies such as a CT scan may be valuable in detecting extraluminal collections of pus or fluid. Isotopic imaging studies such as an indium-labeled white blood cell study or gallium scan, however, may be falsely negative in the presence of severe leukopenia.

Treatment

While the indications for surgery are the same in the HIV-infected and non–HIV-infected patient, the expected results may differ. One should anticipate a need for a longer course of antibotics in HIV-infected patients, the possibility of unusual pathogens, and the possibility of impaired wound healing. The reported incidence of postoperative complications and mortality is high, but this is due, at least in part, to the seriousness of the underlying illness and other complications. It is important to bear in mind that recovery after surgery is possible and may be followed by prolonged survival.

Many centers have approached the question of laparotomy in AIDS patients with caution. Early clinical observations indicated substantial short- and long-term post-operative mortality, although deaths appeared to be related to progression of underlying disease, rather than the results of surgery. Other studies showed that specific subgroups of patients, such as patients undergoing splenectomy for refractory thrombocytopenia, had an acceptable postoperative mortality. Further experience has shown that with the appropriate indication and clinical status, laparotomy can be carried out with expectation of clinical benefit. Laparoscopic surgery can also be performed and lead to significant clinical benefit.

Operating on a patient with AIDS entails extra risk to members of the surgical team, both from injuries and from contact with blood or body secretions by mucous membranes. The occupational risk of nosocomial infection by hepatitis, tuberculosis, or other illnesses during surgery has long been recognized. Potential risks to the surgical team can be minimized by double-gloving, using face masks or other devices to shield the mucous membranes from splattering of fluids, separating needles from suture material, and removing them and other sharp instruments from the immediate surgical field and using laparoscopic techniques when possible. Such types of protection measures are increasingly being adapted for all surgical patients regardless of whether or not HIV status is known.

SUGGESTED READING

Benhamou Y, Caumes E, Gerosa Y, Cadranel JF, Dohin E, Katlama C, Amouyal P, Candard JM, Azar N, Hoang C, Charpentier Y, Gentilini M, Opolon P, Valla D. AIDS-related cholangiopathy: critical analysis of a prospective series of 26 patients. *Dig Dis Sci* 1993;38:1113–1118.

Cappell MS. Hepatobiliary manifestations of the acquired immunodeficiency syndrome. *Am J Gastroenterol* 1992;86:1–15.

Clayton F, Cronin WJ, Reka S, Torlakovic E, Sigal S, Kotler DP. Rectal mucosal histopathology in HIV infection varies with disease stage and HIV protein content. *Gastroenterology* 1992;103:919–933.

Dieterich DT, Kotler DP, Busch D, et al. Ganciclovir treatment of cytomegalovirus colitis in AIDS: a randomized, double-blind, placebo-controlled multicenter trial. *J Infect Dis* 1992;167:278–283.

Greenson J, Belitsos P, Yardley J, Bartlett J. AIDS enteropathy: occult enteric infections and duodenal mucosal alterations in chronic diarrhea. *Ann Intern Med* 1991;114:366–372.

Kotler DP. Gastrointestinal complications of the acquired immunodeficiency syndrome. In: Yamada T, ed. *Textbook of Gastroenterology*, Philadelphia: Lippincott, 1991;2086–2103.

Kotler DP, Giang TT, Thiim M, Nataro JP, Sordillo EM, Orenstein JM. Chronic bacterial enteropathy in patients with AIDS. *J Infect Dis* 1994;171:552–558.

Kotler DP, Orenstein JM. Prevalence of intestinal microsporidiosis in HIV-infected individuals for gastroenterological evaluation. *Am J Gastroenterol* 1994;89:1998–2002.

Kotler DP, Reka S, Borcich A, Cronin WJ. Detection, localization and quantitation of HIV-associated antigens in intestinal biopsies from HIV-infected patients. *Am J Pathol* 1991;139:823–830.

Orenstein J, Chiang J, Steinberg W, Smith P, Rotterdam H, Kotler DP. Intestinal microsporidiosis as a cause of diarrhea in HIV-infected patients: a report of 20 cases. *Hum Pathol* 1990;21:475–481.

Parente F, Cernuschi M, Valsecchi L, Musicco M, Lazzarin A, Bianchi Porro G. Acute upper gastrointestinal bleeding in patients with AIDS: a relatively uncommon condition associated with reduced survival. *J Br Soc Gastroenterol* 1991;32:987–990.

Soave R, Johnson WD Jr. Cryptosporidium and *Isospora belli* infections. *J Infect Dis* 1988;157:225–229.

Ullrich R, Zeitz M, Heise M, L'age M, Hoffken G, Rieken EO. Small intestinal structure and function in patients infected with human immunodeficiency virus (HIV): evidence for HIV-induced enteropathy. *Ann Intern Med* 1989;111:15–21.

Wilcox CM, Diehl DL, Cello JP, Margarettan W, Jacobson MA. Cytomegalovirus esophagitis in patients with AIDS. A clinical, endoscopic, and pathologic correlation. *Ann Intern Med* 1991;113:589–593.

Wilcox CM, Schwartz DA. A pilot study of oral corticosteroid therapy for idiopathic esophageal ulcerations associated with human immunodeficiency virus infection. *Am J Med* 1992;93:131–134.

A Clinical Guide to AIDS and HIV,
edited by Gary P. Wormser.
Lippincott-Raven Publishers, Philadelphia © 1996.

8

Neoplastic Complications of HIV Infection

Anil Tulpule, *Parkash S. Gill, and *Alexandra M. Levine

*Department of Medicine, University of Southern California, and Norris Cancer Hospital;
and *Division of Hematology, Department of Internal Medicine,
University of Southern California School of Medicine, Los Angeles, California 90033*

PATHOGENESIS AND TREATMENT OF AIDS-RELATED KAPOSI'S SARCOMA

Prior to the AIDS epidemic, Kaposi's sarcoma (KS) was a rare tumor. It was seen in certain geographic regions in well-defined population groups, such as classic KS in older men from the Eastern European and Mediterranean regions, and in adult men and children from Central Africa. Since the beginning of the AIDS epidemic, KS has been reported in 20% to 50% of AIDS patients. Homosexual and bisexual men with AIDS develop KS more frequently than other HIV-infected populations. It is unclear as to the factors that predispose homosexual men to the development of KS, or why there has been a steady decline in the incidence of KS since the beginning of the epidemic.

This decline may be related to changes in lifestyle that have occurred in the male homosexual population, such as a decrease in high-risk sexual behaviors, number of sexual partners, use of recreational drugs, and occurrence of other sexually transmitted diseases. It is possible that a general diminution in chronic stimuli to the immune system may reduce the incidence of KS, due to a reduction of cytokines, which serve as growth initiation factors for KS liberated from activated T lymphocytes and monocytes. Furthermore, the use of zidovudine (AZT) and other antiretroviral agents may play a significant role in reducing these growth factors through inhibition of HIV, which may act directly and indirectly as a mitogen to those cells that produce the KS growth initiation factors. These possibilities, however, remain speculative at present should be addressed through appropriate scientific inquiry.

It is also possible that the reported decline in incidence of KS may be artifactual, due to more frequent clinical diagnoses of KS, without biopsy confirmation, and to underreporting of KS, when it is diagnosed after an earlier AIDS-defining opportunistic infection. It is clear that formal studies are warranted to confirm the decline in incidence, and to ascertain the cofactors involved in development of KS.

The pathologic characteristics of epidemic, AIDS-associated KS are similar to

KS when it occurs in other epidemiologic settings. The clinical course is different, however, with early visceral involvement and a more rapid course of disease. Although KS causes mortality only in patients with extensive visceral involvement, it contributes significantly to morbidity. Treatment modalities should be guided by tumor burden, immunologic status of the patient, and toxicity potential of the therapy. Early KS, particularly in patients with a relatively intact immune status, can be treated with antiretroviral agents combined with immune modulators (e.g., AZT + α-interferon). Rapidly progressive disease or advanced KS requires systemic chemotherapy alone or in combination with antiretroviral agents. However, bone marrow suppression is a dose-limiting toxicity of such therapy, which may be circumvented with the combined use of hematopoietic growth factors [such as granulocyte colony-stimulating factor (G-CSF)]. Kaposi's sarcoma often relapses following discontinuation of therapy, emphasizing the need for discovery of a safe and effective form of maintenance therapy. Newer experimental modes of therapy employ inhibitors of angiogenesis, and/or growth factors thought to play a role in the pathogenesis of disease.

Pathogenesis

To understand the pathogenesis of KS, a number of issues must be addressed: the origin of the KS cell, the role of autocrine and paracrine growth modulators, and the role of HIV.

Various investigators have attempted to define the cell of origin in KS. KS cells express certain markers of endothelial cells, such as factor VIII–related antigen and Europeus I antigen. However, KS cells have also been shown to express antigens associated with smooth muscle cells, such as alpha actin. Further, dermal dendrocytic markers, such as factor XIIIa, are also expressed. In addition, the spindle cells of KS bear the human progenitor cell antigen (CD 34). It is therefore possible that the KS cell originates from primitive pluripotent or mesenchymal cells that may differentiate into more specialized cell types that share phenotypic characteristics of both endothelial and smooth muscle cells.

Several studies have shown that cytokines such as interleukin (IL)-1β, IL-6, and Oncostatin M are autocrine factors for AIDS-related KS. Both IL-1β and IL-6 are produced by KS cells, and inhibition of their effects whether through blocking the receptors (IL-1 receptor antagonist) or inhibition of gene expression through antisense oligonucleotides (for IL-6) can inhibit growth of KS cells. Oncostatin M expressed in KS cells is also known to induce the growth of these cells. Furthermore, inhibition of Oncostatin-M expression through antisense oligonucleotides can reduce the proliferative potential of AIDS-KS cells. The role of glucocorticoids in KS is also well documented. Use of glucocorticoids leads either to development or progression of KS. The expression of glucocorticoids and their mitogenic effect on KS *in vitro* has been established.

HIV may play an indirect role in the pathogenesis of KS via the aforementioned cytokines. IL-1β, TNF-α, and IL-6 are perturbed as a result of HIV infection. These cytokines could increase the rate of growth of KS lesions. Furthermore, although HIV is not known to infect the KS cell per se, transfection of fertilized eggs from transgenic mice expressing the HIV "tat" protein results in expression of the tat protein in skin alone in the offspring, with development of a tumor, which appears identical to KS, of mouse origin, in 15% of the male offspring. The tumor cells, however, do not express "tat" gene.

Pathology

Skin is the most commonly involved site, but KS lesions can occur in any organ, although rarely in brain or bone marrow. KS is a tumor of mixed cellularity, consisting of spindle-like cells, small vascular spaces, numerous dilated abnormal lymphocytes, blood vessels, and extravasated red cells present in slit-like vascular structures. A variety of mononuclear cells may also be present in these lesions such as T cells, plasma cells, and phagocytic macrophages. Often there is associated edema. Histologically, KS lesions are remarkably similar, regardless of anatomic location (skin, lymph nodes, respiratory tract, and/or intestine).

The cutaneous lesions of KS are classified into patch, plaque, and/or nodular lesions. Early on, KS of the skin begins as a small, flat purple lesions (patch lesion). The lesion may broaden and become elevated to form a plaque. A plaque may enlarge progressively to become a nodule. Histopathologic studies show that earlier lesions are located in the reticular (upper) dermis, with subdermal involvement in some cases.

In very early stages of KS, the lesions may resemble granulation tissue, with patchy distribution in the reticular dermis. Vessel proliferation is composed of irregular jagged vessels dissecting the collagen bundles of the dermis. The nuclei of the endothelial cells are flat, elongated, and darkly stained. They are frequently surrounded by plasma cells and scattered lymphocytes and neutrophils. As the vascular structures proliferate, plaque lesions develop. Nodular lesions are quite different histologically from the patch and plaque lesions, and consist predominantly of spindle cells, giving a sarcomatous appearance. These spindle cells are arranged in interwoven fasciles. The spindle cells themsevles are generally not strikingly atypical, although they are often pleomorphic, and may be seen in mitosis. Areas of necrosis may be observed. Nodular lesions also express extensive perivascular infiltration of lymphocytes, plasma cells, and macrophages. Red cell extravasation into the slit-like spaces among the spindle cells is characteristic of KS lesions, and may help to distinguish them from other lesions.

Clinical Manifestations

The epidemic form of KS is seen predominantly in young homosexual men. The lesions may affect any site of the body, although the skin is the most common site for initial presentation. The lesions are multifocal. Sites of presentation in the absence of skin involvement include lymph nodes, gastrointestinal tract, oral mucosa, conjunctiva, and lungs.

Cutaneous lesions often first appear as small, fleshy, flat lesions that progress to reddish or purple nodules. They are generally painless, nonpruritic, and often linear, following the pattern of cutaneous lymphatic drainage (Fig. 1). The lesions may be associated with local edema; they may coalesce to form large infiltrating lesions, and may even ulcerate and cause local pain. The soles of the feet are often affected, where the lesions appear less purple or red. Interestingly, the palms are rarely involved.

Sites other than skin are frequently involved and correlate with advanced or progressive cutaneous disease. The oral cavity is involved in nearly one-third of cases, often located on the palate and less frequently the gingiva and the tongue (Fig. 2). Although common, the true frequency of lymph node involvement is not known because of the lack of routine node biopsy in all KS cases. Visceral involvement, particularly in the gastrointestinal tract, occurs in nearly 50% of cases with oral KS and may involve the esophagus, stomach, duodenum, colon, and rectum. Advanced

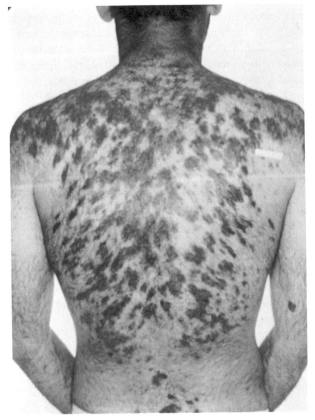

FIG. 1. Raised, reddish-purple cutaneous lesions of Kaposi's sarcoma on the skin. Note the symmetric pattern of distribution.

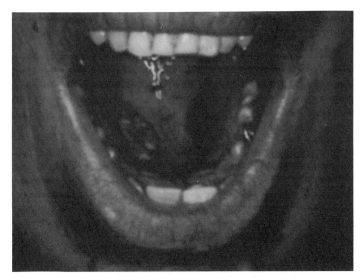

FIG. 2. Kaposi's sarcoma lesion within the mucous membranes of the mouth.

gastrointestinal involvement may cause abdominal pain, early satiety, and even bleeding. Asymptomatic gastrointestinal involvement does not affect survival, and routine evaluation is not needed in the absence of symptoms. However, symptomatic gastrointestinal involvement should be evaluated with endoscopy, since barium contrast studies often produce false-negative findings.

Pulmonary involvement has also been reported with increasing frequency in the past several years, and has occurred in 20% to 50% of KS cases. Pulmonary involvement can often be diagnosed with bronchoscopy without biopsy, due to the classic appearance of these lesions; further, biopsy is often complicated by bleeding. Open lung biopsy is rarely necessary to make the diagnosis. Patients with significant involvement often complain of exertional dyspnea, dry cough, hemoptysis, and (rarely) chest pain. Radiographic findings may be abnormal and include diffuse interstitial infiltrates, mediastinal adenopathy, pulmonary nodules, and/or pleural effusions, in order of decreasing frequency. Patients with advanced pulmonary involvement have a poor prognosis, with a median survival of only 3 months.

Cardiac involvement has rarely been reported, but may lead to cardiac tamponade and death. Nearly all organs have been shown to be involved with KS, including the brain (rarely).

Staging System

Several methods to define the extent and bulk of KS have been proposed, in order to provide guidelines for treatment, prognosis, and uniform response criteria. Several pitfalls exist, due to (1) the multifocal manifestations of disease; (2) the difficulty in objectively determining tumor response because of residual hyperpigmentation even after successful therapy; and, most importantly, (3) the infectious complications of immune deficiency and their impact on tumor response. Most recently, investigators have devised a modified staging system that attempts to incorporate these complex parameters, particularly tumor bulk, with or without local complications; presence of visceral disease; and status of the immune system, particularly the CD4 lymphocyte count; history of opportunistic infection; and the presence or absence of constitutional "B" symptoms.

Prognostic Features

The survival of patients with AIDS/KS is predominantly related to the underlying immunologic status and multiplicity of infectious complications that may have occurred. KS is often the source of serious morbidity, due to cosmetic problems, local edema, pain, and even ulceration. Although visceral KS is often asymptomatic, gastrointestinal and pulmonary involvement can lead to bleeding, organ dysfunction, and death.

Several investigators have defined various prognostic parameters that predict for response and survival. One group has shown that patients with CD4 counts above 400/mm^3 are more likely to respond to α-interferon, while response rates decline rapidly with CD4 counts below 200/mm^3. Another group in a large database of 212 AIDS/KS cases, has shown that significant prognostic variables include the presence of systemic constitutional symptoms ("B" symptoms) ($p = .001$), prior or coexistent opportunistic infections ($p = .02$), and CD4 lymphocyte counts less than 300/mm^3 ($p = .02$). They have suggested that based upon these features, AIDS/KS cases may be subdivided into the following groups:

1. No prior or coexistent opportunistic infections, no systemic symptoms, CD4 $\geq$ 300/mm^3: expected median survival of 31 months;
2. No prior or coexistent opportunistic infections, no systemic symptoms, CD4 < 300/mm^3: median survival of 20 months;
3. No prior or coexistent opportunistic infections, presence of systemic symptoms: median survival of 15 months;
4. Prior or coexistent opportunistic infections: median survival of 7 months.

Treatment

The management of KS should be designed based on consideration of several aspects. First, one must define any complications related to HIV, such as acute opportunistic infections, AIDS dementia complex, status of bone marrow function, and concurrent use of various myelosuppressive agents. Second, one must define the extent of KS, such as the number of cutaneous lesions; local complications, such as edema, ulceration, or superinfections; and visceral sites of involvement and the severity of such involvement. For example, symptomatic pulmonary KS requires immediate attention, with use of systemic cytotoxic therapy. Third, the immunologic status of the patient should be established at baseline, including the number of peripheral blood CD4 lymphocytes, in order to predict response to certain treatment modalities (such as α-interferon) and the risk of opportunistic infections.

Radiation Therapy

The role of radiotherapy in localized cutaneous disease for cosmetic purposes and for local pain control is well established. However, radiation therapy rarely produces complete resolution of large lesions. Furthermore, radiation therapy of KS lesions in the oral cavity may result in severe mucositis and should therefore be used with caution, employing relatively low-dose fractions, and total doses. Normal skin fibroblasts have been found exquisitely sensitive to radiation in HIV-infected individuals.

Other Local Therapies

Various other local therapies including surgical excision, liquid nitrogen, cryotherapy, sclerotherapy, and argon laser therapy may be efficacious. In addition, intralesional injections of vinblastin, vincristine, or interferon have also been effective.

Interferon

Recombinant α-interferon (α-INF) has been studied extensively in the treatment of AIDS/KS, due to its immunoregulatory antitumor, and antiviral activity. Specifically, α-interferon inhibits HIV replication *in vitro*, through interference with viral assembly at the cell membrane. Furthermore, *in vitro*, α-interferon acts synergistically with AZT in HIV inhibition. α-Interferon has been used at a dose of 1 mU to 52 mU per day with response rates ranging between 25% and 50%. Tumor regression begins 4 to 8 weeks after initiation of therapy and major response is achieved in 12 to 24 weeks. Upon analyzing CD4 lymphocyte counts as a parameter to predict response to interferon, it is clear that patients with CD4 counts above $400/mm^3$ are most likely to achieve tumor response. More recently combinations of AZT and α-INF have been shown to be efficacious. Combining 8 to 10 million units SQ daily of α-INF with 500 mg/day of AZT, a response rate of approximately 30% was seen in patients with poor prognostic factors, while those with good prognoses experienced a response rate of 50% to 60%. Most of these are partial responses.

Chemotherapy

Systemic cytotoxic chemotherapy should be reserved for patients with extensive or rapidly progressive KS, symptomatic visceral involvement, pulmonary KS, and those with lymphoedema. Single-agent chemotherapy has been associated with modest responses. Thus, vinblastine used alone has produced responses in less than one third of cases. Other agents used effectively as single agents include etoposide, doxorubicin, and alternating vinblastine and vincristine. As shown by one group, a combination of doxorubicin (20 mg/m^2), bleomycin (10 mg/m^2), and vineristine (2 mg) given every two weeks is well tolerated, with responses in over 80%, while Adriamycin alone at the same dose and schedule produced major responses in just under 50% of the cases. Combinations of bleomycin and vincristine at the above dosages and schedule can be administered, even when patients have compromised bone marrow function, and result in response rates of approximately 70%. Patients with symptomatic pulmonary KS have a predicted survival of approximately 3 months without therapy, but may respond to combination chemotherapy with improved survival. In a retrospective analysis, combinations of AZT with bleomycin and vincristine have been well tolerated with high response rates; predominant toxicity consists of anemia and neutropenia. Prospective studies of chemotherapy and AZT, with or without granulocyte macrophage–colony stimulating factor (GM-CSF) have shown that AZT is very difficult to administer, even with GM-CSF support. Instead, the use of G-CSF in this circumstance may be more effective, with fewer side effects. Studies are currently in progress comparing the efficacy of liposomal daunomycin with the standard doxorubicin, bleomycin, and vincristine combination. Several such preparations of liposomal anthracyclines are currently being evaluated in clinical trials.

A major problem is that KS almost always relapses shortly after discontinuation of chemotherapy. Thus, safe and effective maintenance therapy short of cytotoxic chemotherapy will be needed to maintain tumor response. α-Interferon alone has limited activity in this regard, and studies using combinations of AZT and interferon following chemotherapy are currently in progress.

Several angiostatic compounds have been discovered recently, and are undergoing clinical evaluation. Two such antiangiogenic compounds are Tecogalan (SP-PG or DS-4152) and TNP-470 (a fumagillin analogue). Tecogalan is a 29-kd sulfated polysaccharide, purified from the cell membrane of a bacterium, *Arthrobacter* species AT-25. TNP-470 was first isolated from *Aspergillus fumigatus fresensius*. These two compounds are currently in phase I clinical trials and the results of these studies will form the basis for further study of drug development.

Conclusion

Kaposi's sarcoma occurs in a significant number of HIV-infected individuals. The cell of origin and the etiology of the malignancy are still poorly understood.

However, significant advances have occurred during the last few years regarding the pathogenesis of KS and the role of HIV in its development. In addition, the demonstration of various known autocrine and paracrine growth factors produced by the KS cell, as well as the existence of one or more novel growth factors for KS, has further expanded our understanding of the initiation and progression of this neoplasm. These findings allow for the possibility of novel treatment regimens, which would be designed to block the effects of these various growth factors.

AIDS-ASSOCIATED LYMPHOMA

Although lymphoma primary to the central nervous system was considered one of the initial criteria for the diagnosis of AIDS, it was not until 1985 that sufficient epidemiologic data was available to indicate a statistical increase in systemic lymphoma as well. Based upon these data, the Centers for Disease Control changed the case definition of AIDS in October 1985, to include cases of intermediate or high-grade B-cell lymphoma in AIDS risk group members. At the present time, such cases in the setting of HIV seropositivity would indicate the development of full-blown AIDS. This delayed recognition of systemic lymphoma as a criterion for AIDS is consistent with the hypothesis that lymphoma is a relatively late manifestation of infection by HIV, a concept that has recently been supported by data from the National Cancer Institute. Thus, as demonstrated by one study, 8 of 116 patients with symptomatic HIV disease have developed lymphoma after having been followed in various antiretroviral trials at the National Cancer Institute. The risk of developing lymphoma was 19% at 36 months in this cohort. Although patient numbers are very small, and the precise incidence of lymphoma over time is yet to be truly defined, it is still apparent that ever-increasing numbers of HIV-infected patients with lymphoma are to be expected. This follows directly from the enhanced patient survival being witnessed, due to effective antiretroviral therapy and prophylaxis, early recognition, and therapy for the various complicating opportunistic infections.

Pathologic Characteristics

Approximately 70% to 90% of patients with AIDS lymphoma are diagnosed with "high-grade" pathologic types of disease, including immunoblastic lymphoma, and/or small noncleaved lymphoma ("undifferentiated"), which may be of the Burkitt or non-Burkitt types. This very unique pathologic spectrum of disease may be appreciated by review of prior experience at the University of Southern California (USC) and the Working Formulation for Clinical Usage. In these very large series of well over 1,000 cases diagnosed prior to the 1980s, immunoblastic or small noncleaved lymphomas comprised approximately 10% of all cases.

Although the vast majority of AIDS lymphomas are immunoblastic or small noncleaved lymphomas, approximately 10% to 30% consist of an "intermediate grade," usually the large noncleaved type. The precise meaning of this distinction is somewhat problematic, especially considering the subtle nature of pathologic distinction, and the well-appreciated difficulties in reproducibility of pathologic diagnosis. Furthermore, although some investigators have found certain clinicopathologic correlates of disease in the intermediate versus high-grade types, these correlates have not been confirmed in other series, and at the present time it is probably justified to consider patients with either intermediate or high-grade disease similarly, with regard to prognosis and therapy.

A small number of patients with underlying HIV infection have also been diagnosed with low-grade lymphomas, including chronic lymphocytic leukemia, multiple myeloma, and small cleaved lymphoma. There are no epidemiologic data to suggest that these cases represent anything other than chance occurrence. Furthermore, these patients appear to behave identically to patients without HIV infection, in regard to prognosis and therapeutic outcome. Likewise, several HIV-infected patients with various types of T-cell lymphoma have also been reported; once again, there is no statistical evidence to indicate that these cases represent anything other than chance occurrence, especially considering the fact that the most commonly reported of these lymphomas, lymphoblastic lymphoma, is expected to occur in young males. Recently, several series of anaplastic Ki-1 positive large cell lymphoma have been reported in HIV infected patients. All clinical and pathologic aspects of lymphomatous disease appear similar to what has previously been reported in patients without HIV infection.

Immunobiologic Features

AIDS lymphomas are expected to be of B-lymphoid origin. In the series from USC of 93 cases, 31% marked as the monoclonal κ immunophenotype; 13% were monoclonal λ; 8% were both κ and λ positive; 14% were other B-cell marker positive; 5% were nonmarking; and the remainder (29%) were not studied. In a series from New York University (NYU), 25/26 patients tested were positive for B-cell antigens, and one had T-cell antigen expression. Seventy-seven percent of small noncleaved lymphomas were common acute lymphocytic leukemia antigen (CALLA) positive, while 13% of the large noncleaved cases expressed the CALLA marker.

Interestingly, immunoglobulin gene rearrangement studies, performed by Southern blot technology, have indicated that, while the majority of cases demonstrate one clonal heavy chain gene rearrangement, consistent with immunogenotypic monoclonality, many cases have multiple clonal B-cell expansions, similar to what has previously been described in transplantation-associated lymphoma. These data have implications related to the etiology and pathogenesis of lymphoma in the setting of underlying immunodeficiency.

Epidemiology

Unlike Kaposi's sarcoma, in which the predominant group affected appears to be homosexual or bisexual men, AIDS-associated lymphoma may be seen equally in any group at risk for HIV infection. Thus, homosexual males, hemophiliacs, intravenous drug users, and transfusion recipients have all been at risk for development of lymphoma. Interestingly, the clinical and pathologic characteristics of disease appear identical in all population groups. Furthermore, as noted above, the incidence of AIDS-related lymphoma is expected to rise in all of these groups over time, as the epidemic proceeds.

Clinical Characteristics

Approximately 70% to 80% of patients with AIDS lymphoma present with systemic "B" symptoms, including unexplained fever, drenching night sweats, and/ or weight loss, in excess of 10% of normal body weight. This type of presentation may be quite problematic, as the clinician searches for the presence of what is assumed to be an occult opportunistic infection, or even considers underlying HIV infection, per se. It is important to recognize that such systemic symptoms may be an indication of underlying lymphomatous disease as well. Conversely, in the patient with known lymphoma, the presence of such symptoms cannot be assumed to be lymphoma related, until a careful evaluation for infection, such as *Mycobacterium avium-intracellulare* infection or others, has been performed.

Patients with AIDS-associated lymphoma classically present with widespread lymphomatous disease, involving multiple extranodal sites. Thus, in the series from USC, 84% of individuals presented with lymphoma in extranodal sites. In one report from several institutions, 95% had evidence of lymphomatous disease in extranodal sites, while investigators at NYU reported such a finding in 87%, and investigators from San Francisco General Hospital noted extranodal presentations in 97% of cases.

The unique nature of such widespread lymphomatous disease at presentation may be appreciated from older experiences published in 1973. In this series of 405 lymphoma patients, all diagnosed prior to the AIDS epidemic, 39% were found to have extranodal lymphoma at the time of initial diagnosis. One of the distinguishing features of AIDS-related lymphoma, then, is the widespread nature of lymphomatous involvement, even at initial presentation. It is not unusual, for example, to see a patient with extensive involvement of the entire gastrointestinal tract, from mouth to anus.

Not only do affected individuals present with extranodal disease, but they are also distinguished by the very unusual sites of lymphomatous involvement that have been reported. Lymphoma in the myocardium, bile ducts, ear lobes, orbit, popliteal fossa, gingiva, appendix, and rectum have been seen. In addition to these sites, other areas of involvement are observed with some regularity. Thus, in the series from USC, central nervous system (CNS) involvement has been noted in approximately 32%; gastrointestinal tract in 26%; bone marrow in 25%; liver in 12%; and kidney and lung in 9% each. Other series have had consistent findings. One of the challenges in treating such individuals is the frequent occurrence of extensive organ involvement and even of organ failure, and the necessity of utilizing chemotherapeutic agents that in themselves may cause organ dysfunction, especially related to the bone marrow and liver.

Staging Evaluation

Approximately 20% of patients can have leptomeningeal disease in the absence of specific signs and symptoms. Therefore, staging evaluation should routinely include a lumbar puncture in addition to computed tomography (CT) and/or magnetic resonance imaging (MRI) of the head; CTS of chest, abdomen, and pelvis; a gallium scan; and bilateral bone marrow examination.

Prognostic Factors for Survival

Several investigators have reported pretherapy characteristics that were found to be associated with shorter survival in patients with HIV-related lymphoma. The results of these various series have been remarkably consistent. As noted in a retrospective, multiinstitutional trial, the presence of an AIDS diagnosis prior to diagnosis of lymphoma predicted shorter survival, a finding also noted by others. In a large retrospective study from the University of California San Francisco, investigators performed multivariate analysis and found that a low CD4 count (less than 100/ mm^3), history of prior AIDS, Karnofsky performance status (KPS) of 70% or less, and presence of extranodal disease each predicted for decreased survival. In a retrospective study of 60 cases of systemic lymphoma in known HIV-seropositive individuals, all of whom were treated with curative intent, we defined three poor prognostic indicators on multivariate analysis, including a KPS less than 70%, an AIDS diagnosis prior to development of lymphoma, and the presence of bone marrow involvement. Lower CD4 counts, on a continuous scale, were also a significant predictor of shorter survival.

Patients with primary CNS lymphoma have a very poor prognosis with median survival of only 2 to 3 months. However, leptomeningeal involvement in patients with systemic lymphoma does not adversely affect prognosis, if appropriate treatment is rendered.

It is apparent from this information that both HIV-related factors (CD4 count, history of prior AIDS, KPS less than 70%) and lymphoma-related factors (bone marrow involvement, presence of extranodal disease) are important in determining prognosis in the HIV-infected patient with systemic lymphoma.

Therapeutic Considerations

In the 1980s, higher dose intensity regimens were studied in attempts to define optimal therapy of the patient with non–HIV-related lymphoma. These regimens have not proven to be superior to the earlier, less intensive cyclophosphamide, hydroxydaunomycin, Oncovin (vineristine), and prednisone (CHOP) regimen.

However, in concert with the concepts of dose intensity in the 1980s, investigators from USC embarked upon an intensive regimen of multiagent chemotherapy, reported in 1987. High-dose cytosine arabinoside, methotrexate, and cyclophosphamide were used, along with other traditional agents, in an attempt to provide early CNS therapy, as well as to give attention to systemic sites of disease. Despite the known efficacy of these agents in other settings, the regimen was essentially ineffective in patients with HIV-related disease, associated with a complete remission (CR) rate of only 33%, and evidence of CNS progression in 66%. Furthermore, the regimen was simply too toxic in these individuals, with complicating opportunistic infections developing in 78%, leading to demise in all. Due to these results the trial was terminated early.

Other investigators have also noted poor treatment results after use of very intensive regimens. Thus, the NYU group reported a 20% CR rate after use of the intensive ProMACE-MOPP regimen, which also required extensive delays and dose reductions, due to the underlying HIV-related immunodeficiency. Furthermore, investigators treated 38 patients with COMET-A, consisting of high-dose cytosine arabinoside, cyclophosphamide, methotrexate, and other agents. Median survival for patients treated with this regimen was significantly shorter than that for patients who had received other, less-intensive regimens.

There has been one published report of the efficacious use of intensive therapy in HIV-infected patients with lymphoma. The MACOP-B regimen was used in 12 patients, 8 of whom (67%) attained complete remission. It is noteworthy that 6/8 had a KPS of 100%, and only one had a KPS less than 80%. Furthermore, only one had a history of AIDS prior to the diagnosis of lymphoma. It is certainly possible, then, that selected individuals, with none of the predictors of poor prognosis, may be able to tolerate such dose-intensive therapy with good response. However, in the majority of individuals with more severe HIV-related disease (history of prior AIDS, low CD4 cells, low KPS), such dose-intensive therapy is likely to be quite toxic, and ineffective, as discussed above.

With these considerations in mind, one group embarked upon a study of low-dose chemotherapy, with early CNS prophylaxis. Using a low-dose modification of the M-BACOD regimen (Table 1), a total of 42 patients were accrued as part of the AIDS Clinical Trials Groups (ACTG) of the National Institute of Allergy and Infectious Diseases (NIAID). With 35 evaluable patients, a complete remission rate of 46% was achieved, with only 4/16 complete remission patients experiencing relapse, after a median follow-up period of over 14 months. The median survival of complete responders has not yet been reached, but will be in excess of 14 months. Although nadir granulocyte counts less than $500/mm^3$ were seen in approximately 20%, only one patient experienced bacterial sepsis, and a total of approximately 20% developed opportunistic infections, consisting of *Pneumocystis carinii* pneumonia (PCP) in all. Prior series of chemotherapy-treated patients with AIDS-related lymphoma or Kaposi's sarcoma have reported the development of PCP in between 40% and 78% of treated

TABLE 1. *Treatment protocols for lymphoma[a] in HIV-infected patients*

	Current regimen	M-BACOD regimen
Bleomycin	4 mg/m^2, day 1 IV	4 mg/m^2, day 1, IV
Doxorubicin	25 mg/m^2, day 1 IV	45 mg/m^2, day 1, IV
Cyclophosphamide	300 mg/m^2, day 1 IV	600 mg/m^2, day 1, IV
Vincristine	1.4 mg/m^2, day 1 IV (not to exceed 2 mg)	1.0 mg/m^2, day 1, IV
Dexamethasone	3 mg/m^2 days 1–5, po	6 mg/m^2, days 1–5, po
Methotrexate (MTX)	500 mg/m^2 day 15, IV with folinic acid rescue, 25 mg po Q6H × 4, beginning 6 hours after completion of MTX	3,000 mg/m^2, day 14, IV with folinic acid rescue, 10 mg/m^2 IV or po Q6H for 72 hours, beginning 24 hours after completion of MTX
Cytosine arabinoside	50 mg, intrathecal, days 1, 8, 21, 28	0
Helmet field radiotherapy	2,400 cGy with marrow involvement; 4,000 cGy with known CNS involvement	0
Zidovudine (AZT)	200 mg every 4 hours for 1 year; starting after chemo	0
Total treatment	4–6 cycles, at 28-day intervals	10 cycles, at 21-day intervals

[a]Excluding primary central nervous system lymphoma.

subjects. Thus, although the results with low-dose M-BACOD are still not optimal, the regimen appears tolerable and associated with the likelihood of long-term, lymphoma-free survival, even in patients presenting with a history of prior AIDS, low CD4 count, low KPS, and/or bone marrow involvement.

It is important to know that even though long-term lymphoma-free survival was achieved in this study, patients were still at risk for development of additional HIV-related illness, including opportunistic infections and/or HIV wasting syndrome, after completion of all chemotherapy. It is thus apparent that long-term, "event-free" survival will require not only effective chemotherapy, but effective anti-retroviral therapy as well. To this end, several ongoing therapeutic trials are now studying the use of concomitant chemotherapy and antiviral therapy, with or without the use of hematopoietic growth factor support. The results of these studies are awaited with interest. The effect of growth factor support (G-CSF or GM-CSF) and intensification of chemotherapy on response rates is currently being studied. Other strategies including the delivery of chemotherapy by continuous intravenous infusion have shown efficacy as well. Furthermore, the use of methylglyoxal bisguanyl-hydrazone (MGBG) by a newer schedule given every 2 weeks, and the use of immunotoxins, such as anti-B4 blocked ricin, are currently being evaluated, with some responses reported in patients with refractory/relapsed disease.

Primary Central Nervous System Lymphoma

Primary CNS lymphoma usually presents with one or two mass lesions in the brain; any parenchymal area may be involved. Symptoms include seizures, focal neurologic dysfunction, headache, and/or cranial nerve palsies. Interestingly, affected patients may present with altered mental status, even of a very subtle nature, as the only clinical manifestation of disease.

Radiographic evaluation usually reveals one or two relatively large (2–4 cm) homogeneous or heterogeneous lesions within the parenchyma. Ring enhancement may be seen on double-dose contrast studies, and, in general, the lesions are enhancing. Although CT scans of the brain may be similar in patients with cerebral toxoplasmosis, these individuals often have multiple, smaller lesions than those seen in primary CNS lymphoma. It is not unusual for such patients to receive empiric therapy for cerebral toxoplasmosis, with repeat of the CT scan within 1 to 2 weeks. With definite improvement documented, the patient may be safely assumed to have cerebral toxoplasmosis. However, with similar or worsening disease parameters after this period of empiric therapy, a brain biopsy is indicated to confirm the diagnosis of primary CNS lymphoma, or some other pathologic process.

The prognosis of the HIV-infected patient with primary CNS lymphoma is quite poor. In fact, in our retrospective series, the survival of these individuals, even when treated, was significantly shorter than that for patients with systemic HIV-related lymphoma. Interestingly, patients with primary CNS disease had significantly more severe underlying HIV-related disease, as reflected by the fact that 73% had a prior diagnosis of AIDS, and the median CD4 count at diagnosis of lymphoma was only 34/mm^3.

Although radiation therapy may be associated with complete remission in approximately 50% of these patients, median survival is only 2 to 3 months, with death due to intercurrent opportunistic infections and the presence of multiple ongoing neuropathologic processes. Of importance, however, CNS radiation may be associated with significant improvement in the quality of life in approximately 75% of treated patients. Clearly, effective antiretroviral therapy must be a part of future therapeutic trials, used early in the treatment schema. Also, the use of cytotoxic chemotherapy in addition to radiation must be explored.

CERVICAL CANCER

The relative risk of cervical cancer is known to be approximately 14-fold higher than expected in organ transplant recipients. In these immunocompromised individuals, the median incubation period between transplantation and cervical cancer is approximately 107 months. With the recognition that immunocompromise might predispose to cervical cancer, the development of this malignancy in HIV-infected women became an issue. In fact, the anticipated increase in cervical cancer with prolonged survival in HIV disease has now been confirmed; this malignancy became an AIDS-defining condition on January 1, 1993.

It has recently become clear that human papilloma virus (HPV) is associated with the development of cervical intraepithelial neoplasia (CIN) in women and anal intraepithelial neoplasia (AIN) in homosexual men. Further, certain HPV serotypes, such as 16, 18, 30, 31, 33, and 35, are more likely to be associated with subsequent neoplasia. Several studies have also demonstrated an increasing incidence of HPV infection in women infected by HIV. In these dually infected women, an increasing incidence of infection by HPV types 16 and 18, with increasing likelihood of CIN, has been reported as the immune status deteriorates, with falling CD4 counts. CIN developing in HIV-infected women tends to be more difficult to eradicate, and more likely to relapse after definitive therapy, when compared with the same disease in non–HIV-infected patients. Furthermore, invasive cervical carcinoma has been associated with a 100% relapse and a median survival of only 7 months in one study of HIV-infected women, representing a significantly more aggressive course than would be expected in *de novo* cervical carcinoma. For all these reasons, it would seem intuitively obvious that early detection of infection by HPV types 16 and 18 would be important in HIV-infected women, as part of their routine gynecologic care. With discovery of such HPV infection, early evaluation by colposcopy might be indicated, despite the presence of a normal Pap smear. The recent Centers for Disease Control (CDC) guidelines, omitting such considerations, may serve to delay our true understanding of the nature of cervical neoplastic disease in HIV-infected women, as well as the optimal means to prevent development of invasive cervical cancer. The significance of this issue is likely to expand in the years ahead, as ever-increasing numbers of women with HIV/AIDS are diagnosed.

MISCELLANEOUS CANCERS

Hodgkin's Disease

Although there are no epidemiologic data to demonstrate a statistical increase in Hodgkin's disease since the onset of AIDS, it is apparent that the course of disease in an HIV-infected patient is altered. This is fully consistent with the previously understood relationship between host immunity and the specific clinicopathologic characteristics of Hodgkin's disease in a given patient.

In the patient with underlying HIV infection, Hodgkin's disease is likely to be widespread, often involving extranodal sites, such as bone marrow, liver, and/or lung. Although unusual sites of disease have been described, such as the rectum, clearly this is the exception, in contrast to the experience with AIDS-associated lymphoma. Aside from widespread disease, affected patients are often symptomatic ("B" symptoms), with fever, night sweats, and/or unexplained weight loss. Mixed cellularity and lymphocyte depletion subtypes are seen most frequently.

Therapy of such patients may be problematic, due to underlying bone marrow dysfunction secondary to HIV, or in some cases, due to involvement by Hodgkin's disease itself. Multiagent chemotherapy may further compromise hematologic parameters, with the risk of neutropenia and resulting bacterial and/or opportunistic infections (which may occur even in the patient without underlying HIV infection). Despite all of the potential difficulties of multiagent chemotherapy in this setting, the likelihood of symptomatic, disseminated disease is so high that the majority of these patients do require such therapeutic intervention. The median survival of HIV-infected patients with Hodgkin's disease has been in the range of 2 years, in comparison with the strong likelihood of cure in the majority of such patients who are not infected by HIV. Clearly, alternative strategies are required, such as the concomitant use of chemotherapy with hematopoietic growth factors. Such trials are currently under way.

MISCELLANEOUS SOLID CANCERS

Miscellaneous cancers have been reported in patients with HIV infection, and although there is no statistical evidence to suggest an epidemic of these tumors, it is wise to follow such cases and gather statistics over time, to ascertain their true incidence and significance.

Experience in patients with organ transplantation provides a model for the development of such cancers. Presumably because of iatrogenically induced immunosuppression, organ transplantation recipients are at increased risk for a variety of cancers, including Kaposi's sarcoma, lymphoma, squamous cell carcinomas of the mouth and skin, and carcinomas of the vulva and perineum, kidney, and hepatobiliary tract, as well as various sarcomas. Interestingly, the degree of immunosuppression may be predictive of the specific type of malignancy that develops, with the more immunosuppressive regimens more likely to be associated with lymphomas, occurring relatively early in the posttransplantation period. In general, the average interval between renal transplantation and the development of Kaposi's sarcoma is approximately 20 months, while that of lymphoma is 33 months, miscellaneous other tumors is approximately 67 months, and cancers of the vulva and perineum occur approximately 107 months after transplantation.

Patients with underlying HIV infection have now been described with squamous cell carcinomas of the skin and oral and anogenital regions, basal cell carcinomas of the skin, melanomas, germinal testicular tumors, gastric adenocarcinomas, and others. Since the transplantation model would predict ever-increasing numbers of these cancers in the years ahead, it is important to document such cases, with information obtained regarding specific immune status, clinical and pathologic correlates, presence of coinfections such as papilloma virus infection, and therapeutic outcome.

SUGGESTED READING

Ballerini P, Gaidano G, Gong JZ, et al. Multiple genetic lesions in AIDS-related non-Hodgkin's lymphoma. *Blood* 1993;81:166–176.
Baumgartner JE, Rachlin JR, Beckstead JH, et al. Primary CNS lymphomas: natural history and response to radiation therapy in 55 patients with AIDS. *J Neurosurg* 1990;73:206–211.
Chang Y, Cesarman E, Pessin MS, et al. Identification of Herpesvirus-like DNA sequences in AIDS-associated Kaposi's sarcoma. *Science* 1994;266:1865–1869.

Fruchter RG, Maiman M, Sillman FH, et al. Characteristics of cervical intraepithelial neoplasia in women infected with the human immunodeficiency virus. *Am J Obstet Gynecol* 1994;171:531–537.

Kaplan L, Straus D, Testa M, Levine AM. Randomized trial of standard dose mBACOD with GM-CSF versus reduced dose mBACOD for systemic HIV-associated lymphoma: ACTG 142. (abstract). *Annual Society of Clinical Oncology (ASCO)* 1995;14:288.

Levine AM. AIDS-related malignancies: the emerging epidemic (review). *J Natl Cancer Inst* 1993; 85:1382.

Levine AM, Sullivan-Halley J, Pike MC, et al. HIV-related lymphoma: prognostic factors predictive of survival. *Cancer* 1991;68:2466–2472.

Lilenbaum RC, Ratner L. Systemic treatment of Kaposi's sarcoma: current status and future directions. *AIDS* 1994;8:141–151.

Maiman M, Fruchter RG, Guy L, et al. Human immunodeficiency virus infection and invasive cervical carcinoma. *Cancer* 1993;71:402–406.

Miles SA. Pathogenesis of HIV-related Kaposi's sarcoma. *Curr Opin Oncol* 1994;6:497–502.

Miles SA, Wang H, Elashoff R, Mitsuyasu RT. Improved survival for patients with AIDS-related Kaposi's sarcoma. *J Clin Oncol* 1994;12:1910–1916.

Rabkin CS. Epidemiology of AIDS-related malignancies. *Curr Opin Oncol* 1994;6:492–496.

Shibata D, Weiss LM, Hernandez AM, Nathwani B, Bernstein L, Levine AM. Epstein Barr virus associated non-Hodgkin's lymphoma in patients infected with the human immunodeficiency virus. *Blood* 1993;91:2102–2109.

Sparano JA, Wiernik PH, Strack M, et al. Infusional cyclophosphamide, doxorubicin, and etoposide in HIV and HTLV-1 related non-Hodgkin's lymphoma: a highly active regimen. *Blood* 1993;81:2810.

Williams A, Darragh T, Vranizan K, et al. Anal and cervical human papillomavirus infection and risk of anal and cervical epithelial abnormalities in human immunodeficiency virus-infected women. *Obstet Gynecol* 1994;83:205–211.

A Clinical Guide to AIDS and HIV,
edited by Gary P. Wormser.
Lippincott-Raven Publishers, Philadelphia 1996.

9

Infection Control Considerations in HIV Infection

Jerome I. Tokars and *William J. Martone

*Hospital Infections Program; Centers for Disease Control and Prevention,
Atlanta, Georgia 30333; and *National Foundation for Infectious Diseases,
Bethesda, Maryland 20814*

The primary modes of transmission of HIV, the virus that causes AIDS, are sexual contact, exposure to infected blood or blood components, and perinatal transmission from mother to neonate. HIV has been isolated from blood and a number of other body fluids, including semen, vaginal secretions, saliva, tears, breast milk, cerebrospinal fluid, amniotic fluid, bronchoalveolar-lavage fluid, and urine. However, epidemiologic evidence has implicated only blood, semen, vaginal secretions, and breast milk in transmission. Although instances of HIV transmission in households have been reported, transmission of HIV through ordinary social or occupational contact with HIV-infected persons or through air, water, or food has not been demonstrated. The mode of transmission of HIV is similar to that of hepatitis B virus, although the potential for hepatitis B virus transmission is greater.

In the health-care setting, blood is the single most important source of HIV, and transmission has been documented only after exposure to blood, bloody pleural fluid, or culture medium containing concentrated virus. Percutaneous inoculation has been the route of infection in most instances of nosocomial HIV transmission; however, transmission by mucutaneous contact has also been reported.

This chapter outlines infection control measures to prevent nosocomial transmission of blood-borne pathogens such as HIV and of other pathogens that occur frequently in HIV-infected patients. Precautions designed to prevent transmission of blood-borne pathogens, referred to as "universal precautions," should be applied to all patients. Prevention of transmission of certain other pathogens require additional precautions.

DISINFECTION, STERILIZATION, AND ENVIRONMENTAL HYGIENE

An important infection control issue is whether routine sterilization and disinfection procedures are adequate for preventing HIV transmission. A number of laboratory studies using various experimental conditions and assays for viral inactivation suggest that HIV does not possess unusual resistance properties. In these studies, HIV was inactivated by many chemical germicides at concentrations below those commonly used. In one study, HIV was rapidly inactivated by drying, but continued to be detectable after 1 to 3 days. Another study showed survival of HIV for several weeks when suspended in serum and several days when dried on a glass coverslip. However, in these studies, HIV was used in concentrations of 10^7 to 10^8 tissue culture infective doses (TCID) per milliliter, a much higher concentration than that estimated to be present in the blood of HIV-infected persons (60–7000 TCID per milliliter). Studies performed at the Centers for Disease Control and Prevention (CDC) have shown that HIV is reduced in concentration by 1 to 2 logs (90–99%) within several hours when allowed to dry. Instruments, devices, or other items contaminated with blood or other body fluids from persons infected with HIV may be disinfected and sterilized according to standard procedures.

Critical, Semicritical, and Noncritical Items

The rationale for cleaning, disinfection, and sterilization can be more readily understood if medical devices, equipment, and surgical materials are divided into three general categories: critical items (e.g., surgical instruments, cardiac catheters, and implants), which are introduced directly into the bloodstream or into normally sterile areas of the body; semicritical items (e.g., flexible and rigid fiberoptic endoscopes, endotracheal tubes, anesthesia breathing circuits, and cystoscopes), which come in contact with intact mucous membranes but do not ordinarily penetrate body surfaces; and noncritical items (e.g., crutches, bed boards, and blood pressure cuffs), which do not ordinarily touch the patient or touch only intact skin.

Disinfection and Sterilization

Disinfection and sterilization procedures for critical, semicritical, and noncritical items and for environmental surfaces are presented in the CDC Guideline for Handwashing and Hospital Environmental Control, 1985, and are summarized in Table 1. It is important that all items and surfaces be cleaned to remove debris prior to disinfection or sterilization.

Chemical germicides classified as sterilants or disinfectants are regulated and registered by the Environmental Protection Agency (EPA). The EPA requires testing under specific and standardized protocols of chemical germicides formulated as general disinfectants, hospital disinfectants, and disinfectants applied to other environments. EPA-registered tuberculocidal "hospital grade" disinfectants will inactivate HIV. The EPA has also approved a standard testing protocol that allows manufacturers to claim that a product inactivates HIV specifically. When using chemical germicides, the manufacturer's instructions for use, length of treatment, and specifications for compatibility of the medical device with chemical germicides should

TABLE 1. *Disinfection and sterilization procedures*[a]

Sterilization
Destroys: All forms of microbial life, including high numbers of bacterial spores.
Methods: Steam under pressure (autoclave), gas (ethylene oxide), dry heat or immersion in EPA-approved chemical "sterilant"[b] for prolonged period of time (e.g., 6–10 hr) or according to manufacturers' instructions. *Note:* Liquid chemical "sterilants" should be used *only* on those instruments that are impossible to sterilize or disinfect with heat. After use and before sterilization, surgical instruments should be decontaminated with a chemical germicide rather than just rinsed with water.
Use: Critical items.[c] Disposable invasive equipment eliminates the need to reprocess critical items.
High-level disinfection
Destroys: All forms of microbial life *except* high numbers of bacterial spores.
Methods: Hot-water pasteurization (80–100°C, 30 min) or exposure to an EPA-registered "sterilant"[b] chemical as above, except for a short exposure time (10–45 min or as directed by the manufacturer).
Use: Semicritical items.[c]
Intermediate-level disinfection
Destroys: *Mycobacterium tuberculosis*, vegetative bacteria, most viruses (including hepatitis B and HIV), and most fungi; does *not* kill bacterial spores.
Methods: EPA-registered "hospital disinfectant"[b] chemical germicides that have a label claim for tuberculocidal activity; commercially available hard-surface germicides or solutions containing at least 500 ppm free available chlorine (a 1:100 dilution of common household bleach—approximately ¼ cup bleach per gallon of tap water.)
Use: Noncritical[c] items that have been visibly contaminated with blood.
Low-level disinfection
Destroys: Most bacteria, some viruses, some fungi, but *not M. tuberculosis* or bacterial spores.
Methods: EPA-registered "hospital disinfectants"[b] *without* a label claim for tuberculocidal activity.
Use: Noncritical[c] items or surfaces *without* visible blood contamination.
Environmental disinfection
Methods: Any cleaner or disinfectant agent that is intended for environmental use.
Use: Environmental surfaces such as floors, woodwork, and countertops that have become soiled but *not* contaminated with visible bood.

[a]*Important:* To ensure the effectiveness of any sterilization or disinfection process, items and surfaces must first be cleaned of all visible soil.
[b]The manufacturer's instructions for use, length of treatment, and specifications for compatibility of the medical device with chemical germicides should be followed.
[c]See text for definition of critical, semicritical, and noncritical items.

be followed. Information on specific label claims of commercial germicides can be obtained by writing to the Disinfectants Branch, Office of Pesticides, Environmental Protection Agency, 401 M Street, S.W., Washington, DC 20460.

Cleaning and Decontaminating of Spills of Blood and Body Fluids

When spills of blood or body fluids occur in the patient-care setting, visible material should first be removed and then the area disinfected. With large spills of cultured or concentrated infectious agents in the laboratory, the contaminated area should be flooded with a liquid germicide before cleaning, then disinfected with fresh germicidal chemical. In both patient-care and laboratory settings, gloves should be worn during the cleaning and decontaminating procedures. Disinfection can be accomplished with chemical germicides that are approved for use as "hospital disinfectants" and are tuberculocidal when used at recommended dilutions, or with a 1:100 solution of household bleach.

Housekeeping

Environmental surfaces such as walls and floors are not associated with transmission of infections to patients or health-care workers. Therefore, extraordinary efforts to disinfect or sterilize these environmental surfaces are not necessary. However, cleaning and removal of soil should be done routinely. Disinfectant-detergent formulations registered by the EPA can be used for cleaning environmental surfaces, but the actual physical removal of microorganisms by scrubbing is probably at least as important as any antimicrobial effect of the cleaning agent used. Therefore, cost, safety, and acceptability by housekeepers can be the main criteria for selecting any such registered agent. The manufacturers' instructions for appropriate use should be followed.

Laundry

Although soiled linen is a source of large numbers of certain pathogenic microorganisms, the risk of actual disease transmission is negligible. Rather than rigid procedures and specifications, hygienic and common-sense storage and processing of clean and soiled linen are recommended. Soiled linen should be handled as little as possible and with minimum agitation to prevent gross microbial contamination of the air and of persons handling the linen. All soiled linen should be bagged at the location where it was used. Linen soiled with blood or body fluids should be placed and transported in bags that prevent leakage.

Infective Waste

No epidemiologic evidence suggests that most hospital waste is any more infective than residential waste or that improper disposal of hospital waste has caused disease in the community. However, it appears prudent to take special precautions in disposal of blood specimens or blood products and waste from microbiology and pathology laboratories. Such waste should either be incinerated or autoclaved before disposal in a sanitary landfill. Bulk blood, suctioned fluids, excretions, and secretions may be carefully poured down a drain connected to a sanitary sewer. Sanitary sewers may also be used to dispose of other infectious wastes capable of being ground and flushed into the sewer. In all cases, appropriate local and state regulations should be followed.

Sharp items should be considered as potentially infectious and should be handled and disposed of with extraordinary care to prevent accidental injuries (see Prevention of Percutaneous Injury, below).

UNIVERSAL PRECAUTIONS

In 1987, the CDC developed the strategy of "universal blood and body fluid precautions" to address concerns regarding transmission of HIV in the health-care setting. This concept, now referred to simply as universal precautions, stresses that *all patients should be assumed to be infectious for HIV and other blood-borne pathogens*. Such an approach is necessary because patients with blood-borne infection cannot always be identified by history, physical examination, or readily available laboratory tests. The basic components of universal precautions are (a) barrier precautions to prevent contact with blood and infectious fluids, (b) handwashing, and (c) prevention of percutaneous injuries (e.g., needlesticks, cuts from sharp objects). Hepatitis B vaccination is also stressed as an important measure in prevention of blood-borne disease.

Fluids to Which Universal Precautions Apply

Universal precautions apply to (a) blood, which is the single most important source of HIV, hepatitis B, and other blood-borne pathogens in the occupational setting; (b) visible bloody fluids; (c) semen and vaginal secretions, which have been implicated in the sexual (but not occupational) transmission of hepatitis B and HIV; (d) fluids for which the risk of transmission of hepatitis B and HIV is undetermined, including amniotic, pericardial, peritoneal, pleural, synovial, and cerebrospinal fluids; (e) laboratory specimens that contain hepatitis B or HIV (e.g., suspensions of concentrated virus); and (f) saliva in the dental setting, where contamination with blood is likely. Universal precautions do not apply to feces, nasal secretions, sputum, sweat, tears, urine, and vomitus, since these fluids have not been associated with transmission of hepatitis B or HIV.

Saliva positive for hepatitis B surface antigen (HBsAg) has been shown to be infectious when injected into experimental animals and in human bite exposures, but not through contamination of musical instruments or cardioresuscitation dummies used by hepatitis B carriers. In addition, epidemiologic studies of nonsexual household contacts of HIV-infected patients, including several small series in which HIV transmission failed to occur after bites or after percutaneous inoculation or contamination of cuts and open wounds with saliva, suggest that the potential for salivary transmission of HIV is remote. A case of possible HIV transmission after a human bite has been reported. However, the bite did not break the skin or result in bleeding and the date of seroconversion is unknown, so the role of the bite and of saliva in transmission is unclear. Universal precautions do not apply to saliva, except in the dental setting, where saliva is predictably contaminated with blood.

Barrier Precautions

Barrier precautions, such as gloves, masks, protective eyewear, and gowns, should be used to protect the health-care worker's skin and mucous membranes from contact with fluids to which universal precautions apply. Barrier precautions appropriate to the situation should be employed whenever such contact is anticipated.

Gloves should be worn when touching (a) blood and other fluids to which universal precautions apply, (b) items or surfaces contaminated with such fluids, (c) a patient's mucous membrane, or (d) a patient's body tissues. Gloves should be changed and hands washed after contact with each patient.

Medical gloves include those marketed as sterile surgical or nonsterile examination gloves made of vinyl or latex. There have been conflicting reports that latex gloves are superior to vinyl gloves in integrity and ability to exclude virus. It is unknown whether such differences, if substantiated, would be of practical importance as long as the glove is intact during use. Thus the type of gloves selected should be appropriate for the task being performed. Medical gloves should be discarded after use and not be washed or disinfected for reuse, because washing with surfactants may cause enhanced penetration of liquids through undetected holes in the gloves ("wicking"), and disinfecting agents may cause deterioration.

During phlebotomy, gloves reduce the chance of blood contact with skin but cannot prevent penetrating injuries such as needlesticks. Gloves should be made available to health-care workers performing phlebotomy and should be used if the health-care worker has breaks in his/her skin, is performing a finger or heel stick on an infant or child, is being trained in phlebotomy, or is working in other situations where the worker judges that hand contamination may occur. In other circumstances, the decision on glove use during phlebotomy should be based on (a) the prevalence of infection with blood-borne pathogens in the patient population, (b) the skill and technique of the worker, (c) the frequency with which the worker performs phlebotomy, (d) any circumstances of the phlebotomy that may increase the risk of hand contamination, such as phlebotomy on an uncooperative patient or in an emergency situation.

Masks and protective eyewear or face shields should be worn during procedures (i.e., endotracheal intubation, bronchoscopy, and endoscopy) that are likely to generate splashes of blood or fluids to which universal precautions apply, and during many common dental procedures. Precautions during other procedures should be determined on an individual basis. Gowns or aprons should be worn during procedures that are likely to generate splashes of blood or other potentially infective sources.

Efficacy of Universal Precautions

Use of universal precautions has been shown to reduce the number of blood contacts. After implementation of universal precautions, the mean number of contacts with blood or body fluids decreased from 5.07 to 2.66 exposures per month among physicians at two acute-care hospitals, and from 35.8 to 18.1 per year among workers at the Clinical Center, National Institutes of Health. A study in emergency rooms revealed that use of gloves was associated with a reduction in the adjusted blood contact rate from 11.2 to 1.3 per 100 procedures.

Handwashing

Handwashing is the single most important procedure for preventing nosocomial infections. Universal precautions dictate that hands and other skin surfaces should be washed immediately and thoroughly if contaminated with blood or other body fluids to which universal precautions apply.

For general infection control purposes, hands should be washed (a) after taking care of a patient(s), even if gloves are used; (b) after touching excretions (i.e., feces and urine) or secretions (e.g., from wounds or skin infections) and before touching any patient again; (c) after touching materials soiled with excretions or secretions; (d) before performing invasive procedures, touching wounds, or touching immunocompromised patients; and (e) immediately after gloves are removed, even if the gloves appear to be intact. When handwashing facilities are not available, a waterless antiseptic hand cleanser may be used according to the manufacturer's recommendations. A crossover study of handwashing efficacy showed a greater reduction in nosocomial infections in intensive-care units when an antimicrobial agent (chlorhexidine) was used than when alcohol and soap were used, possibly because of better compliance with chlorhexidine.

Prevention of Percutaneous Injury

Among occupational exposures, percutaneous injuries, such as needlesticks and cuts from sharp instruments and objects, have been most frequently implicated in occupational transmission of blood-borne pathogens. Precautions to prevent such injuries must therefore be implemented by all health-care workers during procedures, when cleaning used instruments, during disposal of used needles, and when handling sharp instruments after procedures. Used needles should never be recapped or otherwise manipulated using both hands or any other technique that involves directing the point of a needle toward any part of the body. Either a one-handed "scoop" technique or a mechanical device designed for holding the needle sheath should be employed. Workers should not remove used needles from disposable syringes by hand, and should not bend, break, or otherwise manipulate needles by hand. Used disposable syringes and needles, scalpel blades, and other sharp items should be placed in appropriate puncture-resistant containers located as close as is practical to the area in which the items were used.

A study at a university hospital revealed that one third of all needlesticks were related to recapping and that devices requiring disassembly had the highest rates of injury, suggesting the need for continued education of health-care workers as well as for development of devices providing for safer covering of contaminated sharps (e.g., self-sheathing needles) and disassembling of devices.

Resuscitation Equipment

Although saliva has not been implicated in HIV transmission, the need for mouth-to-mouth resuscitation should be minimized by placing mouthpieces, resuscitation bags, or other ventilation devices in areas where the need for resuscitation is predictable.

Health-Care Workers with Nonintact Skin

Health-care workers with exudative lesions or weeping dermatitis should refrain from all direct patient care and from handling patient-care equipment until the condition resolves.

Serologic Testing

For the medical benefit of the patients, routine voluntary HIV counseling and testing should be considered in hospitalized patients in age groups deemed to have a high prevalence of HIV infection. The utility of routine HIV serologic testing of patients as an infection control measure to protect health-care workers is unknown; drawbacks include the unavailability of results in some emergency or outpatient settings and the inability to detect HIV antibody in some recently infected patients. In addition, it is uncertain whether health-care workers who are using universal precautions can further reduce their risk of exposure to blood and body fluids even if they know that a patient is HIV infected.

Personnel in some hospitals have advocated serologic testing of patients in settings in which exposure of health-care workers to large amounts of patients' blood may be anticipated. Specific patients for whom serologic testing has been advocated include those undergoing major operative procedures and those undergoing treatment in critical-care units, especially if they have conditions involving uncontrolled bleeding. Decisions regarding the need to establish testing programs for patients should be made by physicians or individual institutions. In addition, when deemed appropriate, testing of individual patients may be performed on agreement between the patient and the physician providing care.

In addition to the universal precautions recommended for all patients, certain additional precautions during the care of HIV-infected patients undergoing major surgical operations have been proposed by personnel in some hospitals. For example, surgical procedures on an HIV-infected patient might be altered so that hand-to-hand passing of sharp instruments would be eliminated; stapling instruments rather than hand-suturing equipment might be used to perform tissue approximation; electrocautery devices rather than scalpels might be used as cutting instruments; and, even though uncomfortable, gowns that totally prevent seepage of blood onto the skin of members of the operative team might be worn. While such modifications might further minimize the risk of HIV infection for members of the operative team, some of these techniques could result in prolongation of operative time and could potentially have an adverse effect on the patient. Observational studies done in operating rooms to date have not demonstrated that fewer blood exposures occur during surgical procedures performed on patients known to be HIV seropositive.

The CDC recommends these guidelines for HIV testing at acute-care facilities:

1. Patients should be asked about their risks for HIV infection, and should be offered HIV counseling and testing if at risk.
2. Hospitals with an HIV seroprevalence rate of ≥1% or an AIDS diagnosis rate (= 1000 × annual number of individual AIDS patients diagnosed and reported to the health department/annual number of discharges) ≥1.0 should strongly consider offering HIV counseling and testing routinely to patients ages 15 to 54 years. The AIDS diagnosis rate should be calculated using figures from prior to January 1, 1993, when the AIDS case definition was changed; this is likely to be a reasonable estimate of prevalence for the next several years since overall hospital prevalence is not likely to change significantly.
3. Testing should be confidential and voluntary, with documentation of informed consent. In all cases, local and state regulations regarding confidentiality and reporting of HIV test results and patient-care information should be observed.
4. Persons who are HIV-antibody positive or who decline testing should not be denied needed medical care or provided suboptimal care.
5. The HIV testing program must not be used as a substitute for universal precautions and other infection-control techniques.

Among 561 hospitals responding to a survey in 1989, 83% had formal written policies about HIV testing. Among hospitals with written policies, 78% required pretest informed consent and 75% required that seropositive patients be informed of their result; 56% required that test results appear in patient records, and 38% required a review of treatment plans for patients with positive HIV test results.

In a voluntary HIV screening program at a large private hospital, 51% of 8,868 admitted patients not previously known to be HIV infected consented to HIV screening. Twelve seropositive patients were found (seroprevalence rate 0.26%), 10 of whom were known to be in a high-risk group at the time of admission. The authors concluded that although the testing program may have benefited patients, there was no evidence that it reduced the risk of nosocomial HIV transmission. The potential efficacy of screening programs as an infection control measure might depend in part on the HIV seroprevalence among hospital inpatients not known to be HIV positive, which is highly variable among hospitals.

The Role of the Occupational Safety and Health Administration

CDC recommendations for universal precautions are guidelines that should be interpreted according to local policies and needs. Statutory authority to regulate health-care facilities and other workplaces to protect the health of workers rests with the Occupational Safety and Health Administration (OSHA). On December 6, 1991, OSHA published a set of regulations, termed a "standard," regarding protection of health-care workers from occupational exposure to blood-borne pathogens. Components of the standard include the following:

1. A plan to control exposures to blood and other potentially infectious materials; the plan includes a list of all job classifications where some or all workers may have occupational exposures and a schedule for implementing other requirements.
2. Methods of compliance, including use of universal precautions, engineering, and work practice controls (e.g., facilities for handwashing and safe disposal of sharps), and personal protective equipment (e.g., eyewear, gowns, gloves); and housekeeping to provide a clean and sanitary worksite.
3. Hepatitis B vaccination, which should be offered free to all employees covered by the standard, and postexposure evaluation and follow-up for employees with occupational exposures.
4. Communication of hazards to employees, through warning labels and training sessions.
5. Record keeping, including records of training and documentation of postexposure evaluations.

Management of Occupational Exposures

The Public Health Service has provided guidelines on management of occupational HIV exposures, including considerations regarding zidovudine postexposure use. Information is also available on the toxicity and documented failure of postexposure zidovudine.

Blood or Tissue Aerosols

Aerosols are inspirable airborne particles less than approximately 100 μm in diameter and should be distinguished from larger, noninspirable droplets or spatter. Aerosols are not known to present a risk of transmission of HIV, hepatitis B virus, or other blood-borne pathogens in the health-care setting. In studies conducted in dental operatories and hemodialysis centers, hepatitis B virus could not be detected in the air during the treatment of infected patients, including during procedures known to generate aerosols. This suggests that detection of HIV in aerosols in clinical settings would also be uncommon, since the concentration of HIV in blood is generally lower than that of hepatitis B virus. Additionally, aerosols of blood can be generated only with considerable mechanical energy (e.g., power equipment) and are unlikely to be present in most clinical situations. It is uncertain whether surgical power tools can generate aerosols containing infective blood-borne pathogens in clinical situations. Hemoglobin was detected in aerosols collected from the breathing zone outside of the surgical mask of surgeons during certain procedures. However, hemoglobin molecules cannot be considered a reliable surrogate for particles containing infective blood-borne pathogens. In a laboratory study that used blood to which HIV had been added, certain power instruments produced aerosols that in some instances contained infective HIV. The clinical significance of this experiment is unclear.

Body Substance Isolation

An alternate system of infection control in the health-care setting, body substance isolation, has been proposed. Unlike universal precautions, which apply only to fluids that may transmit HIV and certain other blood-borne pathogens, body substance isolation includes precautions to prevent contact with all body substances, including blood, secretions, and other moist body substances (feces, urine, sputum, saliva, wound drainage, and other body fluids). Gloves and other barrier precautions are used for anticipated contact with any of these body substances, or with mucous membranes or nonintact skin. Hands are washed only when visibly soiled. Additional measures, such as private rooms, are used for patients with infections transmitted by the airborne route.

The fact that handwashing is not routinely required when gloves are changed between patients is a theoretical disadvantage of body substance isolation. Only a few reports have addressed the efficacy of body substance isolation, and this issue requires further study.

PRECAUTIONS FOR INFECTIOUS DISEASES OCCURRING WITH HIGH FREQUENCY IN HIV-INFECTED PATIENTS

Universal precautions, which should be followed during care of all patients, are designed to prevent transmission of blood-borne pathogens. When patients are known or suspected to be infected with pathogens transmitted by other than the blood-borne route, additional precautions should be followed.

Table 2 lists isolation precautions for many microorganisms that commonly infect AIDS patients. Appropriate precautions will prevent transmission of these micro-

TABLE 2. *Category-specific isolation precautions for microorganisms causing opportunistic infections in patients with AIDS*

Microorganism	Syndrome	Precautions
Bacteria		
Mycobacteria, nontuberculous (atypical)	Pulmonary	None
	Wound	Drainage/secretion
Mycobacterium tuberculosis	Extrapulmonary, draining lesion	Drainage/secretion
		None
	Extrapulmonary, meningitis	Tuberculosis
	Pulmonary	
Nocardia asteroides	Draining lesions	None
	Other	None
Salmonella species	Gastroenteritis	Enteric
	Bacteremia	Enteric[a]
Listeria monocytogenes	Infection at any site	None
Legionella species	Pneumonias, cellulitis	None
Streptococcus pneumoniae	Pneumonia	None
Haemophilus influenzae	Adults	None
	Infant/children	Respiratory
Staphylococcus aureus	Skin, wound, or burn infection	
	Major	Contact
	Minor or limited	Drainage/secretion
	Pneumonia or draining lung abscess	Contact
Shigella species	Gastroenteritis	Enteric
	Bacteremia	Enteric[a]
Viruses		
Cytomegalovirus	Infection at any site	Pregnant personnel may need special counseling
Herpes simplex	Encephalitis	None
	Mucocutaneous, disseminated or primary, severe (skin, oral, and genital)	Contact
	Mucocutaneous, recurrent (skin, oral, and genital)	Drainage/secretion
Herpes zoster (varicella zoster)	Localized in immunocompromised patient, or disseminated	Strict
Epstein-Barr	Infectious mononucleosis	None
Adenoviruses	Respiratory infection in infants and young children	Contact
Parasites		
Pneumocystis carinii	Pneumonia	None
Toxoplasma gondii	Encephalitis, brain abscess	None
Cryptosporidium species	Gastroenteritis	Enteric
Fungi		
Candida species	Infection at any site, including mucocutaneous (thrush, moniliasis)	None
Cryptococcus neoformans	Infection at any site	None
Histoplasma capsulatum	Infection at any site	None
Aspergillus species	Infection at any site	None

[a]Unless stool culture negative.

organisms in health-care settings. Detailed instructions for isolation precautions are outlined in the "CDC Guideline for Isolation Precautions in Hospitals."

Private Versus Multiple-Bed Rooms for HIV-Infected Patients

A private room is not necessary for patients infected with HIV unless the patient's hygiene is poor or the presence of other infections makes a private room necessary (e.g., infection with *Mycobacterium tuberculosis*). However, if HIV-infected patients or other immunosuppressed patients are placed in the same room, cross-infection with opportunistic pathogens may occur. If intensive-care unit (ICU) care is required, HIV-infected patients without infections requiring a private room may be placed in an open ICU. Otherwise, an isolation room is desirable.

Tuberculosis

Transmission of tuberculosis in the health-care setting has been well documented. Concern about nosocomial transmission of tuberculosis has been heightened by recent outbreaks in health-care settings, including outbreaks involving multidrug-resistant strains of *M. tuberculosis* in HIV-infected patients.

Nosocomial transmission of tuberculosis is most likely to occur from patients with unrecognized pulmonary or laryngeal tuberculosis who are not on effective antituberculous therapy and have not been placed in tuberculosis isolation. Recognition of tuberculosis in HIV-infected persons may be delayed because of impaired response to tuberculin skin testing, atypical clinical or radiographic presentations, simultaneous occurrence of other pulmonary infections, low sensitivity of sputum smears for detecting acid-fast bacilli (AFB), and overgrowth of cultures with *Mycobacterium avium* complex among patients with dual infections.

The guideline for the prevention of tuberculosis transmission in health-care settings in the United States was revised in 1994. The new guideline retains the basic elements of tuberculosis infection control. However, precautions are grouped into the following hierarchy:

1. Administrative measures to reduce generation of infectious airborne particles, e.g., rapid detection, isolation, diagnostic evaluation, and treatment of persons likely to have tuberculosis.
2. Engineering (environmental) controls to prevent the spread and reduce the concentration of infectious droplet nuclei, e.g., tuberculosis isolation rooms with air exhausted directly to the outside, negative pressure with respect to the hallway, and at least six air exchanges per hour. Additional recommendations for ventilation of rooms used for tuberculosis isolation have been published.
3. Personal respiratory protective equipment (e.g., respirators) in areas where there is still a risk of exposure to *M. tuberculosis*, such as tuberculosis isolation rooms.

The draft also provides criteria for categorization of health-care facilities, or areas within facilities, as high, intermediate, and low risk for nosocomial transmission of tuberculosis. The suggested frequency of health-care worker tuberculin skin testing, evaluation of the tuberculosis infection control program, and detailed engineering evaluation of tuberculosis isolation rooms depends on the level of assessed risk for nosocomial transmission of tuberculosis.

Cytomegalovirus

Many patients with AIDS are infected with and excrete cytomegalovirus (CMV). Although CMV has been found in nearly all body fluids and secretions, transmission usually results only from close intimate contact. In health-care facilities, transmission has been documented to occur from patient to patient, but not from patient to health-care worker. A practical approach to reducing the risk of infection with CMV among health-care workers is to stress careful handwashing after all patient contacts and to avoid contact with materials that are potentially infective. Because of risk to the fetus, all pregnant patient-care personnel should at least be counseled about precautions for preventing acquisition of CMV. Other measures, such as serologic screening of pregnant personnel, with reassignment of those susceptible, are controversial.

Pneumocystis Carinii

Pneumocystis carinii is usually thought to be ubiquitous, and CDC guidelines do not recommend isolation of patients infected with this organism. However, clusters of *P. carinii* infection have been noted in immunosuppressed persons, and a cluster in elderly immunocompetent patients has recently been reported. Such reports have led some authors to recommend isolation of patients infected with this organism.

ISOLATION GUIDELINE UPDATE

In 1996 the CDC's Hospital Infection Control Practices Advisory Committee published a revised and updated system of infection control that encompasses concepts of both universal precautions and body substance isolation in a set of precautions to be termed "standard precautions." Under standard precautions, precautions are indicated to prevent contact with all body fluids, secretions, excretions, nonintact skin, and mucous membranes of all patients. In addition to standard precautions, transmission-based precautions will be used for specific patients documented or suspected to be infected with highly transmissible or epidemiologically important pathogens for which additional precautions are needed (e.g., airborne precautions for patients with infectious pulmonary tuberculosis).

PRECAUTIONS FOR SPECIFIC SETTINGS

Dental and Oral Surgical Procedures

Most microorganisms known to be human pathogens have been isolated from oral secretions. General infection-control precautions and disinfection and sterilization procedures for dentistry have been described.

Blood, saliva, and gingival fluid from all dental patients should be considered potential sources of blood-borne pathogens requiring universal precautions. In addition to wearing gloves for contact with oral mucous membranes of all patients, dental workers should wear surgical masks and protective eyewear or chin-length plastic face-shields during procedures in which splashing or splattering of blood, saliva, or gingival fluids is likely. Rubber dams, high-speed evacuation, and proper patient positioning, when appropriate, should be used to minimize generation of droplets and spatter.

Although an instance of probable transmission of HIV from a dentist to patients has been reported, adherence to basic infection control principles (e.g., sterilization and disinfection, universal precautions) will prevent transmission of HIV and other blood-borne pathogens in the dental setting.

Hemodialysis and Peritoneal Dialysis

Patients infected with HIV may occasionally require hemodialysis or peritoneal dialysis. In 1992, 1.5% of U.S. hemodialysis patients were reported to be HIV infected, and 0.7% were reported to have AIDS. An HIV serosurvey among hemodialysis patients at 28 dialysis centers found that none of 254 seronegative patients became HIV-positive during a one-year follow-up period. Transmission of HIV infection in U.S. hemodialysis centers has not been reported. HIV-infected patients can be dialyzed in hospital-based or free-standing dialysis units using conventional infection-control precautions. Universal precautions should be used when dialyzing all patients. Procedures for disinfecting the fluid pathways of the hemodialysis machine are targeted to control bacterial contamination and need not be changed for dialyzing patients infected with HIV.

When HIV-infected patients receive peritoneal dialysis, peritoneal dialysis bags and other disposable items can be disposed of in the same fashion as other solid waste. Bags containing peritoneal dialysis fluid should be handled with care, but extraordinary precautions are not needed. Disposable gloves should be worn when handling bags containing peritoneal dialysis fluid. In the home environment, the peritoneal dialysis fluid can be carefully poured down a toilet. The empty bag should be wrapped securely in an impervious plastic bag or double bagged and discarded in the conventional trash system.

Surgical Procedures

Surgical personnel should routinely use barrier precautions, such as gloves, masks, and gowns or aprons; protective eyewear or face shields should be used during procedures likely to cause splashes or droplets of blood and body fluids, or to generate bone chips. Observational studies have reported percutaneous injuries such as needlesticks and cuts during 1.3% to 6.9% of surgical procedures, and blood contacts of any type (percutaneous injuries, blood–skin contacts, and blood–mucous membrane contacts) during 6.4% to 46.6% of procedures. Because many blood contacts are caused by perforations in surgical gloves, use of two pairs of gloves ("double-gloving") has been suggested. Use of instruments, such as a forceps, to manipulate suture needles may help minimize the number of percutaneous injuries during surgery. Careful adherence to guidelines will help to minimize blood contacts during surgery, but innovative approaches to this problem may also be required.

Laboratories

Universal precautions should be observed when handling specimens of blood, other fluids to which universal precautions apply, and tissues from all patients. Specimens should be placed in secure containers for transport. Laboratory workers processing blood and body fluid specimens should wear gloves, and a mask and protective eyewear should be worn if generation of droplets or splashes is likely. Mouth pipetting should not be done, and use of needles and syringes should be limited to situations in which there is no alternative. After completion of laboratory activities, protective clothing should be removed and hands washed.

Postmortem Care

Universal precautions should be followed during postmortem procedures on all patients. In addition, gloves, masks, protective eyewear, gowns, and waterproof aprons should be worn, and instruments and surfaces that become contaminated during the procedure should be disinfected with an appropriate chemical germicide.

OTHER INFECTION CONTROL CONSIDERATIONS

Pregnant Health-Care Workers

Pregnant health-care workers are not known to be at greater risk of contracting HIV infection than health-care workers who are not pregnant; however, if a health-care worker develops HIV infection during pregnancy, the infant is at risk of infection from perinatal transmission. Therefore, pregnant health-care workers should be especially familiar with and strictly adhere to precautions to minimize the risk of HIV transmission.

Immunosuppressed Health-Care Workers

Health-care workers with defective immune systems are not known to be at greater risk of acquiring HIV infection than workers with normal immune systems. However, they may have an increased risk of acquiring or experiencing serious complications from other infectious diseases. Of particular concern is the risk of severe infection following exposure to patients infected with HIV who may be infected with microorganisms that are easily transmitted if appropriate precautions are not adhered to (e.g., *M. tuberculosis*). Health-care workers with defective immune systems should be counseled about the potential risk associated with taking care of patients with transmissible infections and should follow existing recommendations for infection control to minimize their risk of exposure to other infectious agents.

Blood and Blood Products

The risk of acquiring HIV infection from transfusion of blood and blood products has been significantly reduced by voluntary deferral of blood donation by those with HIV risk factors and screening of donated blood for HIV since 1985. The risk from screened blood has been estimated by statistical models to be 1:38,000 to 1:153,000 per unit, and by prospective studies to be approximately 1:60,000 per unit. Strategies that have been suggested to minimize the risk include increased use of blood from female donors, use of blood from a smaller group of donors who make frequent donations and consequently have been repeatedly tested for HIV, transfusion of fewer units, and, in any one patient, use of blood from as small a number of donors as possible.

Factor concentrates that have been heat-treated or otherwise treated to reduce the risk of transmission of infectious agents are available for treatment of persons with hemophilia. Instances of HIV seroconversion associated with the use of heat-treated products are now rare; the rate of HIV seroconversion among those using such products appears to be less than 1 per 1,000 persons per year.

Two types of hepatitis B vaccines are licensed in the United States: recombinant vaccine produced in yeast cultures and vaccine derived from human plasma. Although plasma-derived vaccines have not been associated with disease transmission, they are no longer produced in the United States, and there use is now limited to hemodialysis patients, other immunocompromised hosts, and persons with known allergy to yeast.

Transmission of HIV has not been associated with use of immune globulin preparations.

CONCLUSION

Health-care institutions should develop educational programs regarding the epidemiology of HIV and precautions recommended to prevent transmission of bloodborne infection. Universal precautions, a set of precautions to prevent transmission of HIV and other blood-borne pathogens, should be followed during care of all patients. Additional disease-specific or category-specific precautions should be used if patients have infectious diseases transmitted by non–blood-borne routes. Adherence to routine procedures for disinfection, sterilization, and environmental hygiene is adequate during care of persons with HIV infection.

ACKNOWLEDGMENTS

We gratefully acknowledge the assistance of David M. Bell, M.D., Mary E. Chamberland, M.D., M.P.H., Martin S. Favero, Ph.D., and Julie Garner, R.N., M.S., Hospital Infections Program, Center for Infectious Diseases, CDC, in preparation of this chapter.

SUGGESTED READING

Beekman SE, Vlahov D, Kozoil DE, McShalley ED, Schmitt JM, Henderson DK. Temporal association between implementation of universal precautions and a sustained, progressive decrease in percutaneous exposures to blood. *Clin Infec Dis* 1994;18:562–569.

CDC. Public health service statement on management of occupational exposure to human immunodeficiency virus, including considerations regarding zidovudine postexposure use. *MMWR* 1990; 39(RR-1).

CDC. Human immunodeficiency virus transmission in household settings—United States. *MMWR* 1994;43:347,353–356.

Centers for Disease Control and Prevention. Guidelines for preventing the transmission of *Mycobacterium tuberculosis* in health-care facilities—1994. *MMWR* 1994;43(RR-13).

Ciesielski C, Marianos D, Ou CY, et al. Transmission of human immunodeficiency virus in a dental practice. *Ann Intern Med* 1992;116:798–805.

Favero MS. Dialysis associated diseases and their control. In: Bennett JV, Brachman PS, eds. *Hospital infections*, 2nd ed. Boston: Little, Brown, 1985;267–284.

Garner JS. Guidelines for isolation precautions in hospitals. *Infect Control Hosp Epidemiol* 1996;17:54–80.

Gerberding JL. Management of occupational exposures to blood-borne viruses. *N Engl J Med* 1995; 332:444–451.

Health Resources and Services Administration. *Guidelines for construction and equipment of hospital and medical facilities*. Rockville, MD: US Department of Health and Human Services, Public Health Service, 1984; PHS publication no. (HRSA) 84-14500.

Jagger J, Hunt EH, Brand-Elnaggar J, Pearson RD. Rates of needlestick injury caused by various devices in a university hospital. *N Engl J Med* 1988;319:284–288.

Janssen RS, Bolyard EA. Considerations for programs for routine, voluntary HIV counseling and testing of patients in acute-care hospitals. In: Schochetman G, George JR, eds. *AIDS testing*, 2nd ed. New York: Springer-Verlag, 1994.

Jarvis WR. Nosocomial transmission of multidrug-resistant *Mycobacterium tuberculosis*. *Res Microbiol* 1993;144:117–122.

Rhodes RH, Bell DM, eds. Prevention of transmission of bloodborne pathogens in surgery and obstetrics. *Surg Clin North Am* 1995;75:1047–1241.

Robert LM, Bell DM. Human immunodeficiency virus transmission in health care settings: risk and risk reduction. *Infect Dis Clin North Am* 1994;8:319–329.

Tokars JI, Marcus R, Culver DH, et al. Surveillance of HIV infection and zidovudine use among health-care workers after occupational exposure to HIV-infected blood. *Ann Intern Med* 1993;118:913–919.

A Clinical Guide to AIDS and HIV,
edited by Gary P. Wormser.
Lippincott-Raven Publishers, Philadelphia © 1996.

10

Antiretroviral Chemotherapy

Robert T. Schooley

*Infectious Disease Division, University of Colorado Health Sciences Center,
Denver, Colorado 80134*

Antiretroviral chemotherapy is at a crossroads on the 15th anniversary of the initial description of AIDS. Over the past decade, the etiologic agent for AIDS, human immunodeficiency virus type-1 (HIV-1), as been isolated, and multiple isolates have been sequenced. Much has been learned at the molecular level about replicative and regulatory mechanisms of HIV-1. This knowledge, coupled with a deepening appreciation of HIV pathogenesis, has led to an increasing array of potential approaches to therapeutic intervention. At this writing, four antiretroviral drugs have been approved by the Food and Drug Administration. The expansion of treatment investigational new drug (IND) programs, the increasing availability of drugs from "underground" sources, and the trend toward more widespread application of combination chemotherapy have added further complexity to management of the antiretroviral aspects of therapeutic regimens for individuals with HIV infection. This chapter outlines a reasonable current approach to antiretroviral chemotherapy and provides insight into the directions likely to be followed by the field over the next several years.

RATIONAL DESIGN OF ANTIRETROVIRAL CHEMOTHERAPEUTIC AGENTS

The rational development of antiretroviral chemotherapy compounds is based on the development of agents that are directed at aspects of the viral replicative cycle that are not shared by the host. In the case of HIV-1, additional complexity is added by the wide variety of cell types in which the virus replicates, artifacts that are introduced by the *in vitro* cultivation of the virus in continuous cell lines, and the highly error-prone process of reverse transcription. The high rate of errors introduced into the replicative process results in major strain diversity at the population level and in a propensity in individual patients for the emergence of strains with reduced susceptibility to antiretroviral agents following prolonged exposure to antiviral drugs. Finally, HIV-1 poses unique problems of drug delivery, both in terms of general pharmacokinetic principles, which must take into account the probable need for the continuous maintenance of therapeutic levels of drug and the need for penetration of the central nervous system, and in terms of the intracellular site of action for many of the currently contemplated agents.

The initial step in replication of HIV-1 involves its use of the CD4 molecule as its major ligand for interaction of the viral envelope of glycoprotein, gp120, with susceptible cells. This high-affinity interaction, which accounts for much of the selectivity of the virus for cells of the CD4 surface phenotype, has led to several major efforts directed at interfering with gp120–CD4 binding.

After gaining entry into a susceptible cell, the virus is confronted with the problem of converting its genetic information, which is contained in two identical strands of single-stranded RNA, into double-stranded DNA. This conversion requires reverse transcription of the viral genomic RNA in the hostile milieu of the cellular cytoplasm. This reverse transcription is mediated by an RNA-dependent DNA polymerase known as reverse transcriptase. This enzyme has, so far, served as the major target for antiretroviral drug development. Inhibition of reverse transcription is the mechanism of action for all the nucleoside analogues currently approved or in development (zidovudine [AZT], didanosine [ddI], zalcitabine [ddC], stavudine [D4T]), as well as for the class of allosteric inhibitors known as nonnucleoside reverse transcriptase inhibitors (NNRTs).

The double-stranded DNA that results from reverse transcription may exist in a free form within the cytoplasm of the cell for several days, or it may be integrated into the host cell DNA. Cellular activation favors integration, which is catalyzed by another viral enzyme termed integrase. Systems have been developed to screen for inhibitors of integrase activity, but no compounds have yet emerged from these screening attempts into later stages of drug development. After integration, the virus may remain within the host cell in latent form for long periods of time. Viral transcription is controlled by the long terminal repeat (LTR) sequence of the virus. Activation of the viral LTR sequence is, like integration, favored by cellular activation. HIV-1 has evolved a complex regulatory strategy to control its replication. This regulatory process includes several HIV-1 gene products that interact to control splicing and intracellular trafficking of viral RNA. *Tat* is an 86-kd protein that binds to a short segment to of viral messenger RNAs. *Tat* binding segments of viral messenger RNAs, which are termed the trans-acting responsive (TAR) region, are located in the 5' end of all HIV-1 messenger RNAs. Binding of these segments by *tat* protein enhances the efficiency of viral replication by several thousandfold.

Rev is another regulatory gene of HIV-1 that plays a critical role in determining the success of the virus in production of its structural genes, especially the viral envelope. *Rev* encodes a protein that binds to messenger RNA encoding the viral envelope and that is required for efficient translation of the viral envelope mRNA. No prototypic drugs have yet been developed that inhibit the action of the *rev* protein, but it is clear that both *tat* and *rev* will receive increasing attention as potential targets of both chemotherapeutic and genetic approaches to antiretroviral therapy.

Several other viral genes including *nef, vif, vpu,* and *vpr* with regulatory properties or properties affecting efficiency of cell-to-cell transmission of HIV have also been identified. At this point several investigative groups are attempting to delineate in more detail the function of these genes using molecular biologic approaches. The demonstration of the importance of *nef* in determining the clinical virulence of simian immunodeficiency virus type 1 suggests that interference with the function of the *nef* gene product might pose an excellent target for antiretroviral drug development.

Translation of the viral gag–pol messenger RNA results in a large fusion polyprotein that must be cleaved into separate gag and pol proteins. This cleavage is mediated by a viral proteinase, which is located within the polyprotein near the gag–pol junction. This proteinase activity, which cleaves the large gag–pol fusion polyprotein into the polymerase component and into four separate gag polypeptides, is essential for the production of viral structural proteins that are capable of being assembled into infectious viral particles. Several groups have developed compounds that are capable of inhibiting the viral proteinase with a high degree of selectivity.

The envelope glycoprotein of HIV-1 is heavily glycosylated by cellular glycosidation enzymes. Inhibition of this process results in a significant reduction in viral infectivity. This approach has been demonstrated to be extremely effective *in vitro*, but because the target for such inhibition is cellular, rather than viral, in origin, there have been no reported clinical trials that have demonstrated antiviral activity in the absence of unacceptable toxicity.

After synthesis of viral structural proteins has occurred, viral genomic RNA is packaged with the structural elements of the virus at the cell membrane. Viral packaging is a complex process that is dependent on the recognition of specific sequences within the RNA. Inhibition of this recognition process has been put forward as a potential antiviral strategy, but a practical means of achieving this goal has not yet been developed. Inhibition of packaging has also been hypothesized to be one of the sites of action of interferon-α, although it is not yet clear whether this is the primary mechanism by which interferons mediate antiretroviral activity. Evidence has been developed that the *vif* gene product plays a role in maintaining integrity of the viral particle and thus increasing the infectivity of the free viral particle.

Thus many potential steps in the viral replicative cycle have been identified that might serve as excellent candidates for the rational development of effective antiretroviral agents. This chapter focuses primarily on approaches that have progressed to clinical trials and practice, namely, inhibition of binding or entry, reverse transcription, viral proteinase activity, glycosylation, and packaging.

INHIBITORS OF REVERSE TRANSCRIPTION

Up to now, the greatest success in the development of antiretroviral drugs has been derived from agents directed at inhibiting reverse transcription. The prototype

TABLE 1. *Selected antiretroviral agents classified by putative mechanism of action*

A. Inhibitors of binding or entry
  1. Recombinant soluble CD4
  2. CD4/immunoglobulin conjugates
  3. Dextran sulfate
  4. Carbomethoxycarbonyl-pyrolyl-phenalanine esters (CPFs)
B. Reverse transcriptase inhibitors
  1. Nucleoside analogues
    a. Zidovudine (AZT, Retrovir)
    b. Zalcitabine (dideoxycytidine, ddC)
    c. Didanosine (dideoxyinosine, ddI)
    d. Stavudine (3'-Deoxythymidin-2'-ene, D4T)
    e. 3TC
  2. Nonnucleoside analogues
    a. Tetrahydro-imidazol (4-5 1-j,k) (1,4) benzodiazepin-2-(1H)-one ("TIBO")
    b. Dipyridodiazepinone (BI-RG-587)
    c. Other pyridinone derivatives (L-697, 661)
    d. Foscarnet (Foscavir)
C. TAT inhibitors
D. Protease inhibitors
E. Glycosylation inhibitors
  1. Castanospermine
  2. *l*-deoxynojirimycin (*N*-butyl-DNJ)
F. Interferons

drug in this class, zidovudine (AZT, Retrovir), made its debut as an antineoplastic agent in the 1960s and was resurrected as an antiretroviral drug in 1985. Zidovudine is capable of inhibiting HIV replication in cell lines at concentrations in the range of 0.1 μm. Zidovudine and the other nucleoside analogues currently in development as antiretroviral agents serve as competitive inhibitors of reverse transcription (Table 1). In each case these nucleoside analogues are taken up by cells susceptible to HIV infection and phosphorylated by kinases of the host cell to triphosphate derivatives of the parent compound. These nucleotides are incorporated by the reverse transcriptase enzyme as the viral RNA template is used to construct complementary DNA (Fig. 1). This incorporation prevents further elongation of the DNA and terminates reverse transcription. Thus, because such agents serve primarily to protect susceptible cells from initial infection with HIV, these agents have no effect on previously infected cells.

Zidovudine

Demonstration of Efficacy

Zidovudine was initially found to have antiretroviral activity against murine retroviruses in the 1960s. Broder and his colleagues noted that zidovudine also had

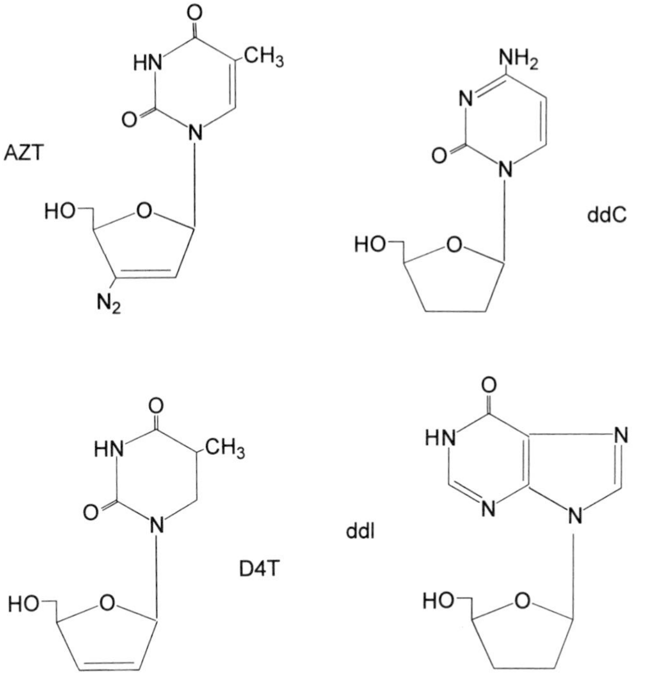

FIG. 1. Comparison of chemical structures of four nucleoside analogue reverse transcriptase inhibitors: zidovudine (AZT), zalcitabine (ddC), didanosine (ddI), and stavudine (D4T).

activity against HIV-1 in tissue culture and initiated a small phase I escalating dose tolerance trial of zidovudine in individuals with advanced HIV infection in 1985. This trial demonstrated that the drug could be tolerated in doses of up to 15 to 20 mg/kg/day, but that hematologic toxicity limited further dose escalation.

Based on these results, a placebo-controlled trial was designed that subsequently enrolled 282 subjects with AIDS or advanced AIDS-related complex (ARC). This trial chose the maximally tolerated zidovudine dose that had been determined with the phase I trial (1,500 mg/day). This study was terminated by a Data Safety and Monitoring Board after 4 months when it became apparent that there was a significant excess in morbidity and mortality in study participants receiving placebo. The initial placebo-controlled trial of zidovudine also exhibited significant toxicity. The major dose-limiting toxicity was hematologic. Forty-five percent of study participants receiving zidovudine experienced hematologic toxicity; more than 30% of zidovudine recipients required transfusions. In addition to hematologic toxicity, zidovudine recipients were more likely to experience fatigue, anorexia, and mild to moderate headaches. This study resulted in approval of zidovudine by the Food and Drug Administration in July 1987 for individuals with AIDS or with symptoms of HIV infection and less than 200 CD4 cells/mm^3 in the peripheral blood.

Dose Modification and Extension to Earlier Stages of HIV Infection

The past 4 years have witnessed a host of clinical trials that have provided a better understanding of optimal dosing for zidovudine and that have extended its use to earlier phases of the illness. Shortly after the completion of the initial placebo-controlled trial, three additional studies conducted by the National Institutes of Health (NIH)-sponsored AIDS Clinical Trials Group (ACTG) provided important insights into both dosing of zidovudine and the utility of antiretroviral chemotherapy at earlier stages in the disease process. ACTG 002 compared a 1,200-mg daily dose of zidovudine to a regimen that included a 6-week "induction" phase of 1,500 mg daily followed by 100 mg every 4 hours. This study demonstrated that the higher dose of zidovudine conferred no advantages in terms of survival or prevention of recurrent *Pneumocystic carinii* pneumonia. Those receiving the lower daily dose of zidovudine were able to be maintained on zidovudine therapy for a significantly longer period of time than those randomized to the 1,200-mg daily dose arm. On the basis of this trial and a subsequent dose-finding study in patients in earlier stages of the disease process (ACTG 019), the highest recommended daily dose of zidovudine was reduced to 500 to 600 mg daily. A small pilot study has demonstrated that serum levels of HIV-1 p24 antigen can be suppressed by as little as 300 mg of zidovudine daily. This study has been widely misinterpreted to suggest that equal clinical efficacy has been demonstrated at this dose of zidovudine as with the currently accepted 500- to 600-mg daily dose. The pilot study was conducted with the primary goal of determining the dose of zidovudine that would be just below that which would decrease serum HIV-1 p24 antigen. Participation in the study was restricted by the FDA to individuals with more than 200 CD4 cells/mm^3 and serum HIV-1 p24 antigen levels of more than 700 pg/ml. In this highly selected patient population, which included less than 70 participants, serum HIV p24 antigen levels were suppressed as effectively by 300 mg of zidovudine daily as by doses of up to 1,200 mg daily. The study did not examine clinical endpoints or include individuals with more advanced disease. At this point it is premature to conclude that the 300-mg daily dose of zidovudine is equivalent to the currently recommended 500- to 600-mg daily dose in terms of clinical efficacy.

Two large-scale studies examined the role of zidovudine in individuals with less advanced disease. ACTG 016 enrolled 711 participants who had one or two early signs of HIV infection. These study participants were stratified into a group with more than 500 CD4 cells/mm^3 at entry and a second group with 200 to 500 CD4 cells/mm^3 and randomized to receive either 1,200 mg of zidovudine daily or a placebo. This study was terminated when it was determined that study participants receiving placebo entering the trial with less than 500 CD4 cells/mm^3 progressed to AIDS or late AIDS-related complex at roughly three times the rate of those receiving zidovudine. Too few individuals entered the study with more than 500 CD4 cells/mm^3 to detect differences in the progression rate in this stratum of study participants.

A parallel study was also conducted that recruited 3,200 asymptomatic HIV-infected individuals. This study had a similar design in that participants were randomized to receive zidovudine or placebo. In this study, however, individuals were stratified into a group with less than 200 CD4 cells/mm^3 at entry, another with 200 to 500 CD4 cells/mm^3, and a final group with more than 500 CD4 cells/mm^3. Participants in each CD4 cell stratum were then randomized to received a placebo or one of two daily doses of zidovudine (500 or 1,500 mg daily). This study demonstrated that zidovudine at either dose level decreased by half the rate of clinical progression to AIDS or advanced ARC among trial participants entering the study with less than 500 CD4 cells/mm^3. Hematologic toxicity was significantly more likely (12%) in the 1,500-mg daily dose group than in those receiving 500 mg daily (3%). With the decreased hematologic toxicity of the 500-mg daily dose of drug, and that observed in the aforementioned ACTG 002 study, the recommended daily dose of zidovudine has been reduced to 500 to 600 mg administered daily in three divided doses.

Use of Zidovudine in Earlier Stages of HIV-1 Infection

Considerable controversy remains as to the optimal stage at which antiretroviral therapy should be initiated. From the theoretical standpoint, and by analogy with other infectious diseases, it would seem most logical to initiate therapy as soon as infection is detected. This strategy has yet to be supported in controlled clinical trials. The use of antiretroviral therapy in primary infection has been examined in a randomized, double-blinded, placebo-controlled clinical trial. This study, undertaken by a consortium of European and Australian investigators, enrolled individuals within an average of one month following the onset of symptoms of primary HIV-1 infection. Study participants were randomized to a regimen of zidovudine (250 mg bid) or a matching placebo for a period of 6 months, and were observed for an additional year during which most study participants were on no antiretroviral therapy. This trial revealed that treatment during primary HIV-1 infection is associated with fewer clinical manifestations of HIV-1–associated immunodeficiency (herpes zoster, oral thrush, hairy leukoplakia), and that those receiving drug had significantly greater CD4 cell counts one year following the blinded period of the study. Coupled with the absence of either significant drug toxicity in the treated group or the emergence of viral isolates with reduced susceptibility to zidovudine, the study has lent support to the concept that earlier therapy might be indicated in certain settings. The routine use of antiretroviral therapy during primary infection has been complicated by the finding that there is an increased incidence of transmission of zidovudine-resistant isolates in a study undertaken in several European, American, and Australian cities.

Until 1993, most North American clinicians recommended the initiation of antiretroviral therapy in HIV-1–infected individuals when CD4 cells dropped below 500 cells/mm^3. With the publication of the British/French Concorde study, however, a considerable amount of debate has arisen concerning these recommendations. The Concorde study was initiated prior to the completion of the ACTG trials (ACTG 016 and 019) that defined 500 CD4 cells as the threshold for the initiation of antiretroviral therapy of HIV-1–infected individuals. As originally conceived, the Concorde study sought to compare the strategy of immediate initiation of zidovudine therapy in asymptomatic individuals with that of delaying therapy until HIV-1–related symptoms developed. According to the original Concorde design, asymptomatic HIV-1–infected individuals were randomly assigned to receive zidovudine (500 mg bid) upon enrollment (immediate therapy), or to a matching placebo (delayed therapy). Upon the onset of HIV-1–related symptoms, zidovudine therapy was to be offered to those initially assigned to placebo. The primary endpoints of the study were to be death or the onset of an AIDS-defining illness.

Enrollment in the Concorde study was still under way when the ACTG studies were completed that demonstrated zidovudine therapy resulted in a delay in the progression of HIV-1 disease in individuals with less than 500 CD4 cells/mm^3. Concorde investigators then decided, for ethical reasons and because of the wish to retain the study subject population, to alter the trial design to allow any participant with <500 CD4$^+$ cells/mm^3 to elect open-label zidovudine if he or she had been in the trial for more than 6 months. This option was elected by most study participants who dropped below 500 CD4 cells/mm^3. At the completion of the study, the trial was analyzed according to the initially assigned group. With the significant degree of use of open-label zidovudine by study participants most likely to progress (those with <500 CD4 cells/mm^3), this analysis resulted in the comparison of two groups of study participants that received overlapping therapeutic regimens. As in ACTG studies 016 and 019, disease progression was delayed for the first 12 to 18 months of the trial. However, no differences were noted between the two arms with respect to survival or the onset of AIDS at the end of the full 3 years of the trial. Because of the modification of the trial design, the question posed by Concorde investigators (the benefits of immediate vs. delayed therapy) was not addressed in a straightforward fashion, and it is difficult to draw definitive conclusions from the study.

Another difficulty in assessing the Concorde study is that the three additional antiretroviral drugs that are now available were not routinely offered to Concorde study participants. Since it is clear that additional benefits of antiretroviral therapy may be obtained by the substitution or addition of these agents in the management of individuals with prior zidovudine experience, the Concorde study does not directly address the most critical question regarding initiation of therapy, namely the optimal time to initiate antiretroviral therapy, rather than the more restricted issue related to the initiation of zidovudine therapy.

A final study of earlier antiretroviral therapy, which utilized a design similar to that initially envisioned for the Concorde study, has recently been reported. This trial, however, sought to determine whether early therapy would delay the onset of "softer" signs of HIV-1 infection such as oral thrush, hairy leukoplakia, or herpes zoster. The study recruited asymptomatic HIV-1–infected study subjects without regard to CD4$^+$ count at entry. The mean CD4 cell count at entry was in the range of 600 cells/mm^3. The primary endpoints of the trial included the first detection of an HIV-1–related symptom, or a fall in CD4$^+$ cells to 350/mm^3 or less. In this study, immediate institution of zidovudine therapy was associated with slower progression to the onset of symptomatic HIV-1 disease, or to a CD4$^+$ cell count of 350 cells/mm^3. Thus, the study demonstrated full immunologic and clinical benefits in individuals treated at earlier stages of the illness.

The collection of the ACTG studies, the Concorde trial, and the European-Australian Cooperative study has left clinicians and patients somewhat confused about the most appropriate time for the initiation of antiretroviral therapy. The availability of ddI, ddC, and D4T renders the earlier studies of the optimal time for initiation of zidovudine less relevant. The potential benefits of antiretroviral therapy must be weighed against the risks in each patient, and patient preference must be taken into account in that such considerations have a strong impact on compliance. At this writing, it seems prudent to offer antiretroviral therapy to symptomatic HIV-1–infected individuals, and to most asymptomatic individuals with <500 CD4 cells/mm^3. As additional studies are completed, and as additional antiretroviral chemotheraputic studies become available, this issue will warrant continuing reevaluation.

Effects of Zidovudine on Other Manifestations of HIV Infection

Zidovudine has also been demonstrated to exhibit beneficial effects on several other complications of HIV infection. At the time the initial efficacy trials were being conducted, there was great concern that zidovudine might have positive effects on viral replication in the periphery, and thus lead to immune restoration and morbidity reduction, but that it would achieve insufficient levels in the central nervous system to reduce the impact of the virus there. This has not proved to be the case. In the initial placebo-controlled trial of zidovudine, an analysis of neuropsychological function demonstrated an improvement in cognitive function among zidovudine recipients. A more recently completed double-blinded randomized study of zidovudine in individuals with HIV encephalopathy as the major clinical manifestation of HIV infection has also demonstrated benefits of zidovudine in this setting (ACTG 005). This study indicated a slightly more beneficial effect with dosing of zidovudine as high as 2 g/day, but the number of individuals in each of the dosing arms of this study is insufficient to recommend this dose of zidovudine on a routine basis for AIDS-dementia complex. Indeed, as zidovudine has achieved wider use in the early phases of the disease process, epidemiologic surveys have indicated a decrease in the incidence of the AIDS-dementia complex.

Thrombocytopenia is commonly encountered in the setting of HIV infection. HIV-associated thrombocytopenia may be encountered in AIDS, or it may be the presenting manifestation of the illness in an individual who otherwise has no HIV-related symptoms. The mechanism(s) by which HIV causes thrombocytopenia remains to be fully elucidated. The two mechanisms that have received the most attention are direct involvement of platelet precursors in HIV-infected individuals and an immune-based mechanism by which immune complexes bind to platelets and enhance clearance by the reticuloendothelial system. A number of approaches to the management of HIV-associated thrombocytopenia including corticosteroids, immune globulin, and splenectomy have been used. Zidovudine has also been shown to be useful in the management of HIV-related thrombocytopenia in both open label and crossover-designed studies.

Zidovudine has not proved useful as a primary therapy for Kaposi's sarcoma, despite anecdotal reports of regression of Kaposi's sarcoma with its use. Zidovudine has been combined with interferon-α in several clinical trials of the efficacy of this combination in the management of Kaposi's sarcoma. In this setting, hematologic toxicity may require dose reduction of the zidovudine to 300 mg daily, but in these trials individuals tolerating zidovudine and interferon-α frequently demonstrated both antitumor effects and rises in CD4 cells in the peripheral blood.

Zidovudine is not efficacious in the management of HIV-associated lymphoma and may complicate the hematologic toxicity of combination chemotherapy. A report from the National Cancer Institute raised concerns that prolonged nucleoside analogue therapy for HIV infection might contribute to the development of non-Hodgkin's lymphoma. A much larger retrospective analysis has not confirmed this observation and suggests a more likely alternative possibility, namely, that prolonged survival associated with antiretroviral chemotherapy and more effective management of HIV-associated opportunistic infections allows the development of lymphoma in individuals who previously would have succumbed to other HIV-related complications.

As noted earlier, zidovudine has been shown to decrease the incidence of HIV-associated opportunistic infections in several placebo-controlled trials. Anecdotal reports have noted the occurrence of temporary remissions of several HIV-associated opportunistic infections including cytomegalovirus retinitis, hairy leukoplakia, molluscum contagiosum, cryptosporidiosis, and progressive multifocal leukoencephalopathy. It is likely that these benefits are mediated in individual cases by partial restoration of pathogen-specific immune responses, although the drug itself has been demonstrated to have efficacy in a murine *Escherichia coli* or *Salmonella dublin* model. Another setting in which reversal of the HIV-associated immune dysfunction by zidovudine has been of demonstrated utility is in the management of HIV-associated psoriasis.

Zidovudine in Children and Special Patient Populations

Zidovudine has also undergone extensive investigation in pediatric populations. These studies, which have included both continuous intravenous and oral administration, have demonstrated similar effects of the drug on disease manifestations, immunologic function, and virologic activity as that seen in adult populations. Because HIV infection has a particularly heavy impact on the neurologic and physical development in children, several of these studies have focused on the effects of zidovudine on neuropsychometric testing, CNS glucose metabolism, or physical growth. These studies have demonstrated both the utility of zidovudine in terms of these measures of HIV-associated morbidity and the suitability of these parameters in the assessment of efficacy of antiretroviral chemotherapy in clinical trials involving children.

An important study has recently examined the effects of zidovudine therapy on perinatal transmission of HIV-1. Natural history studies have demonstrated that HIV-1 is transmitted to about 25% of neonates born to HIV-1–infected mothers. Transmission rates are increased in mothers with more advanced immunologic dysfunction or increased viral load. In an effort to determine whether perinatal transmission can be reduced by antiretroviral therapy, a multicenter study recruited 850 HIV-1–infected pregnant women with >200 CD4 cells/mm^3 to a randomized, blinded, placebo-controlled trial of the effects of zidovudine administration on perinatal HIV-1 transmission. The treated group received oral zidovudine during the third trimester of pregnancy, and intravenous zidovudine during delivery. Children born of mothers randomized to receive zidovudine during pregnancy and delivery were treated with zidovudine for the first 6 weeks of life. An identical group of mothers and children received a parallel placebo regimen. Upon completion of the study, it was determined that zidovudine reduced the transmission rate of HIV-1 from 25% to 8%. This study provided definitive data that antiretroviral therapy reduces perinatal transmission. At this point, however, it is not clear whether all three components of the regimen (oral and intravenous zidovudine for the mother, and postnatal zidovudine for the child) are required to effect this reduction in HIV-1 transmission, and the appropriate approach to women with extensive prior antiretroviral therapy has not yet been delineated.

A study of zidovudine among individuals with early HIV infection initially raised questions as to whether zidovudine's clinical benefits might be restricted to white, non-Hispanic populations. The study revealed a decrease in the rate of occurrence of AIDS-defining opportunistic infections among zidovudine recipients, but a post hoc analysis revealed an apparent increase in the death rate of black and Hispanic study participants who received early zidovudine therapy. The apparent increase, however, included a significant number of deaths unrelated to AIDS, such as suicides and motor vehicle accidents. A much more extensive analysis of the survival experience of the HIV-infected population of Maryland between 1983 and 1989 has revealed survival benefits among minority group members who were treated with zidovudine. In this analysis, non-Hispanic whites had a more prolonged survival than minority group members, but this difference appeared to be primarily related to access to medical care. In addition, an analysis of a much larger experience in NIH-sponsored studies has failed to confirm the concerns raised by the VA CSG 398 study. Thus, at this point, there is no evidence that there is a cultural difference in the responsiveness to antiretroviral chemotherapy.

Zidovudine Toxicity

The major dose-limiting toxicity of zidovudine is suppression of bone marrow function. Bone marrow toxicity is a function both of the stage of disease and the zidovudine dose. Dose-limiting anemia or granulocytopenia is unusual in asymptomatic individuals receiving 500 mg of zidovudine daily. In this setting, discontinuation of the drug or dose reduction is required in less than 3% of individuals. Hematologic toxicity in individuals with AIDS or late ARC taking 1,200 to 1,500 mg daily may occur in over one third of cases.

As experience with granulocytopenia in the setting of HIV infection has accumulated, it has become clear that bacterial sepsis attributable to granulocytopenia is seen less frequently than might be expected from the experiences with cytotoxic chemotherapy. Thus, it is often reasonable to tolerate granulocyte counts of 500 to 750/mm^3 in the setting of HIV infection. Zidovudine-related bone marrow toxicity is almost always reversible. Management of an initial bout of granulocytopenia is approached by withholding the drug temporarily and resuming therapy at a lower dose (generally 300 mg daily). In individuals in whom the granulocyte count does not recover over the course of 7 to 10 days, consideration should be given to other possible causes for the granulocytopenia, including other drugs or involvement of the bone marrow with an infectious organism such as *Mycobacterium avium-intra-cellulare*.

If the granulocytopenia recurs after resumption of reduced dose zidovudine, alternative antiviral agents such as didanosine (ddI), zalcitabine (ddC), or stavudine (D4T) should be considered.

If the granulocytopenia persists despite replacement of zidovudine with ddC or ddI, another option involves the use of granulocyte monocyte–colony stimulating factor (GM-CSF) or granulocyte colony stimulating factor (G-CSF). Although both GM-CSF and G-CSF stimulate production of granulocytes, G-CSF is generally better tolerated than GM-CSF and does not have the theoretical concern that has been raised about stimulation of HIV-1 replication with GM-CSF.

Zidovudine administration is associated with macrocytosis in virtually all individuals who take the drug for more than 6 weeks; this has been used as an indicator of compliance in blinded controlled trials of zidovudine. Anemia, like granulocytopenia, is a dose-related toxicity that occurs more frequently in individuals with more advanced disease. If anemia is encountered in the setting of zidovudine therapy, other causes of anemia, such as hemolysis or bone marrow suppression from other drugs or infection involving the marrow, should be ruled out. As in the case of granulocytopenia, substitution of zidovudine with ddI, d4T, or ddC should be considered if it is determined that the anemia is secondary to zidovudine therapy. With the availability of these alternative agents, there is less rationale for the continued use of zidovudine if transfusions or erythropoietin are required for hematologic support.

In addition to bone marrow toxicity, zidovudine is also associated with several subjective complaints. In the initial randomized placebo-controlled trial of zidovudine, anorexia, mild to moderate headaches, and insomnia were reported significantly more frequently by zidovudine recipients than by those receiving placebo. In practice, anorexia and headache are the subjective complaints that most frequently trouble patients to the extent that discontinuation of the drug is contemplated. In most cases these symptoms subside despite continuation of the drug over the first 2 to 3 weeks of therapy. In situations in which anorexia, nausea, or headache are particularly troublesome, symptomatic relief may be offered with antiemetics, aspirin, or nonsteroidal antiinflammatory agents.

Zidovudine is rarely associated with confusion or more serious alteration of consciousness. The mechanism for this complication of zidovudine therapy has not been delineated, but it is more frequently seen in individuals with underlying CNS dysfunction or in individuals who are taking other drugs with CNS effects. A final toxicity that has been reported with zidovudine is a myositis-like syndrome that is associated with muscle tenderness and wasting. It has been hypothesized that this complication of zidovudine therapy is a manifestation of inhibitory effects of zidovudine on mitochondrial DNA polymerase.

Drug Interactions

Zidovudine undergoes glucuronidation in the liver. Zidovudine and zidovudine glucuronide are both excreted by the kidney. The hepatic metabolism of zidovudine coupled with an apparent increased rate of hematologic toxicity in zidovudine recipients who also received acetaminophen in controlled trials raised concerns about adverse interactions between acetaminophen and zidovudine. This was not confirmed in a subsequent study. The major adverse drug interactions involve zidovudine and other agents that suppress the bone marrow such as interferons, ganciclovir, or cytotoxic chemotherapeutic agents.

Decreased Susceptibility of HIV-1 Isolates to Zidovudine

Over the past several years it has become apparent that antiretroviral therapy is associated with the emergence of viral isolates with reduced susceptibility to the drugs that are employed. In the case of zidovudine, this was first demonstrated by Richman and colleagues, who obtained serial viral isolates from participants in the initial placebo-controlled study of zidovudine. A subsequent *in vitro* analysis revealed a progressive decrease in zidovudine susceptibility in isolates of HIV-1 obtained 12 to 18 months after initiation of zidovudine therapy. Isolates obtained from two trial participants after this period of therapy were 100- to 1,000-fold less susceptible to zidovudine in an *in vitro* plaque-forming assay than were isolates obtained prior to the initiation of therapy. Subsequent studies revealed that the decrease susceptibility to zidovudine is associated with the stepwise appearance of mutations of four amino acids of the reverse transcriptase enzyme. Isolates of HIV-1 with reduced susceptibility to zidovudine exhibit cross-resistance to 3'-azido-2',3'-dideoxyuridine (AZdu), but not to non-azido group containing nucleoside analogue antiretroviral drugs, such as ddC, ddI, or D4T, or to drugs with other mechanisms of antiretroviral activity. Other investigative groups have confirmed and extended these findings, and a polymerase-chain-reaction-based assay for detection of genotypic changes in *pol* associated with the resistant phenotype has been developed. Recently, isolates of HIV-1 that exhibit decreased susceptibility to dideoxyinosine have been obtained from patients receiving ddI. ddI resistance has been detected primarily among isolates obtained from individuals who were first treated for a prolonged period with zidovudine, after which ddI was administered as monotherapy. In one of these reports, the ddI resistance was associated with an amino acid change in the viral reverse transcriptase at a position remote from those that conferred zidovudine resistance. The change related to ddI resistance was associated with restoration of susceptibility to zidovudine. It has been demonstrated that the rate at which isolates with decreased *in vitro* zidovudine susceptibility emerge is a function of disease stage. This is presumably a reflection of increased viral load in individuals with more advanced immunodeficiency.

The clinical significance of the emergence of viral isolates with reduced *in vitro* susceptibility to zidovudine is complex. Individuals with isolates that are sensitive to antiretroviral drugs *in vitro* may exhibit disease progression. Conversely, the emergence of resistant viral isolates does not always signal progression of the illness. This complexity is a reflection of several factors. First, resistance is a multistep phenomenon. Second, in the case of certain agents, mutations incorporated by the virus may be associated with a viral quasi-species that is less vigorous in its replicative capacity. Disease progression also correlates with a number of additional variables, such as viral load and phenotype, that interact with viral susceptibility in a complex fashion. In addition, even in the presence of fully susceptible viral isolates, substantial viral replication continues, and immunologic damage proceeds. Disease progression, when assessed by clinical endpoints, is a somewhat stochastic process that requires the presence of a potential opportunistic pathogen in the absence of effective prophylaxis. Although at least two studies have demonstrated a relationship between resistance to zidovudine and disease progression, no study has yet demonstrated that a change in therapy prompted by the emergence of resistance is associated with an improved clinical outcome. At present there are no data to support the routine use of *in vitro* susceptibility testing in the management of individual patients.

Use of Zidovudine Following Nosocomial Exposure

Transmission of HIV-1 to health-care workers after percutaneous or mucosal exposure to virus-containing material is infrequent. The administration of zidovudine has been recommended after "significant" nosocomial exposure to HIV-1. Such recommendations have been made despite several anecdotal reports of the failure of postexposure prophylaxis to prevent infection, and the absence of animal model data that administration of drug after viral exposure prevents infection. Prevention of infection by administering therapy after exposure is a formidable task. The therapeutic agents currently available merely prevent infection of uninfected cells and must be present in the cytoplasm as triphosphate derivatives of the parent compound at the time of reverse transcription. In addition, many hospitalized patients from whom the infectious virus might have arisen are likely to be in the later stages of infection and thus to have had extensive zidovudine experience. Therefore, it is possible that prophylaxis will be compromised by the fact that the transmitted virus will exhibit less susceptibility to the agent used for prophylaxis. Nonetheless, it is prudent to offer zidovudine after significant nosocomial exposure for several reasons. First, anecdotal reports of transmission following postexposure treatment with zidovudine do not address whether the incidence of infection is decreased by prophylaxis. Second, it is possible that, while early therapy might not prevent infection, a decrease in the early burst of viral replication in the setting of primary infection might be of benefit to the host. Finally, and perhaps most important, the establishment of a comprehensive postexposure counseling and testing service is essential from the standpoint of employee support and of risk management.

Zalcitabine [Dideoxycytidine (ddC)]

Zalcitabine (ddC) is another nucleoside analogue with potent and selective antiretroviral activity. The agent is roughly tenfold more active against HIV-1 *in vitro* than is zidovudine. As with the case with zidovudine, ddC must be phosphorylated intracellularly by cellular kinases. Preclinical studies with ddC revealed that the drug exhibited significantly less hematopoietic toxicity than zidovudine. These findings prompted an escalating dose tolerance trial of ddC, which revealed that the drug exhibited antiviral effects *in vivo*, as ascertained by decreases in the serum HIV-1 p24 antigen levels; however, significant dose-related toxicities were encountered. These included painful peripheral neuropathy, oral ulcerations, a cutaneous eruption, and thrombocytopenia (Table 2). A larger multicenter dose-ranging study was subsequently completed that further refined the relationships among ddC dosage, effects on surrogate markers for antiviral activity, and toxicity. This study revealed that daily doses of ddC in the range of 0.005 to 0.01 mg/kg/day were

TABLE 2. *Pharmacologic characteristics and toxicities of nucleoside analogue reverse transcriptase inhibitors*

Agent	Terminal serum $T_{1/2}$	Intracellular triphosphate $T_{1/2}$	Major toxicities
Zidovudine (AZT)	45–60 min	3 hr	Granulocytopenia, anemia, nausea, headaches, confusion, myositis
Didanosine (ddI)	65–75 min	12 hr	Pancreatitis, peripheral neuropathy, nausea, diarrhea, confusion, gastrointestinal distress
Zalcitabine (ddC)	35–40 min	3 hr	Peripheral neuropathy, stomatitis, cutaneous eruption, pancreatitis
Stavudine (D4T)	75 min	3 hr	Peripheral neuropathy, hepatitis

required for suppression of serum HIV-1 p24 antigen. Peripheral neuropathy was encountered in all patients receiving 0.01 mg/kg/day; the neuropathy was so severe at doses of 0.03 mg/kg/day that discontinuation of medication was frequently required at this dose level. Fewer patients receiving 0.005 mg/kg/day or less required dose modification.

The neuropathy associated with ddC may be relatively sudden in onset and may be extremely severe. Nonetheless, it is almost always reversible if the drug is discontinued promptly. Patients usually note the bilaterally symmetrical onset of painful paresthesias, which are burning in character. These paresthesias may progress to be almost incapacitating if drug administration is continued and may progress to motor involvement. This toxicity, which has proved to be dose-limiting very near the threshold for demonstration of efficacy using surrogate virologic markers, has severely limited the therapeutic niche of ddC.

Several clinical trials have been designed to define the clinical utility of ddC. In a comparison with zidovudine monotherapy as initial therapy, ddC recipients experienced more rapid disease progression, a higher death rate, and a greater number of dose-limiting toxic reactions. Thus, ddC is not recommended for initial therapy of HIV-1–infected individuals. A parallel study of individuals who were clinically stable but who had been on zidovudine for more than a year was terminated prematurely, but suggested that ddC might be as effective as continued zidovudine in this patient population. In a study of individuals who were intolerant of zidovudine or had experienced disease progression despite therapy, ddC appeared to be at least as effective as ddI. Taken together, these studies support the use of ddC monotherapy in advanced stage patient populations that are progressing on other agents or who are intolerant of these agents. Precise recommendations regarding the relative efficacy of ddC and D4T in this setting cannot be made because the two drugs have not been compared directly. Although each drug is well tolerated in advanced disease, it is the clinical impression of many that D4T should be preferentially utilized in this setting if all other factors are equal. In addition to its use in late-stage patients, ddC has found use in combination with zidovudine (see below).

Didanosine [Dideoxyinosine (ddI)]

Didanosine (ddI) is another nucleoside analogue with antiretroviral activity *in vitro*, which followed zidovudine and ddC into clinical trials in 1988. ddI administration is associated with decreases in viral HIV-1 p24 antigen, decreased proviral HIV-1 DNA in peripheral blood mononuclear cells, and increased numbers of CD4 cells. ddI has a serum half-life of 30 to 90 min, but the intracellular half-life of the active metabolite of ddI, dideoxyadenosine triphosphate, is several hours (Table 2). The prolonged intracellular half-life of ddI has prompted the 8- to 12-hour dosing regimen that has been used in most of the phase II/III clinical trials. Pancreatitis is the major toxicity to ddI requiring discontinuation of therapy. The experience in pediatric populations is very similar to that in adults in terms of both efficacy and toxicity. In the expanded access program, pancreatitis associated with ddI was much more frequently encountered in individuals with prior pancreatitis or with clinical or immunologic evidence of advanced disease. Neuropathy is also reported with ddI and may be rapidly encountered in individuals who have experienced ddC-associated neuropathy. Other reported toxicities of ddI include encephalopathy, seizures, optic neuritis, hypokalemia, and hepatitis.

ddI is used primarily as second-line therapy in individuals who have been previously treated with zidovudine or in combination regimens. The largest controlled experience with ddI was obtained by the ACTG in a series of studies that compared it with zidovudine in individuals with varying amounts of prior zidovudine experience. In these studies, zidovudine was superior to ddI in previously untreated individuals with fewer than 300 CD4 cells/mm^3 in terms of prevention of disease progression. In individuals with at least 16 weeks of prior zidovudine therapy, ddI was superior to zidovudine. In individuals with intermediate months of prior zidovudine, the drugs were roughly equivalent in efficacy. The relatively rapid reversal of efficacy to favor the use of ddI in individuals with as little as 16 weeks of prior zidovudine therapy cannot be explained simply on the basis of resistance to zidovudine. Individuals with viral isolates that were sensitive to zidovudine at study entry were only 60% as likely to progress to more advanced disease regardless of treatment assignment to ddI or zidovudine. In a similar fashion, high viral load at entry and the presence of a syncytium including viral phenotype were also associated with more rapid disease progression, regardless of treatment assignment.

Despite the difficulty in crafting a cohesive biologic explanation for these studies, they have led to a relatively strong consensus that zidovudine be used as first-line therapy in most settings. The exact time at which ddI should be substituted for zidovudine in individuals who are tolerating zidovudine, and who are doing well clinically, is less clear. Given the difficult formulation of ddI, and the general reluctance in clinical medicine to change therapy when individuals are doing well, a rigid approach whereby all patients are switched to ddI after exactly 16 weeks of zidovudine therapy cannot be strongly advocated. A strategy in which ddI is used only in those with clear-cut clinical or immunologic failure is likewise difficult to justify. These studies have, nonetheless, significantly lowered the threshold for substituting ddI for zidovudine, or for adding ddI to zidovudine in settings in which combination therapy is warranted.

Stavudine [3′-Deoxythymidin-2′-ene (D4T)]

Stavudine (D4T) exhibits significant antiretroviral activity *in vitro* and is less cytotoxic to bone marrow progenitor cells *in vitro* than is zidovudine. From the subjective standpoint, the drug is extremely well tolerated by most individuals. The major toxicities that have been reported in completed trials of D4T are peripheral neuropathy and hepatitis, both of which occur in 15% to 20% of individuals. In most cases peripheral neuropathy and hepatitis are reversible with discontinuation of the drug, and resumption of dosing at a lower dose. D4T was approved under the Food and Drug Administration's accelerated approval process in 1994 on the basis of an interim analysis of surrogate marker data from a trial comparing D4T to zidovudine in a group of individuals with an average of 18 months of prior zidovudine therapy. In this study individuals randomized to D4T maintained CD4 cells at a higher level, and experienced a more significant decline in viral load than those randomized to zidovudine. This study continues at this writing with plans for an analysis of clinical events during 1995. As was initially the case with ddI, clinicians and patients are confronted with a need to make decisions about the appropriate use of D4T without definitive clinical data. The FDA's approval suggested that the drug should be used by individuals who are experiencing advancing HIV-1 disease despite therapy with other approved agents, or for whom other forms of therapy are inappropriate. In practice, D4T is used primarily in individuals with relatively advanced disease after experience with zidovudine and ddI, and, sometimes, ddC. The use of D4T in combination regimens is controversial in that it utilizes the same intracellular kinases as zidovudine for phosphorylation, and, thus, could antagonize the antiviral activity of zidovudine. *In vitro* studies on this point have yielded conflicting results, and the *in vivo* interaction has not yet been studied rigorously.

3TC, Lamivudine

3TC is another nucleoside that is currently undergoing clinical development. The drug is a nucleoside analogue reverse transcriptase inhibitor with potent antiretroviral activity that has been well tolerated in initial clinical trials. The major difficulty with the development of 3TC lies in the rapid rate at which viral isolates with reduced 3TC susceptibility arise both *in vitro* and *in vivo*. Of potential major interest is the fact that 3TC induces a point mutation at position 180 of the HIV-1 reverse transcriptase gene product that appears to inhibit the emergence of the position 215 mutation characteristic of zidovudine resistance. This finding, coupled with the excellent tolerance of the drug in preliminary studies, has kindled interest in using the drug in combination with zidovudine to take advantage of this interaction between the two drugs with respect to resistance. Preliminary trials utilizing this strategy have, indeed, yielded extremely promising results, suggesting that 3TC might have an important role in combination therapy, despite its limitations as a single agent.

Nonnucleoside-Based Reverse Transcriptase Inhibitors

Several investigative groups have independently discovered a series of nonnucleoside compounds that exhibit potent inhibitory activity against the HIV-1, but not the HIV-2, reverse transcriptase enzyme. The agents are collectively known as nonnucleoside reverse transcriptase inhibitors (NNRTIs). These compounds are superficially quite dissimilar in terms of structure but exert antiretroviral activity by the same allosteric mechanism of action. Each group of agents is extremely selective for HIV-1. The agents exhibit activity against strains of HIV-1 that show reduced zidovudine susceptibility. NNRTIs exhibit synergistic antiretroviral activity with nucleoside analogue antiretroviral agents. The clinical utility of NNRTIs has not yet been demonstrated. The major difficulty with the use of these agents resides in the rapid emergence of resistance both *in vitro* and *in vivo*. The excellent pharmacokinetic profile and the relatively good tolerance of this class of drugs in clinical trials has raised the possibility that one or more of these agents will still find clinical utility if regimens are utilized that result in higher serum levels of the drugs.

Foscarnet (phosphonoformate, PFA) is a pyrophosphase analogue that exhibits activity against both retroviruses and herpes group viruses, including cytomegalovirus. The antiretroviral activity is mediated by inhibition of reverse transcriptase activity and is demonstrable *in vitro* at concentrations of drug in serum that are attainable following intravenous administration. Although suppression of serum HIV-1 p24 antigen has been demonstrated in clinical trials, this activity has required intravenous administration of the drug. The poor absorption of foscarnet after oral administration limits its potential clinical utility except in selected settings.

HIV-1 PROTEASE (PROTEINASE) INHIBITORS

As noted earlier, the HIV-1 gag–pol fusion polyprotein is cleaved by a viral proteinase (protease) that is contained within the gag–pol polyprotein. The viral protease enzyme has been expressed in *E. coli* and found to be a dimeric aspartic protease. The definition of structure–activity relationships for the viral protease has greatly enhanced insights into mechanisms of action of this enzyme, and into directed approaches to the development of inhibitors. Several investigative groups have developed prototypic compounds that inhibit the HIV-1 protease and that exhibit significant antiretroviral activity *in vitro*.

HIV-1 protease inhibitors entered clinical trials in 1991. The extremely low aqueous solubility of several members of this class of antiretroviral drugs has posed a significant problem in clinical development because bioavailability has been extremely limited. Nonetheless, antiviral activity has been demonstrated in phase I/II clinical trials of at least three prototypical HIV-1 protease inhibitors. In the case of at least two of these agents, the reduction in plasma HIV-1 RNA copy number has been of a magnitude equal to or in excess of that observed with nucleoside analogue reverse transcriptase inhibitors. These studies have proven the concept that HIV-1 protease inhibition is a viable therapeutic strategy. Unfortunately, over the initial 6 months of therapy, isolates with reduced susceptibility to these agents have been observed. Genotypic and phenotypic analyses of viral isolates with reduced susceptibility to HIV-1 protease inhibitors have demonstrated that resistance to a single agent does not imply resistance to all agents in the class. This finding has raised the possibility that these agents will be of more prolonged benefit in the setting of combination therapy.

COMBINATION ANTIRETROVIRAL CHEMOTHERAPY

Over the past several years, increasing attention has been directed toward combination chemotherapy. This approach is attractive for several conceptual reasons. The first is the possibility that concurrent use of two or more antiretroviral agents will exhibit increased antiviral activity. Second, the demonstration of emergence of resistant strains of HIV-1 following prolonged monotherapy with zidovudine or ddI has greatly increased interest in the use of combination chemotherapy as a means to retard the development of resistance to antiviral agents. Third, reduction in the dose-related toxicities associated with currently used agents would be desirable if equivalent antiviral activity could be demonstrated with lower doses of antiretroviral agents. Finally, pharmacokinetic considerations such as issues related to tissue tropism, serum half-life, or CNS penetration might suggest combination regimens that would exhibit increased effectiveness over single-agent regimens.

As the number of antiretroviral agents grows, the number of possible combinations of antiretroviral drugs will also proliferate exponentially, especially as combinations of three or more drugs are considered. The planning of antiretroviral regimens should rest on firm rationale and *in vitro* data. Although it has been suggested that combination regimens might be optimal if different steps in the viral life cycle are targeted, in fact, combinations of reverse transcriptase inhibitors such as zidovudine and ddI or zidovudine and L-697,661 may also exhibit considerable additive or synergistic antiviral activity. It is also important to emphasize that some combinations of antiretroviral agents are antagonistic, as has been demonstrated with zidovudine and ribavirin.

Clinical trials of combination chemotherapy may include either sequential or concurrent designs. In general, selection of agents with nonoverlapping toxicities should permit concurrent, rather than sequential, administration of antiretroviral drugs. Combinations of zidovudine and ddC and zidovudine and ddI have been shown to be well tolerated in phase I/II clinical trials and to exhibit evidence of *in vivo* activity as manifested by decreases in serum HIV-1 p24 antigen and increases in circulating CD4 cells. The clinical investigation of combination regimens from the standpoint of clinical endpoints is a resource-intensive endeavor that will require careful planning over the next several years.

CURRENT CLINICAL APPROACH TO
ANTIVIRAL CHEMOTHERAPY

The field of antiretroviral chemotherapy is changing rapidly and it is likely that it will be in continuous evolution for the foreseeable future. This rapid evolution is both enormously exciting and desperately needed. The pace of these changes, however, poses a significant challenge to physicians in that antiretroviral chemotherapeutic agents are often widely available at significantly earlier stages of development than for other drugs. This, coupled with a rapidly changing database regarding the pathogenesis of HIV-1 infection, requires that clinicians stay abreast of a wide body of data, and necessitates therapeutic decisions that are based on fewer data from formal clinical trials than in the case of more traditional infectious diseases. Given the complexity of the disease process and the wide variety of objective and subjective factors that must be considered in therapeutic decision making, the rigid algorithm that is valid in all situations cannot be recommended. Nonetheless, from the available data, a general approach can be developed that provides a reasonable framework from which to base therapeutic decisions in individual patients (Fig. 2).

At this point, it seems reasonable to offer zidovudine monotherapy to most HIV-1–infected individuals as CD4 cells decline below 500 CD4 cells/mm^3. It should be emphasized that the decision to initiate antiretroviral chemotherapy is one that should be taken in the context of a disease that has an average span of a decade or more, and it is more important to reach consensus with a patient that he or she wishes to embark on antiretroviral therapy than it is to initiate therapy at the precise moment that an individual reaches 500 CD4 cells/mm^3. The decision to initiate antiretroviral chemotherapy is clearly influenced by the willingness of the patient to experience toxicity of currently available agents, the optimism that agents currently under development will prove to be efficacious, and the rate of disease progression. As a general rule, therapeutic decisions should not be made on the basis of a single CD4 cell count. If an individual does not tolerate zidovudine, substitution of ddI or D4T is a reasonable alternative.

In the case of HIV-1–infected individuals who present on the basis of the devel-

Antiretroviral Chemotherapy: A Proposed Algorithm

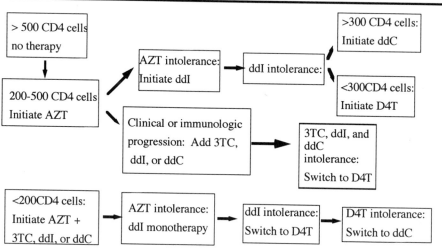

FIG. 2. Proposed framework as basis for therapeutic decision making.

opment of clinical manifestations of HIV-1 infection with CD4 cell counts in the range of 100 to 300/mm^3, it is quite reasonable to offer initial combination therapy with zidovudine and ddI, 3TC, or ddC. As in the case of initial therapy of those with more than 300 CD4 cells/mm^3, monotherapy with ddI or D4T should be considered for those who don't tolerate zidovudine. DDC monotherapy should be reserved for those who do not tolerate either ddI or D4T.

After an individual who has been started on zidovudine therapy develops clinical or immunologic evidence of disease progression, the addition of 3TC, ddI, or ddC should be considered. In that a direct comparison of the agents in this setting has not yet been completed, it is reasonable to make the initial choice of 3TC, ddI, or ddC on the basis of the potential toxicity of the specific agent in the individual patient. If disease progression or drug intolerance is observed following this change of therapy, D4T is an excellent choice for continued therapy. With the progression of HIV-1 disease, the decision as to whether antiretroviral chemotherapy should be continued is often faced. As in the case of decisions about the initiation of antiretroviral therapy, decisions to discontinue therapy should be individualized. In some patients, opportunistic or neoplastic complications of HIV-1 infection will require therapy with agents with toxicities that overlap those of available antiretroviral agents. In these cases, it will be more appropriate to focus on therapy of the opportunistic complication of HIV-1 infection. In settings in which opportunistic complications of HIV-1 disease and/or drug toxicity do not intervene, continuation of antiviral therapy is quite appropriate.

SUMMARY

At present, four antiretroviral drugs have been approved by the FDA. Over the past several years, clinical studies have resulted in a decrease in the recommended dose of zidovudine to 500 to 600 mg/day and have demonstrated its clinical utility in HIV-infected individuals at earlier stages of the disease process. These trials have outlined the long-term toxicity profile of zidovudine and have begun to provide insights into problems related to the emergence of drug-resistant isolates. Three additional nucleoside analogue reverse transcriptase inhibitors (ddC, ddI, and D4T) have been approved by the FDA since the approval of zidovudine. An array of additional antiretroviral agents with several other mechanisms of action are in phase I–III clinical trials.

Since the introduction of zidovudine in 1987, the prognosis for individuals with HIV-1 infection has improved significantly. This improvement has resulted from a combination of the effects of antiretroviral therapy and more insightful use of agents directed at the prophylaxis and therapy of HIV-1–associated opportunistic infections. With the availability of a wider array of antiretroviral chemotherapeutic agents, it is likely that the prognosis of HIV infection will improve further over the next several years. Optimal management of HIV infection requires a thorough familiarity with currently available antiretroviral drugs, as well as ongoing attention to rapidly changing therapeutic approaches in this quickly moving field.

SUGGESTED READING

Concorde Coordinating Committee. Concorde: MRC/ANRS randomised double-blind controlled trial of immediate and deferred zidovudine in symptom-free individuals. *Lancet* 1994;343:871–881.

Erickson J, Niedhart D, VanDrie J, et al. Design, activity, and 2.8 A crystal structure of a c_2 symmetric inhibitor complexed to HIV-1 protease. *Science* 1990;249:527–533.

Fischl MA, Richman DD, Hansen N, et al. The safety and efficacy of zidovudine (AZT) in the treatment of mildly symptomatic human immunodeficiency virus type 1 (HIV) infection: a double-blind, placebo-controlled trial. *Ann Intern Med* 1990;112:727–737.

Kahn JO, Lagakos SW, Richman DD, et al. A controlled trial comparing continued zidovudine with didanosine in human immunodeficiency virus infection. *N Engl J Med* 1992;327:581–587.

Kinloch-de Loes, Hirschel BJ, Hoen B, Cooper DA, Tindall B, Carr A, Saurat J-H, et al. A controlled trial of zidovudine in primary human immunodeficiency virus infection. *N Engl J Med* 1995;333:408–413.

Larder BA, Darby G, Richman DD. HIV with reduced sensitivity to zidovudine isolated during prolonged therapy. *Science* 1989;243:1731–1734.

Larder BA, Kemp SD. Multiple mutations in HIV-1 reverse transcriptase confer high level resistance to AZT. *Science* 1989;246:1155–1158.

Larder BA, Kemp SD, Harrigan R. Potential mechanism for sustained antiretroviral potency of AZT/3TC combination therapy. *Science* 1995;269:696–699.

Roberts N, Martin J, Kinchington D, et al. Rational design of peptide-based HIV proteinase inhibitors. *Science* 1990;248:358–361.

Volberding PA, Lagakos SW, Grimes JM, Stein DS, Rooney J, Meng T-C, et al. A comparison of immediate with deferred zidovudine therapy for asymptomatic HIV-infected adults with CD4 cell counts of 500 or more per cubic millimeter. *N Engl J Med* 1995;333:401–407.

Volberding PA, Lagakos SW, Koch MA, et al., and the AIDS Clinical Trials Group of the National Institute of Allergy and Infectious Diseases. Zidovudine in asymptomatic human immunodeficiency virus infection: a controlled trial in persons with fewer than 500-CD4 positive cells per cubic millimeter. *N Engl J Med* 1990;323:1009–1014.

Wei X, Ghosh SK, Taylor ME, et al. Viral dynamics in human immunodeficiency virus type 1 infection. *Nature* 1995;373:117–122.

A Clinical Guide to AIDS and HIV,
edited by Gary P. Wormser.
Lippincott-Raven Publishers, Philadelphia © 1996.

11

Pharmacology of Drugs Used in the Care of HIV-Infected Patients

John G. Bartlett

Division of Infectious Diseases, The Johns Hopkins University School of Medicine, Baltimore, Maryland 21205

GUIDE TO INFORMATION PROVIDED IN STANDARD FORMAT

Listings are alphabetical usually by name most commonly used in clinical practice. *Trade name* and pharmaceutical company source are provided unless there are multiple providers.

Cost is based on average wholesale price according to Medispan, Hospital Formulary Pricing Guide, April 1995. Prices are often provided for generic and trade name products for comparison.

Pharmacology, Side Effects, and Drug Interactions

Data are from *Drug Information—1995*, American Hospital Formulary Service, Bethesda, MD, pp. 37–587, 1995; *PDR-1995*, Medical Economics Data Production Company, Mintvale, NJ, pp. 402–2642, 1993; and *Drug Evaluations Subscription*, AMA, Chicago, IL (3 volumes), 1994.

Creatinine Clearance

Males: $\dfrac{\text{Weight (kg)} \times (140 - \text{age in years})}{72 \times \text{serum creatinine (mg/dl)}}$

Females: Determination for males × 0.85

Notes:

1. Obese patients—use lean body weight.
2. Formula assumes stable renal function. Assume Cr Cl of 5 to 8 ml/min for patients with anuria or oliguria.

3. Pregnancy and volume expansion: glomerular filtration rate (GFR) may be increased in third trimester of pregnancy and with massive parenteral fluids.

Classification of Controlled Substances

Category	Interpretation
I	*High potential for abuse and no current accepted medical use.* Examples are heroin and LSD.
II	*High potential for abuse.* Use may lead to severe physical or psychological dependence. Examples are opioids, amphetamines, and short-acting barbiturates and preparations containing low quantities of codeine. Prescriptions must be written in ink, or typewritten and signed by the practitioner. Verbal prescriptions must be confirmed in writing within 72 hours, and may be given only in a genuine emergency. No renewals are permitted.
III	*Some potential for abuse.* Use may lead to low-to-moderate physical dependence or high psychological dependence. Examples are barbiturates and preparations containing low quantities of codeine. Prescriptions may be oral or written. Up to five renewals are permitted within 6 months.
IV	*Low potential for abuse.* Examples include chloral hydrate, phenobarbital, and benzodiazepines. Use may lead to limited physical or psychological dependence. Prescriptions may be oral or written. Up to five renewals are permitted within 6 months.
V	*Subject to state and local regulation.* Abuse potential is low; a prescription may not be required. Examples are antitussive and antidiarrheal meds with limited quantities of opioids.

Classification for Use in Pregnancy Based on FDA Categories

Ratings range from "A" for drugs that have been tested for teratogenicity under controlled conditions without showing evidence of damage to the fetus, to "D" and "X" for drugs that are definitely teratogenic. The "D" rating is generally reserved for drugs with no safer alternatives. The "X" rating means there is absolutely no reason to risk using the drug in pregnancy.

Category	Interpretation
A	*Controlled studies show no risk.* Adequate, well-controlled studies in pregnant women have failed to demonstrate risk to the fetus.
B	*No evidence of risk in humans.* Either animal findings show risk, but human findings do not; or, if no adequate human studies have been done, animal findings are negative.
C	*Risk cannot be ruled out.* Human studies are lacking, and animal studies are either positive for fetal risk or lacking. However, potential benefits may justify the potential risk.
D	*Positive evidence of risk.* Investigational or postmarketing data show risk to the fetus. Nevertheless, potential benefits may outweigh the potential risk.

Category	Interpretation
X	*Contraindicated in pregnancy.* Studies in animals or humans, or investigational or postmarketing reports, have shown fetal risk that clearly outweighs any possible benefit to the patient.

Patient Assistance Programs

Usual requirements are lack of a prescription drug plan (including state plans and Ryan White funds) plus income/asset criteria.

ACYCLOVIR

Trade name: Zovirax (Glaxo-Wellcome).
Forms and price: 200 mg caps—$.98/cap; 400 mg tabs (newly available form); 800 mg tabs—$3.68/tab; 200 mg/5 cc suspension—$84.13/473 ml or $.88/200 mg; 500 mg and 1 g vials (IV)—$50.90/500 mg; 5% ointment, 3 g—$15.46; 15 g—$35.74 (utility limited).
Class: Synthetic nucleoside analogue derived from guanine.
Annual cost cap: Eligible patients whose use exceeds 552 g in <1 year may receive free drug up to additional 620 g; call (800) 722-9294.
Patient assistance program—(800) 722-9294: Eligibility based on lack of third-party drug coverage, monthly income criteria using Medicaid guidelines and asset information; forms are reviewed on an individual case basis.
Indications and dose: Regimens suggested are based on *PDR-1995*, *MMWR* 1993; 42:RR-14; Strauss S and Whitely R, *Inf Dis Clin Pract* 1992;2:100; and clinical trials—*JAMA* 1991;264:747; *N Engl J Med* 1983;308:916; 1986;314:144; 1989; 320:293; 1991;325:551; *Ann Intern Med* 1992; 117:358.

Herpes Simplex Virus (HSV)

First episode genital: 200 mg po $5 \times$/day 7–10 days or 5 mg/kg IV q 8 h $\times$ 5–7 days.
Recurrent[1]: 200 mg po $5 \times$/day or 400 mg po tid or 800 mg po bid $\times$ 5 days; AIDS patients pay require higher doses.
Perirectal: 400 mg po $5 \times$/day $\times$ 10 days.
Progressive mucocutaneous: 5–10 mg/kg IV q 8 h $\times$ 7–14 days.
Prophylaxis: 400 mg po bid (this is standard dose in immunocompetent patients;

---

[1]Benefit of therapy for recurrent genital HSV and dermatomal zoster is marginal in immunocompetent hosts and must be started within 24 hours of the exantham with HSV and within 4 days or while new lesions are still forming with dematomal zoster.

400 mg po 3–5 × day may be required by AIDs patients). Prophylaxis is contraindi-cated in pregnancy.

Acyclovir-resistant: Doses up to 10 mg/kg acyclovir IV q 8 hr or by constant infusion (or foscarnet, 40 mg/kg IV q 8 h).

Varicella-Zoster Virus (VZV)

Chicken pox[1]: 800 mg po 5 × /day × 7–10 days.
Dermatomal zoster: 10 mg/kg IV q 8 h × 7 days or 800 mg po 5 × /day × 7 days.
Disseminated zoster: 10 mg/kg IV q 8 h × 7 days.
Acyclovir-resistant: Foscarnet (40 mg/kg IV q 8 h).

Epstein-Barr Virus (EBV)

Oral hairy leukoplakia: 800 mg po 5 × /day × 2–3 weeks.

HIV/Herpes Virus Prophylaxis[2]

800 mg po qid.

Pharmacology

Bioavailability: 15–20% with oral administration.
T1/2: 2.5–3.3 hours; *CSF levels*: 50% serum levels.
Elimination: Renal.

Dose Modification in Renal Failure

Usual dose	Cr. clearance (ml/min)	Adjusted dose
200 mg × 5/day	>10 ml/min	200 mg × 5/day
	<10 ml/min	200 mg q 12 h
800 mg × 5/day	>50 ml/min	800 mg 5 × /day
	10–50 ml/min	800 mg q 8 h
	<10 ml/min	800 mg q 12 h
5–10 mg/kg IV q 8 h	>50 ml/min	5–10 mg/kg IV q 8 h
	10–50 ml/min	5–10 mg/kg q 12–24 h
	<10 ml/min	5–10 mg/kg q 24 h

[2]Efficacy is considered not established. There are six studies: Three showed a survival advantage of AZT + acyclovir, one showed a delay in CD4 cell count decline, and two showed no advantage. None showed a reduction in CMV diseases (*AIDS* 1993;7:197; *AIDS* 1994;8:641; *Ann Intern Med* 1994; 121:100; ACTG 063). Current opinion is mixed; if there is an advantage it is presumably due to acyclovir activity vs. herpes simplex or herpes virus 6. The dose is arbitrary: prospective trials used 3,200–4,000 mg/day, the observational study in Multicenter AIDS Cohort Study (MACS) suggested a dose of 600 mg/day was adequate.

Side effects (infrequent and rarely severe): irritation at infusion site; rash; nausea and vomiting; diarrhea; renal toxicity (especially with rapid IV infusion, prior renal disease and concurrent nephrotoxic drugs), dizziness, abnormal liver function tests; itching; headache. Rare complications are CNS toxicity with encephalopathy, disorientation, seizures, hallucinations; anemia, neutropenia, thrombocytopenia; hypotension.

Pregnancy: Category C. Not teratogenic, but potential to cause chromosomal damage at high doses. Burroughs-Wellcome CDC Registry shows no increased incidence of fetal abnormalities among 601 women for whom pregnancy outcome data were available (*MMWR* 1993; 42:806). The registry may be reached at (800) 722-9292 ext. 58465. The CDC recommendation is to use acyclovir during pregnancy only for life-threatening disease.

Drug interactions: Increased meperidine effect; probenecid prolongs half-life of acyclovir.

ALPRAZOLAM

Trade name: Xanax (Upjohn).
Forms and price: 0.25 mg tab—$.59; 0.5 mg tab—$.74; 1 mg tab—$.98; 2 mg tab—$1.67.
Class: Benzodiazepine, controlled substance category IV.

Indications and Dose Regimen

Anxiety: 0.25–0.5 mg tid; increase if necessary at intervals of 3–4 days to maximum of 4 mg/day.

Panic disorder: 0.5 mg tid with increase at increments of ≤1 mg/day to maximum of 6–10 mg/day.

Dose reduction or withdrawal: Decrease by ≤0.5 mg q 3 days; some suggest decrease by 0.25 mg at 3- to 7-day intervals.

Pharmacokinetics

Bioavailability: >90%.
T1/2: 11 hours, prolonged with obesity and hepatic dysfunction.
Elimination: Metabolized and renally excreted.
Side effects: See Benzodiazepines. Seizures, delirium, and withdrawal symptoms with rapid dose reduction or abrupt discontinuation. Withdrawal symptoms at 18 hours to 3 days after abrupt discontinuation. Seizures usually occur at 24–72 hours after abrupt withdrawal.
Pregnancy: Category D. fetal harm—contraindicated; possible role in cleft lip and heart abnormalities.

Drug interactions: Additive CNS depression with other CNS depressants including alcohol. Disulfiram and cimetidine prolong the half-life of alprazolam.

Relative contraindications: History of serious mental illness, drug abuse, alcoholism, open-angle glaucoma, seizure disorder, severe liver disease.

AMPHOTERICIN B

Generic.
Trade name: Fungisone (Apothecon).
Forms and price: 50 mg vials at $12.61/vial.
Class: Amphoteric polyene macrolide with activity versus nearly all pathogenic and opportunistic fungi.

Indications and Regimens

Condition	Daily dose	Total dose	Comment
Aspergillus	0.5–1.5 mg/kg	30–40 mg/kg	± Flucytosine
Candida			
Stomatitis	0.3–0.5 mg/kg	200–500 mg	Reserved for refractory cases
Esophagitis	0.3–0.5 mg/kg	200–500 mg	Reserved for refractory cases
Line sepsis	0.3–0.5 mg/kg	200–500 mg	Must discontinue line
Disseminated	0.3–0.8 mg/kg	20–40 mg/kg	± Flucytosine
Coccidioidomycosis	0.5–1.0 mg/kg	30–40 mg/kg	Maintenance with itraconazole
Cryptococcosis	0.5–1.0 mg/kg	500–1000 mg	± Flucytosine; maintenance with fluconazole
Histoplasmosis	0.8–1.0 mg/kg	5–20 mg/kg	Maintenance with itraconazole or Ampho B, 1–1.5 mg/kg weekly

Pharmacology

Bioavailability: Poorly absorbed.
CSF levels: 3% of serum concentrations.
T1/2: 24 hours, detected in blood and urine up to 4 weeks after discontinuation.
Elimination: Serum levels in urine; metabolic pathways are unknown.
Dose adjustment in renal failure: None.
Administration: Slow IV infusion; first dose is 1 mg in 350 ml 5% dextrose given over 2–4 hours with monitoring of vital signs q 30 min × 4 hours. Subsequent dose may be increased to 0.3 mg/kg at 4 hours after test dose and given over 2–6 hours; then daily maintenance doses are given. Alternatively, less serious infections may be treated with daily or periodic increases in dose by 5 mg/day or conversion to double doses on alternative days. The daily dose should never exceed 1.5 mg/kg and monitoring should include CBC, serum creatinine, and serum electrolytes. There is no reason to protect infusions from sunlight.

Side effects: Frequent, most are dose-related and less severe with slow administration.

1. Chills, usually 1–3 hours postinfusion and lasts up to 4 hours postinfusion. Reduce with hydrocortisone (10–50 mg added to infusion, but only if necessary due to immunosuppression); alternatives are meperidine or ibuprofen prior to infusion.
2. Hypotension, nausea, vomiting, usually 1–3 hours postinfusion—may be reduced with compazine.
3. Nephrotoxicity in 80% ± nephrocalcinosis, potassium wasting, renal tubular acidosis. Reduce with gradual increase in dose, adequate hydration, avoidance of concurrent nephrotoxic drugs, and, possibly, sodium loading. Discontinue or reduce dose with BUN >40 mg/dl and creatinine >3 mg/ml.
4. Hypokalemia, hypomagnesemia, and hypocalcemia corrected with supplemental K^+, Mg^{2+}, or Ca^{2+}.
5. Normocytic normochromic anemia with average decrease of 9% in hematocrit.
6. Phlebitis and pain at infusion sites—add 1,200–1,600 units of heparin to infusate.

Pregnancy: Category B; harmless in experimental animal studies, but no data for patients.

Drug interactions: Increased nephrotoxicity with concurrent use of nephrotoxic drugs—aminoglycosides, cisplatin, cyclosporine, methoxyflurane, vancomycin; increased hypokalemia with corticosteroids and diuretics.

ANCOBON

See Flucytosine.

ATIVAN

See Lorazepam.

ATOVAQUONE

Trade name: Mepron (Burroughs Wellcome).
Form: 250 mg/5 ml susp.
Cost: Cost of a 21-day course = $523; relative cost for oral TMP-SMX (21 days) = $8.82; oral dapsone + trimethoprim = $36; IV pentamidine = $2,100.
Cost cap program for patients without third-party coverage with use >411 g in ≤1 year may receive free drug: call (800) 722-9294. *Patient assistance program*: (800) 722-9294. Eligibility based on lack of third-party drug coverage, monthly income

criteria using Medicaid guidelines and asset information; forms are reviewed on an individual case basis.

Indications: Oral treatment of mild to moderate PCP (A-a O_2 gradient <45 mm Hg and PaO_2 >60 mm Hg) in patients who are intolerant of trimethoprim-sulfamethoxazole (TMP-SMX).

Dose: 750 mg/5 ml bid *with food.*

Efficacy: Comparative trial with TMP-SMX for mild-moderate *Pneumocystis carinii* pneumonia (PCP) showed TMP-SMX had fewer failures (6% vs. 17%) and more adverse effects requiring drug discontinuation (20% vs. 7%). Decreased efficacy of atovaquone compared to TMP-SMX may be due to reduced bioavailability with oral administration.

Pharmacology

Bioavailability: Increased threefold with 20 g fat (one pad of butter). Administration with food needs emphasis.

T1/2: 2.2–2.9 days.

Elimination: Unchanged in stool; <1% in urine.

CSF/plasma ratio: <1%.

Effect of hepatic or renal disease: No data.

Side effects: Rash (20%), GI intolerance (20%), diarrhea (20%); possibly related—headache, fever, insomnia; life-threatening side effects: none; number requiring discontinuation due to side effects: 7–9% (rash—4%).

Pregnancy: Class C. Not teratogenic in animals; no studies in patients.

Drug interactions: None known.

AVENTYL

See Notriptyline.

AZITHROMYCIN

Trade name: Zithromax (Pfizer).

Form: 250 mg tab.

Price: $6.04/250 mg tabs.

Class: Macrolide.

Forms available through treatment IND for cryptosporidium or toxoplasmosis: (800) 742-3029; 150, 300, and 600 mg tabs; lactose-free tabs available for patients with diarrhea; oral suspension—40 mg/ml; IV form.

Patient assistance program: (800) 646-4455. Physician must write letter stating (1) the drug desired, (2) the diagnosis, and (3) that patient is indigent with no third-party payor including ineligibility for Medicaid. A 3-month supply will be provided.

Activity (in vitro): *S. pneumoniae*, streptococci (not *Enterococcus*), erythromycin-sensitive *S. aureus*, *H. influenzae*, Legionella, *C. pneumoniae*, *Mycoplasma pneumoniae*, *C. trachomatis*, *M. avium*, and *T. gondii*.

Indications and Dosages

Indications	Dose
Sinusitis, bronchitis, and pneumonia[a]	500 mg × 1, then 250 mg po/day × 4 (6 tabs)
Chlamydia trachomatis[a]	1 g po × 1
Toxoplasmosis[b]	900 mg po × 2 on day 1, then 1200 mg/d as single dose × 6 wks, then 600 mg/day (patients <50 kg receive half dose)
Cryptosporidiosis[b]	1200 mg × 2 po on day 1, then 1200 mg/d × 27days, then 600 mg/d
M. avium prophylaxis	1250 mg weekly

[a]FDA approved indications.
[b]Treatment IND: Contact (800) 742-3029.

Pharmacology

Bioavilability: 35–40% reduced by food; take 1 hour before or 2 hours after meals.

T1/2: 68 hours; detectable levels in urine at 7–14 days.

Distribution: High tissue levels; low CSF levels (<0.01 μg/ml).

Excretion: Primarily biliary; 6% in urine.

Dose modification in renal or hepatic failure: Use with caution.

Side effects: GI intolerance (nausea, vomiting, pain)—3%; diarrhea—4%. Frequency of discontinuation in non-AIDS patients receiving standard dose—0.7%. Frequency of discontinuation in AIDS patients receiving high doses: 6%, primarily GI intolerance and reversible ototoxicity (2%); rare—erythema multiforme, increased transaminase.

Contraindication: Hypersensitivity to erythromycin.

Drug interactions: Al and Mg containing antacids and food reduce absorption; increases levels of theophylline and coumadin.

Pregnancy: Category B. Safe in animal studies; no data in humans.

Warnings: (1) Should be taken 1 hour before meals or 2 hours after meals. (2) Use with caution in patients with hepatic disease, especially with prolonged course and high doses.

AZT

See Zidovudine.

BACTRIM

See Trimethoprim-Sulfamethoxazole.

BENZODIAZEPINES

Benzodiazepines are commonly used for anxiety and insomnia. They are also commonly abused, with some studies showing up to 25% of AIDS patients taking these drugs. The decision to use these drugs requires careful consideration of side effects and disclosure of them to the patient:

1. *Dependency* (larger than usual doses or prolonged daily use of therapeutic doses).
2. *Abuse potential* (most common in those with abuse of alcohol and other psychiatric drugs).
3. *Tolerance* (primarily to sedation and ataxia; minimal to antianxiety effects).
4. *Withdrawal symptoms* are related to duration of use, dose, rate of tapering, and drug half-life. Features are (a) recurrence of pretreatment symptoms developing over days or weeks; (b) rebound with symptoms that are similar to but more severe than pretreatment symptoms occurring within hours or days (self-limited); and (c) the benzodiazepine withdrawal syndrome with autonomic symptoms, disturbances in equilibrium, sensory disturbances, etc.
5. *Daytime sedation, dizziness, incoordination, ataxia, and hangover*: Use small doses initially and gradually increase. Patient must be warned that activities requiring mental alertness, judgment, and coordination require special caution; concomitant use with sedatives including alcohol, antihistamines, or marijuana is unusually hazardous.
6. *Drug interactions*: Sedative effects are antagonized by caffeine and theophylline. Erythromycin, cimetadine, omeprazole, and isoniazed may reduce hepatic metabolism and prolong half-life. Rifampin and oral contraceptives increase hepatic clearance to reduce half-life.
7. *Miscellaneous side effects*: Blurred vision, diplopia, confusion, memory disturbance, amnesia, fatigue, incontinence, constipation, hypotension, disinhibition, bizarre behavior.

Selection of agent and regimen: Drug selection is based largely on indication and pharmacokinetic properties (see table below). Drugs with rapid onset are desired when temporary relief of anxiety symptoms is needed. The smallest dose for the shortest time is recommended, and patients need frequent reevaluation for continued use. Short-term use is advised in patients with a history of abuse of alcohol or other sedative-hypnotic drugs. Dose adjustments are usually required to achieve the desired effect with acceptable side effects. Long-term use (more than several weeks) may require an extended tapering schedule over 6 to 8 weeks (20–30% dose reduction weekly) adjusted by symptoms and sometimes facilitated by antidepressants or hypnotics.

Anxiety and Insomnia

Agent	Trade name	Anxiety	Insomnia	T_{max} (hours)	$T_{1/2}$ (hours)	Dose forms	Regimens
Benzodiazepines							
Chlordiazepoxide	Librium	+	−	0.5–4	10	5, 10, 25 mg tabs	15–100 mg/d hs or 3–4 doses
Clorazepate	Tranxene	+	−	1–2	73	3.75, 7.5, 15, 11.25, 22.5 mg tabs	15–60 mg/d hs or 2–4 doses
Diazepam	Valium	+	+	1.5–2	73	2, 4, 10 mg tabs	4–40 mg/d, 2–4 doses
Flurazepam	Dalmane	−	+	0.5–2	74	15, 30 mg caps	30 mg hs
Quazepam	Doral	−	+	2	74	7.5, 15 mg tabs	15 mg hs
Alprazolam	Xanax	+	−	1–2	11	0.25, 0.5, 1, 2 mg tabs	0.25–0.5 mg tid up to 4 mg/d
Lorazepam	Ativan	+	+	2	14	0.5, 1, 2 mg tabs	2–6 mg/d in 2–3 doses
Oxazepam	Serex	+	+	1–4	7	10, 15, 30 mg caps	30–120 mg/d in 3–4 doses
Temazepam	Restoril	−	+	1–1.5	13	15, 30 mg caps	30 mg hs
Triazolam	Halcion	−	+	1–2	3	0.125, 0.25 mg tabs	0.25 mg hs

BIAXIN

See Clarithromycin.

BUSPAR

See Buspirone.

BUSPIRONE

Trade name: Buspar (Mead Johnson).
Forms and price: 5 mg tab—$0.57; 10 mg tab—$1.00.
Class: Nonbenzodiazepine-nonbarbituate antianxiety agent; not a controlled substance.
Indications and dose regimens: Anxiety: 5 mg po tid; increase by 5 mg/day every 2–4 days. Usual effective dose is 15–30 mg/day in 2–3 divided doses. Onset of response requires one week and full effect requires four weeks. Total daily dose should not exceed 60 mg/day.

Pharmacology

Bioavailability: >90% absorbed when taken with food.

T1/2: 2.5 hours.

Elimination: Rapid hepatic metabolism to partially active metabolites; <0.1% of parent compound excreted in urine.

Dose adjustment in renal disease: None or dose reduction of 25–50% with anuria.

Hepatic disease: May decrease clearance and must use with caution.

Side effects: Sleep disturbance, nervousness, headache, nausea, diarrhea, paresthesias, depression, increased or decreased libido, headache, dizziness, excitement. Compared with benzodiazepines dependency, liability to buspirone is nil; it does not potentiate CNS depressants including alcohol, it is usually well tolerated by the elderly, and there is no hypnotic effect, no muscle relaxant effect, less fatigue, less confusion, and less decreased libido, but nearly comparable efficiency for anxiety. Nevertheless, the CNS effects are somewhat unpredictable and there is substantial individual variation; patients should be warned that buspirone may impair ability to perform activities requiring mental alertness or physical coordination such as driving.

Pregnancy: Class B.

CHLORAL HYDRATE

Generic; *Trade name*: Noctect (Apothecon); Aquachloral Supprettes (suppositories).

Forms and price: 325, 500, and 650 mg caps; 500 mg–$0.17/cap; suppositories—$.19/325 mg; syrup with 250 and 500 mg/5 ml syrup—$.32/500 mg.

Class: Nonbenzodiazepine-nonbarbiturate hypnotic, controlled substance category IV.

Indications and dose regimens: Insomnia: 500 mg–1 g po hs; usually produces sleep in 30 min, which lasts 4–8 hours. Sedation: 250 mg po tid.

Note: Tolerance develops within 5 weeks.

Pharmacology

Bioavailability: >90%.

T1/2: Hepatic metabolism to active metabolite (trichloroethanol) with a half life of 4–9.5 hours.

Elimination: Renal excretion of trichloroethanol.

Hepatic or renal disease: Contraindicated.

Side effects: Gastric intolerance; dependence and tolerance with long-term use.

Pregnancy: Category C.
Drug interactions: Potentiates action of oral anticoagulants.

CIPRO

See Ciprofloxacin.

CIPROFLOXACIN

Trade name: Cipro.
Forms: 250, 500, and 750 mg tabs; IV—200 and 400 mg vials.
Price: $2.80/250 mg tab; $3.24/500 mg tab; $5.42/750 mg tab; $28.20/400 mg vial (for IV use).
Class: Fluoroquinolone.
Indications and dose:
   Respiratory infections: 500–750 mg po bid × 7–14 days.
   Gonorrhea: 500 mg × 1.
   Tuberculosis: 500–750 mg po bid.
   Salmonellosis: 500–750 mg po bid 2–4 weeks.
   UTI: 250–500 mg po bid × 3–7 days.

Pharmacology

Bioavailability: 60–70%.
T1/2: 3.3 hours.
Excretion: Metabolized and excreted (parent drug + metabolites) in urine.
Dose reduction in renal failure: cr. clearance >50 ml/min—250–750 mg q 12 h; 10–50 ml/min—250–500 mg q 12 h; <10 ml/min—250–500 mg q 18 h.
Side effects: Usually well tolerated; most common: GI intolerance with nausea—1–2%, diarrhea—1–2%; CNS toxicity—malaise, drowsiness, insomnia, headache, dizziness, agitation, psychosis (rare), seizures (rare), hallucinations (rare); *Candida* vaginitis; contraindicated in persons <18 years due to concern for arthropathy in animals.
Drug interactions: Increased levels of theophylline and caffeine; reduced absorption with cations (Al, Mg in antacids, sucralfate, ddI); gastric achlorhydria does not influence absorption.
Pregnancy: Category C. Arthropathy in immature animals with erosions in joint cartilage; relevance to patients is not known. *Medical Letter* consultants and CDC consider use in pregnant women and persons <18 years contraindicated. This admonition applies to all quinolones.

FLUOROQUINOLONE SUMMARY

	Ciprofloxacin (Cipro)	Olfloxacin (Floxin)	Norfloxacin (Noroxin)	Enoxacin (Penetrex)	Lomefloxacin (Maxaquin)
Oral forms	+	+	+	+	+
IV form	+	+	−	−	−
Price (average wholesale)	$2.92/500 mg	$3.52/400 mg	$2.34/400 mg	$2.60/200 mg	$5.25/400 mg
$T_{1/2}$	3.3 hr	5.0 hr	3.3 hr	4.9 hr	7.8 hr
$T_{1/2}$ renal failure	8 hr	40 hr	8 hr	8 hr	45 hr
Oral bio-availability	65%	95%	45%	95%	95%
Theophylline/ caffeine interactions	+	−	−	+ +	+/−
Activity in vitro					
P. aeruginosa	+ + (90%)	−	−	−	−
S. pneumoniae	+	+	−	−	+
Mycobacteria	+ +	+ +	−	−	+ +
Regimens (oral)[a]					
UTI	250 mg bid	200 mg bid	400 mg bid	200 mg bid	400 mg qd
Gonorrhea	500 mg × 1	400 mg × 1	800 mg × 1	400 mg × 1	−
Respiratory tract	750 mg bid	400 mg bid	−	−	400 mg qd

[a]All fluoroquinolones are active against most *Enterobacteriaceae*, enteric bacterial pathogens (except *C. difficile*), *S. aureus* (resistance increasing), *Neisseria* sp., *H. influenzae*, Legionella; activity vs. *S. pneumoniae* is reduced and no fluoroquinolones should be used for pneumococcal infections; activity vs. anaerobes is poor.

CLARITHROMYCIN

Trade name: Biaxin (Abbott).

Forms and price: 250 mg tab = $3.14; 500 mg tab = $3.14.

Patient assistance program: (800) 688-9118. Patient must have financial need and documented *M. avium* infection.

Class: Macrolide.

Activity: *S. pneumoniae*, erythromycin-sensitive—*S. aureus*, *S. pyogenes*, *M. catarrhalis*, *H. influenzae*, *M. pneumoniae*, *C. pneumoniae*, Legionella, *M. avium*, *T. gondii*, *C. trachomatis*, *U. ureolyticum*.

Indications and Regimens

Indication	Dose regimen
Pharyngitis, sinusitis, otitis pneumonitis, skin and soft tissue infection[a]	250–500 mg po bid
M. avium prophylaxis	500 mg po qd or bid[b]
M. avium treatment[a]	500 mg–1 g po bid[b]

[a]FDA approved for this indication.

[b]Optimal dose is not clearly established. Some patients require dose reduction due to GI intolerance. For treatment of *M. avium* infection, clarithromycin should be combined with clofazamine and/or ethambutol ± rifampin.

Pharmacology

Bioavailability: 50–55%.

T1/2: 3–7 hours.

Elimination: Rapid first pass hepatic metabolism plus renal clearance to 14-hydroxyclarithromycin.

Dose modification in renal failure: Cr cl >30/ml—250–500 mg po bid; Cr clearance <30/ml—250 mg po bid.

Side effects: GI intolerance—4% (compared with 17% with erythromycin); transaminase elevation (1%), headache (2%), pseudomembranous colitis (PMC)—rare.

Pregnancy: Category C. Teratogenic in animal studies and no adequate studies in patients.

Drug interactions: Theophylline, carbamazepine (Tegretol) and seldane terfenadine levels increased; increased levels of seldane may cause fatal arrhythmias.

CLOFAZIMINE

Trade name: Lamprene (Geigy).

Forms: 50 and 100 mg caps.

Price: $0.20/100 mg cap.

Class: Phenozine dye (bright red) with antimycobacterial actvity and antiinflammatory activity.

Indication: *M. avium* infection (in combination with other drugs).

Dose: 50–200 mg po/day, usually 100 mg/day.

Pharmacology

Bioavailability: 45–62%; take with food.

T1/2: 70 days.

Elimination: <1% in urine; hepatic clearance.

Dose modification in renal failure: None.

Side effects: Red-brown discoloration of skin and conjunctivae in 75–100% of patients (dose-related and slowly reversible up to 1–5 years depending on length of use prior to discontinuation); dose-related GI intolerance in up to 58% with doses >100 mg/day, may cause symptoms suggesting bowel obstruction; anticholinergic effect: decreased sweating and tears; photosensitivity; burning of eyes in 24%, GI intolerance-anorexia, nausea, diarrhea in 10–20%; skin changes—dry, rough, or scaly skin—35%, skin rash or pruritis—5%; hepatitis (rare).
Pregnancy: Category C.
Drug interactions: None.
Relative contraindications: Active peptic ulcer disease, idiopathic inflammatory bowel disease, severe liver disease.

CLOTRIMAZOLE

Generic; Trade names: Lotrimin (Schering), Mycelex (Miles), Gyne-Lotrimin, FemCare.
Forms and price: Troche 10 mg—$0.75; topical cream (1%) 15 g—$11.08, 30 g—$18.79; topical solution/lotion (1%) 10 ml—$9.74, 30 ml—$20.28; vaginal cream (1%) 90 g—$31.22; vaginal tablets 100 mg—$1.71 (×7 days = $12); vaginal tablets 500 mg—$12.71 (×1) = $12.71.
Class: Imidazole (related to miconazole).
Spectrum: Active vs. *Candida albicans* and dermatophytes.

Indications and Regimens

Thrush: 10 mg troche 5×/day×14 days.
Dermatophytic infections and cutaneous candidiasis: Topical application of 1% cream, lotion or solution to affected area bid×2–8 weeks; if no improvement, evaluate diagnosis.
Candida vaginitis: Intravaginal 100 mg tab bid×3 days (preferred); alternatives: 100 mg tabs qd×7; 500 mg tab ×1. Vaginal cream: One applicator (about 5 g) intravaginally at hs×7–14 days.

Pharmacology

Bioavailability: Lozenge (troche) dissolves in 15–30 min; administration at 3-hour intervals maintains constant salivary concentrations above MIC of most *Candida* strains. Topical application of 500 mg tab intravaginally achieves local therapeutic levels 48–72 hours. Small amounts of drug are absorbed with oral, vaginal, or skin applications.
Side effects: Topical to skin—(rare) erythema, blistering, pruritis, pain, peeling, urticaria. Topical to vagina—(rare) rash, pruritis, dyspareunia, dysuria, burning,

erythema. Lozenges—elevated AST (up to 15%—monitor LFTs); nausea and vomiting (5%).

Pregnancy: Category C. Avoid during first trimester.

CYTOVENE

See Ganciclovir.

DALMANE

See Flurazepam.

DAPSONE

Generic; *Trade name*: Alvoslfon.

Form and price: 25 mg tab—$.17; 100 mg tabs—$.18. Comparison prices for PCP prophylaxis: dapsone (100 mg/day) = $5.00/mo; TMP-SMX (1 DS/day) = $2.00/mo; aerosolized pentamidine = $100/mo (plus administration costs).

Class: Synthetic sulfone with mechanism of action similar to sulfonamides—inhibition of folic acid synthesis.

Indications and Dose Regimens

Indications	Dose
PCP prophylaxis	100 mg po qd
PCP treatment	100 mg po/day (plus trimethoprim 15 mg/kg/d po or IV) × 3 wks
PCP + toxoplasmosis prophylaxis	50 mg po qd (plus pyrimethamine 50 mg/wk plus folinic acid 25 mg/wk)

Also see Chapters 6 and 9.

Pharmacology

Bioavailability: Nearly completely absorbed.

T1/2: 10–56 hours, average—28 hours.

Elimination: Hepatic concentration, enterohepatic circulation, maintains tissue levels 3 weeks after treatment is discontinued.

Dose modification in renal failure: None.

Side effects: Most common in AIDS patients—rash, pruritis, hepatitis, anemia, and/or neutropenia in 20–40%. Most serious reaction—dose-dependent hemolytic anemia, rare cases of agranulocytosis and aplastic anemia. Suggested monitoring includes screening for G6PD deficiency prior to treatment, especially in high-risk patients including African-American men and men from the Mediterranean area. Some suggest monthly CBCs to detect marrow suppression and hemolytic anemia. GI intolerance—common; may reduce by taking with meals. Infrequent—vomiting, headache, dizziness, peripheral neuropathy. Rare side effect is "sulfone syndrome" after 1–4 weeks of treatment with fever, malaise, exfoliative dermatitis, hepatic necrosis, lymphadenopathy, and anemia with methemoglobinemia (*Arch Dermatol* 1981; 1217:38).

Pregnancy: Category C.

Drug interactions: Decreased levels of dapsone—rifampin and rifabutin; trimethoprim—increased levels of both drugs; coumadin—increased hypoprothrombinemia; pyrimethamine—increased marrow toxicity (monitor CBC); probenecid—increased dapsone levels; primaquine—increased hemolysis due to G6PD deficiency.

Relative contraindications: G6PD deficiency—monitor hematocrit and methemoglobin levels if anemia develops.

DARAPRIM

See Pyrimethamine.

DESYREL

See Trazodone.

ddC

See Dideoxycytidine.

ddI

See Didanosine.

DIDANOSINE (ddI)

Trade name: Videx (Bristol-Myers Squibb).
Forms: 25 mg, 50 mg, 100 mg, and 150 mg wintergreen flavored tabs; 100 mg, 167 mg, 250 mg, and 375 mg buffered provider packets.

Price: 100 mg tab = $1.47; cost/wk (200 mg bid) = $41.35/wk.

Class: Nucleoside analogue.

Financial assistance: (800) 788-0123. For patients without insurance coverage plus financial need.

Indications (based on NIAID/CDC Expert Panel recommendations, *JAMA* 1993; 270:2583): (1) CD4 count <500/mm^3 and progressive disease while receiving AZT. (2) CD4 count <500/mm^3 and intolerance of AZT. (3) CD4 count <300/mm^3 and prior AZT treatment for 2 to >12 months. FDA-approved indication: advanced stage HIV infection and prolonged prior AZT treatment.

Dose Regimen

	Tabs[a]	Powder
Wt≥60 kg	200 mg po bid	250 mg po bid
Wt<60 kg	125 mg po bid	167 mg po bid

[a]Tabs: Must be taken as two tabs in above dose that are chewed thoroughly or crushed and dissolved in one ounce of water or 2–3 ounces of ice cold water. The buffered powder form is citrus flavored and usually used if the tablet form is not tolerated; the contents of one packet are dissolved in four ounces of water. Sodium load is 529 mg/dose with tablet and 1,380 mg/dose with powder.

Minimum effective dose studied: 100 mg (powder) bid.

Pharmacokinetics

Bioavailability: Tablet—40%; powder—30%.

T1/2: 1.6 hours.

Intracellular T1/2: 12 hours.

CNS penetration: 20% of serum levels.

Elimination: Renal excretion—50%.

Renal or hepatic failure: Appears to be associated with increased toxicity, and manufacturer warns that dose reduction should be considered, but specific guidelines are not available. Mg^{2+} load may be a problem with renal failure and sodium load may be problematic for patients requiring sodium restriction.

Side effects:

1. Pancreatitis: Frequency is 5–9% and is fatal in 6% of those with pancreatitis. Frequency is increased in patients with alcoholism, a history of pancreatitis, advanced stage HIV disease, and concurrent meds that cause pancreatitis. Monitor amylase levels at 1 to 2-month intervals, although the value of this in predicting or preventing pancreatitis is not established. Most reduce dose or discontinue ddI if serum amylase level is >1.5–2 × the upper limit of normal.

2. Peripheral neuropathy with pain and/or paresthesias in extremities related to cumulative dose. Frequency is 5–12%. May be persistent and debilitating if ddI is continued despite symptoms of neuropathy.
3. Miscellaneous—GI intolerance, rash, marrow suppression, hyperuricemia, hepatitis.
4. Sodium load: 265 mg/tab and 1,380 mg/packet of powder. Mg load: 15.7 mEg/tab may be problematic in renal failure.

Pregnancy: Category B. No fetal harm in animal studies; no relevant controlled studies in patients.

Drug interactions: Drugs that require gastric acidity for absorption should be given 2 hours before or 2 hours after ddI. These include ketoconazole, tetracyclines, and fluoroquinolones. Drugs that cause pancreatitis (pentamidine) should be avoided; patients should be cautioned about alcohol intake.

DIDEOXYCYTIDINE (ddC)

Trade name: Zalcitabine (Roche).
Forms and price: 0.375 mg—$1.70; 0.75 mg tab—$2.13; cost/week—$44.73.
Class: Nucleoside analogue.
Financial assistance: (800) 285-4484. Patients must not be able to obtain drug from any other source—insurance, Medicaid, or state-sponsored program; no income or asset criteria.
Indications (based on NIAID/CDC Expert Panel recommendations *JAMA* 1993; 270:2583): (1) CD4 count <500/mm^3 and progressive disease despite AZT therapy. (2) CD4 count <500/mm^3 and intolerance to AZT. FDA-approved for use in combination with AZT in patients with advanced stage HIV infection plus progression while treated with AZT.
Regimen: 0.75 mg po tid.

Pharmacology

Bioavailability: 70–88%.
T1/2: 1.2–2 hours.
Intracellular T1/2: 3 hours.
CSF levels: 20% serum levels.
Elimination: Renal excretion—70%.
Dose adjustment in renal failure: CrCl >50 ml/min—0.75 mg po tid; 20–50 ml/min—0.75 mg po bid; <10 ml/min—0.75 mg po qd.
Side effects:

1. The major clinical toxicity is *peripheral neuropathy* noted in 17–31% of patients in initial trials. Features are sensorimotor neuropathy with numbness and burning in distal extremities followed by shooting or continuous pain. Symptoms

usually resolve slowly if the drug is promptly discontinued; with continued use it may be irreversible and require narcotics. Frequency depends on dose and duration of ddC treatment. Pain requiring narcotics or progressive pain for ≥ 1 week represents a contraindication to future use; patients with less severe pain that resolves to mild intensity may be rechallenged with half dose.

2. *Stomatitis and aphthous esophageal ulcers* are relatively common and usually require drug interruption.
3. *Pancreatitis* is noted in <1% of patients, but more frequently in those with a history of prior pancreatitis or elevated amylase levels at time treatment was started.
4. *Hepatitis* with transaminase levels $>5 \times$ upper limit of normal.

Pregnancy: Category C. Teratogenic and embryolethal in doses $>1,000 \times$ those used in patients; no studies in patients.

Interactions: Drugs that cause peripheral neuropathy should be used with caution or avoided—ddI, cisplatin, disulfiram, ethionamide, isoniazid, phenytoin, vincristine, glutethimide, gold, hydralazine, and long-term metronidazole.

DIFLUCAN

See Fluconazole.

DOXYCYCLINE

Generic; Trade names: Vibramycin (Pfizer), Doryx, Doxychel, Vivox.

Forms and Price

Forms and price	Generic	Vibramycin
50 mg cap		$ 1.96
100 mg tab	$ 0.17	$ 3.52
100 mg vial (IV use)	$18.89	$21.07

Dose: 100 mg po bid.
Class: Tetracycline.
Indications:
Chlamydia trachomatis—100 mg po bid $\times$ 7 days.
Common respiratory tract infections (sinusitis, otitis, bronchitis)—100 mg po bid $\times$ 7–14 days.
Bacillary angiomatosis—100 mg po bid $\times$ 6 wks.

Pharmacology

Bioavailability: 93%; complexes with bivalent cations (Ca^{2+}, Mg^{2+}, Fe^{2+}, Al^{2+}, etc.) so milk, mineral preps, cathartics, and antacids with metal salts should not be given concurrently.

T1/2: 18 hours.

Elimination: Excreted in stool as chelated inactive agent independent of renal and hepatic function.

Dose modification with renal or hepatic failure: None.

Side effects: GI intolerance (10% and dose-related, reduced with food), diarrhea; deposited in developing teeth—contraindicated from midpregnancy to term and in children <8 years of age (Committee on Drugs, American Academy of Pediatrics); photosensitivity (exaggerated sunburn); *Candida* vaginitis; "black tongue"; rash.

Pregnancy: Category D; use in pregnant women and infants may cause retardation of skeletal development and bone growth; tetracyclines localize in dentin and enamel of developing teeth to cause enamel hypoplasia and yellow-brown discoloration. Tetracyclines should be avoided in pregnant women and children <8 years unless benefits outweigh these risks.

Drug interactions: Chelation with cations to reduce oral absorption; half-life of doxycycline decreased by carbamazepine (Tegretol), cimetidine, phenytoin, barbiturates; may interfere with oral contraceptives; potentiates oral hypoglycemics, digoxin, and lithium.

DRONABINOL

Trade name: Marinol (Roxane Labs).

Forms: Gelatin capsules of 2.5, 5, and 10 mg.

Cost: $3.12/2.5 mg cap; $6.16/5 mg cap; $12.36/10 mg cap.

Patient assistance program: (800) 274-8651.

Indication: Anorexia associated with weight loss (also used in higher doses as antiemetic in cancer patients).

Class: Psychoactive component of marijuana.

Dose: 2.5 mg bid (before lunch and before dinner). CNS symptoms (dose-related mood high, confusion, dizziness, somnolence) usually resolve in 1–3 days with continued use. If these symptoms are severe or persist, reduce to 2.5 mg before dinner and/or administer at hs. If tolerated and additional therapeutic effect desired, increase dose to 5 mg bid; occasionally patients require 10 mg bid.

Pharmacology

Bioavailability: 90–95%.

T1/2: 25–36 hours.

Elimination: First-pass hepatic metabolism and biliary excretion; 10–15% in urine.

Biologic effects post dose

Onset of action: 0.5–1 h, peak 2–4 h.

Duration psychoactive effect: 4–6 h; appetite effect: ≥24 h.

Side effects (dose-related): CNS with "high"—euphoria (3–10%) paranoia (3–10%), somnolence (3–10%), depersonalization, confusion, visual difficulties; GI intolerance (3–10%); central sympathomimetic effects—dizziness (3–10%), hypotension, palpitations, vasodilation, tachycardia; asthenia.

Pregnancy: Category C.

Drug interactions: Sympathomimetic agents (amphetamines, cocaine, etc.)—increased hypertension and tachycardia; anticholinergic drugs (atropine, scopolamine), amitriptyline, amoxapine, and other tricyclic antidepressants—tachycardia, drowsiness.

Warnings: Dronabinol is an orally psychoactive component of *Cannabis sativa*— marijuana; Schedule II (CII)—*potential for abuse*; use with caution in patients with (1) substance abuse, (2) patients with psychiatric illness (mania, depression, schizophrenia), (3) patients concurrently receiving sedatives, hypnotics, etc., (4) elderly patients (experience limited), (5) cardiac disorder (hypotension). Warn patient: (1) of CNS depression with concurrent use with alcohol, benzodiazepines, barbiturates, etc; (2) to avoid driving, operating machinery, etc. until safety and tolerance is established; (3) of mood and behavior changes.

d4T (STAVUDINE)

Trade name: Zerit (Bristol-Myers Squibb).

Forms and price: 15, 20, 30, and 40 mg caps; 40 mg tab: $2.82.

Class: Nucleoside analogue.

Financial assistance: (800) 788-0123. For patients without insurance coverage plus financial need.

Indications: FDA labeling—advanced HIV infection plus intolerance to approved therapies with proven benefit or significant clinical or immunologic deterioration with these treatments. In practice, d4T is relatively easy to administer (bid dosing) and it is generally well tolerated except for occasional patients with peripheral neuropathy.

Dose regimen:

Wt >60 kg 40 mg po bid

Wt <60 kg 30 mg po bid

Pharmacokinetics

Bioavailability:

T1/2 (serum): 1 hr.

T$_{1/2}$ (intracellular): 3.5 hr.
CNS penetration: 20–30%.
Elimination: Renal.
Dose modification in renal failure: Cr Cl >50 ml/min: 40 mg q 12 h; 26–50 ml/min: 20 mg q 12 h; 10–25 ml/min: 20 mg q 24 h.
Side effects:

1. Peripheral neuropathy: Experience with 13,000 participants in the parallel program and therapeutic trials showed 15–21% developed peripheral neuropathy. Peripheral neuropathy due to HIV infection or alternative nucleoside analogue treatment (ddI, ddC) represents a relative contraindication to d4T.
2. Pancreatitis: 0.5–1%.
3. Elevated transaminase levels—8%; neutropenia (rare).

Drug interactions: (1) AZT: There are conflicting data showing in vitro antagonism; (2) ddI and ddC: Overlapping toxicity with peripheral neuropathy; concurrent use should be avoided; (3) Drugs that cause peripheral neuropathy should be used with caution: cisplatin, disulfiram, ethionamide, isoniazid, phenytoin, vincristine, glutethimide, gold, hydralazine, and long-term metronidazole.

ENOXACIN

See Ciprofloxacin (Fluoroquinolone Summary).

EPOGEN

See Erythropoietin.

ERYTHROPOIETIN (EPO)

Trade name: Epogen (Amgen); Procrit (Ortho Biotech).
Price/vial: 2000 units = $24; 3000 units = $36; 4000 = $48. Usual dose: 30,000 3 × /wk = $360/wk.
Patient assistance program: Procrit-cost sharing—(800) 553-3851; $8,500 cap. Reimbursement appeal—(800) 553-3851; Financial assistance—(800) 553-3851: Patient must have no insurance coverage (or denial after reimbursement hotline is denied) plus physician contace. *Epogen* reimbursement hotline—(800) 272-9376.
Product information: EPO is the human hormone produced by recombinant DNA technology. The naturally occurring agent is a 165 amino acid glycoprotein with a molecular weight of 30.4 kd produced by the kidney.
Indications: Serum EPO level <500 milliunits/ml plus (1) severe anemia ascribed to HIV infection and (2) severe anemia ascribed to AZT treatment (*Ann Intern Med*

1992; 117:739; *J AIDS* 1992; 5:847). If AZT is implicated, it should be reduced in dose or discontinued.

Efficacy: Results of the U.S. trial with recombinant human erythropoietin (r-Hu EPO) initiated in July 1989 with 1,943 evaluable patients showed the following: (1) Inclusion criteria was an EPO serum level of <500 U/L and hematocrit <30%; 75% were receiving AZT at entry; (2) The initial dose was 4000 U SC 6 days/week with subsequent increases to 8000 U SC 6 days/week; mean weekly doses ranged from 22,700–32,500 U/week (340–490 U/kg/week); (3) Response to treatment defined as an increase in baseline hematocrit by siz percentage points (e.g., 30%→36%) with no transfusions within 28 days was achieved in 44%; transfusion requirements decreased from 40% of participants in 6 weeks' pretreatment to 18% at weeks 18–24. The average hematocrit among participants was 28% at entry and 35% at one year (*Arch Intern Med* 1993; 153:2669).

Dose recommendations: Initial dose is 35–200 units/kg IV or subcutaneously $3 \times$ weekly, usually 100 units/kg SC $3 \times$/week. Onset of action is within 1–2 weeks, reticulocytosis is noted at 7–10 days and desired hematocrit is usually attained in 8–12 weeks. Response is dependent on the degree of initial anemia, dose of EPO and available iron stores. The usual target hematocrit is 30–33%. The initial dose is increased by 25 units/kg every 4–8 weeks to a maximum of 300 units/kg $3 \times$/wk. If the hematocrit exceeds 40%, EPO should be stopped and resumed at a 25% dose reduction when the hematocrit is <36%. With failure to respond, consider iron deficiency, occult blood loss, folic acid or B_{12} deficiency, hemolysis, G6PD deficiency, etc.

Pharmacology

Bioavailability: EPO is a 165 amino acid glycoprotein that is not absorbed with oral administration. IV or SC administration is required; SC is preferred.

T1/2: 4–16 hours.

Elimination: Poorly understood but minimally affected by renal failure.

Dose adjustment in renal or hepatic failure: None.

Side effects: Generally well tolerated; serious reactions have not been described. Headache and arthralgias are most common; less common—flu-like symptoms, GI intolerance, diarrhea, edema, fatigue. Hypertension is a rare complication that is much more common in renal failure patients. The most common reactions noted in the therapeutic trial with 1,943 AIDS patients were rash, medication site reaction, nausea, hypertension, and seizures; relationship to EPO was often unclear.

Pregnancy: Class C. Teratogenic in animals; no studies in humans.

ETHAMBUTOL

Generic; Trade name: Myambutol (Lederle).

Forms: 100 and 400 mg tabs.

Price: $1.58/400 mg tab.
Indication: Active tuberculosis or infections with *M. avium* complex or *M. kansasii*.
Dose: 15 mg–25 mg/kg po given as one daily dose, usually 25 mg/kg/day × 1–2 months, then 15 mg/kg/day; maximum dose: 2.5 g/day. Twice weekly treatment: 50 mg/kg; thrice weekly treatment: 25–30 mg/kg.

Pharmacology

Bioavailability: 77%.
T1/2: 3.1 hours.
Elimination: Renal.
Dose modification in renal failure: Cr cl >50 ml/min—15–25 mg/kg q 24 h; 10–50 ml/min—15–25 mg/kg q 24–36 h; <10 ml/min—15–25 mg/kg q 48 h.
Side effects: Dose-related ocular toxicity (decreased acuity, restricted fields, scomata, and loss of color discrimination) with 25 mg/kg dose (0.8%), hypersensitivity (0.1%); peripheral neuropathy (rare); GI intolerance.
Pregnancy: Category C. Teratogenic in animals; no reported adverse effects in women; "use with caution."
Warnings: Patients should be warned to report any vision changes; pretreatment ophthalmologic exam is advocated if there is preexisting ocular abnormality such as cataracts, but not for simple refraction problem. Periodic ophthalmologic exam is not indicated for low-dose treatment (15 mg/kg/day).
Drug interactions: Al^{2+} containing antacids may decrease absorption.

FILGRASTIM

See G-CSF.

FLAGYL

See Metronidazole.

FLOXIN

See Ciprofloxacin (Fluoroquinolone Summary).

FLUCONAZOLE

Trade name: Diflucan (Pfizer).
Forms and price: 50 mg tab—$4.36; 100 mg tab—$6.36; 200 mg tab—$11.20; IV vials of 200 mg—$81.17; IV vials of 400 mg—$118.67.

Patient assistance program: (800) 869-9979. Patients must have no insurance coverage including Medicaid and income criteria ($<$$25,000/yr for single person and $<$$40,000 for married couple). Up to 3-month supply provided.

Class: Triazole related to other imidazoles-ketoconazole, clotrimazole, miconazole; triazoles (fluconazole and itraconazole) have three nitrogens in the azole ring.

Dose Regimen

Indications	Dose regimen[a]	Comment
Candida		
Thrush	50–100 mg po/d × 14 days	Response rates, 80–100%; maintenance therapy often required
Esophagitis	100–200 mg po/d × 2–3 wks	Superior to ketoconazole
Vaginitis	150 mg × 1 or 50 mg/d × 3	Response rates 90–100% in absence of HIV infection
Cryptococcosis		
Nonmeningeal	200–400 mg po/d	Usual initial dose is 400 mg/day × 8 weeks, then 200 mg/day
Meningitis	200 mg po/d (maintenance)	Initial treatment with amphotericin B usually preferred; if fluconazole used initially, the standard dose is 400 mg/day × 8 weeks, then 200 mg/day
Prophylaxis	100–200 mg po/d	Efficacy established for preventing thrush, *Candida* esophagitis and cryptococcosis; concerns are cost, drug interactions, and promotion of azole-resistant *Candida* infections

Note: Use double dose the first day (200–400 mg) when treating established infections.

Pharmacology

Bioavailability: $>$90%.

CSF levels: 50–94% serum levels.

T1/2: 30 hours.

Elimination: Renal, 60–80% of administered dose unchanged.

Dose modification in renal failure: Cr cl $>$50 ml/min—usual dose; 10–50 ml/min half dose; $<$10 ml/min—quarter dose.

Side effects: GI intolerance (1.5–8%, usually does not require discontinuation); rash (5%); transient increases in hepatic enzymes (5%), increases of ALT or AST to $>$8 × upper limit of normal requires discontinuation (1%); dizziness and headache (2%).

Pregnancy: Category C. Animal studies show reduced maternal weight gain and embryolethality of dose $>$20 × comparable doses in people; no studies in patients.

Drug interactions: Increased coumadin effect, phenytoin, oral hypoglycemic and cyclosporine levels; increased levels of terfinadine (Seldane) with ventricular arrhythmias. Fluconazole levels are reduced with rifampin and rifabutin; fluconazole increases levels of rifabutin with increased risk of uveitis.

FLUCYTOSINE

Generic; Trade name: Ancobon (Roche).
Forms: 250 & 500 mg caps.
Price: $1.03/250 mg cap; $1.98/500 mg cap.
Class: Fluorinated purimidime structurally related to fluorouracil.
Indication: Used with amphotericin B to treat serious infections caused by *Candida* sp. and *Cryptococcosis*.
Dose: 25–37.5 mg/kg po q 6 h (100–150 mg/kg/d).

Pharmacology

Bioavailability: >80%.
T1/2: 2.4–4.8 hours.
Elimination: 63–84% unchanged in urine.
CNS penetration: 80% serum levels.
Dose modification in renal failure: Cr cl >50 ml/min—25–37.6 mg/kg q 6 h; 10–50 ml/min—25–37 mg/kg q 12–24 h; <10 ml/min—not recommended.
Therapeutic monitoring: Measure serum concentration 2 hours post–oral dose with goal for peak level of 50–100 mcg/ml.
Side effects: Dose-related leukopenia and thrombocytopenia, especially with renal failure (often secondary to concurrent amphotericin B), levels >100 mcg/ml and concurrent use of other marrow-suppressing agents; GI intolerance; rash; hepatitis; peripheral neuropathy
Pregnancy: Category C. Teratogenic in animals; no studies in patients. Contraindicated in pregnancy unless benefits outweigh potential risks

FLURAZEPAM

Generic; Trade name: Dalmane (Roche), Durapam, Apo-Flurazepam, Som-Pam, Somnol.

Forms and Price

	Dalmane	Generic
15 mg caps	$0.53	$0.05
30 mg caps	$0.58	$0.06

Class: Benzodiazepine antianxiety/hypnotic; controlled substance category IV.

Indications and dose regimen: Insomnia: 15–30 mg po hs; especially useful for *intermittent* treatment of insomnia or for periods up to 4 weeks.

Pharmacology

Bioavailability: >90%.

T1/2: Metabolized to a long-acting metabolite desalkylflurazepam with $T_{1/2}$ of 36–120 hours.

Biologic activity: Hypnotic effect begins 20 min after administration and lasts 7–8 hours; effective for up to 4 weeks.

Elimination: Metabolized to active metabolites, which may accumulate in renal failure.

Side effects: See Benzodiazepines. Major side effects are daytime sedation with drowsiness and impairment of dexterity.

Pregnancy: Category D; Fetal harm—contraindicated.

Drug interactions: See Benzodiazepines.

FOSCAR

See Foscarnet.

FOSCARNET

Trade name: Foscar (Astra).

Forms: Vials of 6,000 mg and 12,000 mg.

Cost (70 kg patient): Induction—$146/day, maintenance—$73/day. Ganciclovir comparison: Induction—$52/day; maintenance—$26/day.

Patient assistance program: (800) 488-3247. Patient must have newly diagnosed CMV retinitis or medical reason to switch from ganciclovir plus lack of insurance. Other indications (acyclovir resistant HSV, CMV colitis, etc.): (800) 388-4148.

Activity: Active versus herpes viruses including CMV, HSV-1, HSV-2, EBV (oral hairy leukoplakia), VZV, HHV-6, most ganciclovir-resistant CMV, and most acyclovir resistant HSV and VZV. Also active *in vitro* vs. HIV.

Indications and Doses

Indications	Regimen
CMV retinitis[a]	Induction: 60 mg/kg IV q 8 h or 90 mg/kg IV q 12 h; Maintenance: 90–120 mg/kg IV qd**
CMV (other)	60 mg/kg IV q 8 h or 90 mg/kg IV q 12 h × 14–21 days; indications for maintenance treatment are unclear

Indications	Regimen
Acyclovir-resistant HSV	40 mg/kg IV q 8 h or 60 mg/kg q 12 h×3 weeks
Acyclovir-resistant VZV	40 mg/kg IV q 8 h or 60 mg/kg q 12 h×3 weeks

*a*FDA appoved.
*b*Survival and time to relapse may be significantly prolonged with maintenance dose of 120 mg/d vs .90 mg/d (*J Infect Dis* 1993; 168:444).

Pharmacology

Bioavailability: 5–8% absorption with oral administration, but poorly tolerated.
T1/2: 3 hours.
CSF levels: 15–70% plasma levels.
Elimination: Renal exclusively.
Administration: Controlled IV infusion using ≤24 mg/ml (undiluted) by central venous catheter of <12 mg/ml (diluted in 5% dextrose or saline) via a peripheral line. No other drug is to be given concurrently via the same catheter. Induction dose of 60 mg/kg is given over ≥1 hour via infusion pump with *adequate hydration*. Maintenance treatment with 90–120 mg/kg is given over ≥2 hours by infusion pump with *adequate hydration*. Many use 90 mg/kg for initial maintenance and 120 mg/kg for maintenance after reinduction for a relapse.

Dose Adjustment in Renal Failure

CrCl (ml/min/kg)	60 mg/kg dose	90 mg/kg dose	120 mg/kg dose
>1.4	60	90	12
1.3	49	78	104
1.1	42	75	100
0.9	35	71	94
0.7	28	63	84
0.5	21	57	76

Side effects:

1. Dose-related renal impairment—37% treated for CMV retinitis have serum creatinine increase to ≥2 mg/dl; most common during second week of induction and usually reversible with recovery of renal function within 1 week of discontinuation. Monitor creatinine 2–3×/week with induction and q 1–2 weeks during maintenance. Modify dose for creatinine clearance changes. Foscarnet should be stopped for creatinine clearance <0.4 ml/min/kg.
2. Changes in serum electrolytes including hypocalcemia (15%), hypophosphatemia (8%), hypomagnesemia (15%), and hypokalemia (16%). Patients should be warned to report symptoms of hypocalcemia: perioral paresthesias, extremity paresthesias, and numbness. Monitor serum Ca^{2+}, Mg^{2+}, K^+, phosphate and

creatinine, usually$\geq 2 \times$/week during induction and $1 \times$/wk during maintenance. If paresthesias develop during infusions with normal electrolytes, measure ionized calcium at start and end of infusion.
3. Seizures (10%) related to renal failure and hypocalcemia.
4. Penile ulcers.

Miscellaneous: Nausea, vomiting, headache, rash, fever, hepatitis, marrow suppression.

Pregnancy: Category C. No adequate studies in animals or patients.

Drug interactions: Concurrent administration with IV pentamidine may cause severe hypocalcemia. Avoid concurrent use of potentially nephrotoxic drugs such as amphotericin B, aminoglycosides, and pentamidine. Possible increase in seizures with imipenem.

FUNGISONE

See Amphotericin B.

GANCICLOVIR

Trade name: Cytovene (Syntex).

Forms and price: 500 mg vial at $34.80 and 250 mg caps at $3.90/cap.

Patient assistance program: (800) 444-4200 or (800) 285-4484. Patient must have CMV retinitis, no insurance coverage, and inability to pay plus outpatient treatment.

Class: Synthetic purine nucleoside analogue of guanine.

Active vs. herpes viruses including CMV, HSV-1, HSV-2, EBV, VZV, and HHV-6. About 10% of patients given ganciclovir ≥ 3 months for CMV will excrete resistant strains that are sensitive to foscarnet (*J Infect Dis* 1991; 163:716, 1991; 163:1348).

Indications and Dose Regimen

CMV retinitis: 5 mg/kg IV q 12 h $\times$ 14–21 days, then maintenance with 5 mg/kg/day IV or 1.0 g tid po. Initial results show time to relapse is somewhat earlier with oral vs. IV ganciclovir, but it avoids the inconvenience cost and complications of the indwelling IV catheter.

Other forms of disseminated CMV: Indications to treat are often not well established; when treated, the usual regimen is the induction dose used for retinitis; need for maintenance therapy is not clear. Oral ganciclovir has been studied only with maintenance therapy of CMV retinitis.

CMV prophylaxis: Initial studies show oral ganciclovir (1 g po tid) significantly reduces rates of CMV disease (primarily retinitis) in AIDS patients with a CD4 count $<50/mm^3$. Concerns are cost (about \$15,000/yr), side effects (neutropenia and anemia), and possible promotion of ganciclovir resistance.

Pharmacology

Bioavailability: ≤7% absorption with oral administration.

CSF concentrations: 24–70% of plasma levels.

T1/2: 2.5–3.6 hours.

Elimination: 90–99% excreted unchanged in urine.

Dose modification in renal failure (IV form): Cr cl ≥80 ml/min—5 mg/kg q 12 h; 50–79 ml/min—2.5 mg/kg q 12 h; 25–49 ml/min—2.5 mg/kg q 24 h; <25 ml/min—1.25 mg/kg q 24 h.

Administration: On December 28, 1993, Syntex published a product warning stating crystals of an antioxidant from rubber stoppers were noted in reconstituted vials. An in-line filter with a 0.22-micron filter (preferred) or a 5-micron filter is now required. The drug should be reconstituted immediately before use and unused portions should be discarded. Infusions should be given over one hour.

Side effects: IV form: (1) Neutropenia with ANC $<500/mm^3$ (25–40%) requires discontinuation of drug in ≥20%; alternative is administration of G-CSF; discontinuation or reduced dose will result in increased ANC in 3–7 days. Monitor CBC 2–3 × /wk and discontinue if WBC $<500/mm^3$ or platelet count $<25,000/mm^3$; (2) thrombocytopenia in 2–8%; (3) CNS toxicity in 10–15% with headaches, seizures, confusion, coma; (4) hepatotoxicity (2–3%); (5) GI intolerance (2%). Oral form: Neutropenia (20%), anemia (15%), possible renal insufficiency.

Pregnancy: Category C. Teratogenic in animals in concentrations comparable to those achieved in patients; should be avoided unless need justifies the risk.

Drug interaction: AZT increases the risk of neutropenia and concurrent use is not recommended. Antagonizes in vitro activity of ddI versus HIV in H9 cells; clinical relevance is unknown. Additive or synergistic activity with foscarnet *in vitro* versus CMV and HSV. Use with caution with drugs that inhibit replication of rapidly dividing cells—dapsone, pentamidine, pyrimethamine, flucytosine, cytotoxic anti-neoplastic drugs (vincristine, vinblastine, doxorubicin), amphotericin B, trimethoprim-sulfa, and nucleoside analogues.

G-CSF (FILGRASTIM)

Trade name: Neupogen (Amgen).

Price: 300 mcg—\$148.30.

Reimbursement assistance/appeal: (800) 272-9376; *patient assistance*: (800) 272-9376. Patient must lack prescription drug insurance and demonstrate financial need.

Product information: A 20-kilodalton glycoprotein produced by recombinant technique that stimulates granulocyte precursors.

Indication: Neutropenia with ANC <500–750/mm^3 ascribed to (1) zidovudine (AZT) (*Blood* 1991; 77:2109); (2) other drugs such as ganciclovir; (3) cancer chemotherapy (lymphoma or Kaposi sarcoma; or (4) HIV infection.

Dose: Initial dose is 1 mcg/kg/day subcutaneously (lean body weight). This may be increased by 1 mcg/kg/day after 5–7 days up to 10 mcg/kg/day. Monitor CBC 2×/wk and reduce dose 50% weekly for maintenance to keep ANC >750–1500/mm^3. Usual maintenance dose is 1 mcg/kg/day (0.3–3 mcg/kg/day). If unresponsive after 7 days at 10 mcg/kg/day, treatment should be discontinued.

Pharmacology

Absorption: Not absorbed with oral administration. G-CSF must be given IV or SC; SC is usually preferred.

T$_{1/2}$: 3.5 hours (subcutaneous injection).

Elimination: Renal.

Side effects: Medullary bone pain is the only important side effect, noted in 10–20% and usually controlled with acetaminophen. Rare side effects: mild dysuria, reversible abnormal liver function tests, increased uric acid, and increased LDH.

Pregnancy: Category C. Caused abortion and embryolethality in animals at 2–10× dose in humans; no studies in patients.

Drug interactions: Should not be given within 24 hours of chemotherapy.

Note: GM-CSF is also available from three suppliers as Leucoman (Sandoz), Leukine (Immunex), and Prokine (Hoechst-Roussel). This may also be used for neutropenia in same dose and same indications, but there is an as yet unsubstantiated concern for stimulation of the monocyte cell line (which harbors HIV) as well as the granulocyte series.

HALCION

See Triazolam.

HUMATIN

See Paromomycin.

INTERFERON

Trade name: Roferon (Hoffmann-LaRoche), Intron (Schering).

Forms and price: Interferon Alfa 2a (Roferon): vials of 3, 18, and 26 million units = $29.87/3 mil units. *Patient assistance program* (Roferon): (800) 443-6676; cap program (983 million units ≤1 year): (800) 443-6676.

Interferon Alfa 2b (Intron): vials of 3, 5, 10, 18, 25, and 50 million units; $31.51/3 million units. *Patient assistance program* (Intron): (800) 521-7157.

Class: Interferon alfa is a family of highly homogeneous species-specific proteins of human origin (using donor cells, cultured human cell lines or combinant techniques with human genes) with complex antiviral, antineoplastic and immunomodulating activities. The alfa 2a and alfa 2b refer to similar subtypes prepared by recombinant techniques.

Activity: Broad spectrum antiviral agent with *in vitro* activity versus HIV, HPV, HBV, HCV, HSV-1 & 2, CMV, VZV, etc.

Indications and regimen (Interferon Alfa 2b)

Hepatitis C: 3 mil units IM or SC $3 \times$/wk $\times$ 6 mo.
Hepatitis B: 5 mil units IM or SC daily or 10 mil units $3 \times$/wk $\times$ 4 mo.
Kaposi sarcoma: 30–36 mil units IM or SC ($3–7 \times$/wk) until KS lesions resolve, toxicity precludes further treatment or rapid progression of KS (average 7 months). Best response rates (40–50%) in patients with CD4 counts >200/mm^3 and no "B symptoms"; dose related.
Genital and anal warts: Intralesion injection of 1 mil units $3 \times$ weekly $\times$ 3 weeks with a maximum of five warts (5 mil units).

Pharmacology

Bioavailability: Protein with 165 amino acids and molecular weight of 18,000–20,000; absorption with oral administration is nil, bioavailability with SC or IM administration is (?) 80%.
T1/2: 2–5.1 hours.
CSF level: None detected.
Elimination: Metabolized by kidney.
Side effects: All patients have side effects and especially with doses$\geq$18 mil units. Most side effects diminish in frequency and severity with continued administration:

1. Flu-like syndrome (50–98%): Fever, chills, fatigue, headache, and arthralgias, usually within 6 hours of administration lasting 2–12 hours. (Reduced with non-steroidal antiinflammatory agents).
2. GI intolerance (20–65%) with anorexia, nausea, vomiting, diarrhea, metallic taste, and abdominal pain.
3. CNS toxicity with delirium or obtundation.
4. Marrow suppression with neutropenia, anemia, or thrombocytopenia.
5. Hepatotoxicity (10–50%) with increased transaminase.
6. Dyspnea and cough.
7. Rash $\pm$ alopecia (25%).
8. Proteinuria (15–20%).

Pregnancy: Category C. Abortifacient in animals with doses 20–500×doses in humans. No data for patients. Use in pregnancy only when need justifies risk.

Drug interactions: AZT-increased hematologic toxicity; increased levels of theophylline, barbiturates.

INTRON

See Interferon.

ISONIAZID

Generic; Trade names: Isotamine, Laniazide, Teebaconin, Rifamate, Nydrazid.
Forms: 50, 100, and 300 mg tabs; solution for injection.
Combinations: Caps with rifampin: 150 mg INH + 300 mg rifampin.
Price: $0.02/300 mg tab.
Indications: Prophylaxis and treatment of tuberculosis.

Dose

	Daily	DOT
Prophylaxis	300 mg	900 mg 2×/wk
Treatment	300 mg	900 mg 2–3×/wk

Pharmacology

Bioavailability: 90%.

T1/2: 1–4 hrs; 1 hr with rapid acetylators.

Elimination: Metabolized and eliminated in urine. Rate of acetylation is genetically determined. Slow inactivation reflects deficiency of hepatic enzyme N-acetyltransferase and is found in about 50% of whites and African-Americans. Rate of acetylation does not effect efficacy of standard daily or DOT regimens.

Dose modification in renal failure: Half dose with creatinine clearance <10 ml/min in slow acetylators.

Side effects: Hepatitis rates by age (Med Clin North Am 1988; 72:661)

	25 yrs	35 yrs	45 yrs	55 yrs	65 yrs
Definite	1.3%	5.9%	10.9%	17.5%	10.5%
Probable	6.3%	12.7%	20.4%	31.4%	25.5%

Peripheral neuropathy due to increased excretion of pyridoxine is dose related and rare with usual doses; it is prevented with concurrent pyridoxine (10–50 mg/day), which is recommended for diabetics, alcoholics, pregnant patients, AIDS patients, and malnourished patients. Miscellaneous reactions: rash, fever, adenopathy, GI intolerance. Rare reactions: psychosis, arthralgias, optic neuropathy, marrow suppression.

Drug interactions: Increase effects of coumadin, benzodiazepines, carbamazepine, cycloserine, ethionamide, phenytoin, theophylline; INH decreased with Al containing antacids; hepatitis: increased frequency with excessive alcohol; ketoconazole: decreased ketoconazole effect; food: decreases absorption; tyramine (cheese, wine, some fish); rare patients develop palpitations, sweating, urticaria, headache, and vomiting.

Pregnancy: Category C. Embryocidal in animals; not teratogenic. No adverse effects noted in patients. AAP recommendation is that pregnant women with positive PPD plus HIV infection should receive INH; begin after first trimester if possible.

ITRACONAZOLE

Trade name: Sporanox (Janssen).
Forms and price: 100 mg caps at $5.37/100 mg cap. Price for histoplasmosis (200 mg bid): $21.48/day. Price for thrush (100–200 mg/day): $5.37–$10.74/day. Price comparison for thrush: nystatin (5cc 5 × /d) = $1.40/day; ketoconazole (200 mg/d) = $2.76/day; fluconazole (100 mg/d) = $6.87/day.
Patient assistance program: (800) 544-2987. Patient must have no insurance and income/asset eligibility, which are individually reviewed. Drug is available for off-label indications.

Indications and Dose Regimen

Indication	Dose
Histoplasmosis[a]	300 mg po bid × 3 days, then 200 mg po bid indefinitely (induction with 1 g amphotericin B preferred for moderately severe disseminated disease) (*Ann Intern Med* 1993; 118:610)
Candida[b]	
Thrush	200 mg po/day, maintenance: 100 mg/day
Vaginitis	100–200 mg po bid × 1 day or 100–200 mg/day × 2–3 days
Esophagitis	100–200 mg po bid
Aspergillus[b]	200 mg po bid (amphotericin B often preferred)
Cryptococcosis[b]	200 mg po tid × 3 days, then 200 mg po bid (fluconazole preferred)

[a]FDA approved.
[b]Alternative agents usually preferred.

Class: Triazole (like fluconazole) with three nitrogens in the azole ring; other imidazoles have two nitrogens.

Activity: *In vitro* activity vs. *H. capsulatum*, *B. dermatitidis*, *Aspergillus*, *Cryptococcus*, *Candida* sp.

Pharmacology

Bioavailability: 55%, improved when taken with food and reduced with gastric achlorhydria.

T1/2: 64 hours.

Elimination: Metabolized by liver to metabolites including hydroxyitraconazole, which is active *in vitro* vs. many fungi. Renal excretion is 0.03% of parent drug and 40% of administered dose as metabolites.

Dose modification with renal failure: None.

Dose modification with liver disease: No data; manufacturer suggests monitoring serum levels.

Side effects: Hepatitis (3/2,500) including one case of fulminant fatal hepatitis. Hepatic enzymes should be monitored in patients with prior hepatic disease and patients should be warned to report symptoms of hepatitis. Most common side effects are GI intolerance (3–10%) and rash (1–9%, most common in immunosuppressed patients).

Pregnancy: Category C; teratogenic to rats, no studies in people.

Interactions: Increases levels of terfenadine (seldane) to cause life-threatening cardiac arrhythmias. Possible serious interaction with astemizole. Increased levels of cyclosporine, oral hypoglycemia, and digoxin. Decreased itraconazole levels with administration of rifampin, rifabutin, isoniazid, phenytoin, and H_2 antagonists.

KETOCONAZOLE

Trade name: Nizoral (Janssen).

Form and price: 200 mg tabs—$2.71; 2% cream 30 g—$22.63.

Class: Azole antifungal agent.

Patient assistance program: (800) 544-2987.

Indications:
Thrush: 200 mg po 1–2 × /day.
Candida esophagitis: 200–400 mg po bid.
Candida vaginitis: 200–400 mg/day po × 7days or 400 mg/day × 3 days.

Pharmacology

Bioavailability: 75% with gastric acid; decreased bioavailability with hypochlorhydria (common in AIDS patients).

Administration with hypochlorhydria: Each 200 mg should be dissolved in 4 ml of 0.2 N hydrochloric acid or taken with 200 ml 0.1 N HCl. Use straw to avoid contact with teeth. Alternatives are concurrent administration 580 mg glutamic acid hydrochloride.

T1/2: 6–10 hrs.

Elimination: Metabolized by liver, but half-life is not prolonged with hepatic failure.

Dose modification in renal failure: None.

Side effects: Gastrointestinal intolerance; temporary increase in transaminase levels (2–5%); dose-related decrease in steroid and testosterone synthesis with impotence gynecomastia, oligospermia, reduced libido, menstrual abnormalities (usually with doses≥600 mg/d for prolonged periods); headache, dizziness, asthenia; rash; abrupt hepatitis with hepatic failure (1:15,000); rare cases of hepatic necrosis; marrow suppression (rare); hypothyroidism (genetically determined); hallucinations (rare).

Drug interactions: Important interactions: H_2-antagonists—decreased ketoconazole absorption (use sucralfate or antacids given >2 hours before); ddI—decreased ketoconazole absorption (give≥2 hours apart); INH—decreased ketoconazole effect; rifampin—decreased activity of both drugs; seldane—ventricular arrhythmias (avoid concurrent use). Others: Alcohol—possible disulfiram-like reaction; antacids—decreased ketoconazole absorption; oral anticoagulants—increased hypoprothrombinemia; corticosteroids—increased methylprednisolone effect; cyclosporine—increased cyclosporine activity; phenytoin—altered metabolism of both drugs; theophylline—increased theophylline activity.

Pregnancy: Category C. Embryotoxic and teratogenic in experimental animals with large doses; no studies in patients; use with caution.

LAMPRENE

See Clofazimine.

LOMAFLOXACIN

See Ciprofloxacin (Fluoroquinolone Summary).

LORAZEPAM

Generic; Trade name: Ativan (Wyeth-Ayerst).

Forms and Price

	Ativan	Generic
0.5 mg tab	$ .60	$.02
1.0 mg tab	$ .78	$.02
2.0 mg tab	$1.98	$.03

Oral soln (Atrivan) 2 mg/ml—$12.67/2 mg and $12.67/4 mg; soln (IV) 2, 4, 20, 40 mg vials (2 or 4 mg/ml) $12.01/2 mg vial; $133.74/40 mg vial.

Class: Benzodiazepine, controlled substance category IV.

Indications and Dose Regimens

Anxiety: 1–2 mg 2–3 × /day; increase to usual dose of 2–6 mg/day in 2–3 divided doses.

IV administration: 2 mg.

Insomnia plus anxiety: 2–4 mg hs.

Pharmacology

Bioavailability: >90%.

T1/2: 10–25 hours.

Elimination: Renal excretion of inactive glucuronide metabolite. Not recommended with severe hepatic and/or renal disease.

Side effects: See Benzodiazepines. Additive CNS depression with other CNS depressants including alcohol. Warn patient of prolonged sedation and decreased recall for >8 hours. Injected lorazepam may reduce physical coordination for 24–48 hours.

Pregnancy: Category D; fetal harm—contraindicated.

LOTRIMIN

See Clotrimazole.

MARINOL

See Dronabinol.

MEGACE

See Megestrol Acetate.

MEGESTROL ACETATE

Trade name: Megace (Bristol-Myers).
Form and price: 20 mg tab—$.70; 40 mg tab—$1.24; oral suspension 40 mg/ml (8 oz.).
Financial assistance program: (800) 788-0123 for patients without insurance coverage plus financial need.
Class: Synthetic progestin related to progesterone.
Indications: Appetite stimulant to promote weight gain in patients with HIV infection or neoplastic disease.
Usual regimen: 80 mg po qid; up to 800 mg/day. Oral suspension—800 mg (20 m) in one daily dose.
Efficacy: Average weight gain in uncontrolled study—0.5 kg/wk with average total weight gain 6.3 kg. However, treatment failures are noted with up to 650 mg/day.

Pharmacology

Bioavailability: >90% absorbed.
T1/2: 30 hours.
Elimination: Completely metabolized by liver and metabolites excreted in urine.
Side effects: Rare—carpal tunnel syndrome, thrombosis, nausea, vomiting, edema, vaginal bleeding, hyperglycemia, rash, and alopecia; high dose (480–1,600 mg/day)—hyperpnea, chest pressure, mild increase in blood pressure, dyspnea, congestive heart failure.
Pregnancy: Progestin with possible adverse effects on fetus during first 4 months of pregnancy.

MEPRON

See Atovaquone.

METHADONE

Generic; Trade name: Dolophine.
Forms: 5 mg tab—$0.07.
       10 mg tab—$0.12.
       5 mg/5 ml (500 ml)—$.26/5 mg.
       10 mg/5 ml (500 ml)—$.45/10 mg.

Usual yearly cost of medication for methadone maintenance averages $180.

Class: Opiate agonist schedule II. The FDA limits access to methadone to patients who attend specially approved methadone clinics.

Indications

Detoxification for substantial opiate-agonist abstinence symptoms: Initial dose is based on opiate tolerance, usually 15–20 mg; additional doses may be necessary. Daily dose—40 mg usually stabilizes patient; when stable 2–3 days, then decrease dose 20%/day. Must complete detoxification <180 days or treatment is considered maintenance.

Maintenance as oral substitute for heroin or other morphine-like drugs: initial dose 15–39 mg depending on extent of prior use, up to 40 mg/day. Subsequent doses depend on response. Usual maintenance dose is 40–100 mg/day, but higher doses are sometimes required. Most states limit the maximum daily dose at 80–120 mg/day.

Note: During first 3 months, all patients receiving >100 mg/day, must be observed 6 days/week; with good compliance and rehabilitation, clinic attendance may be reduced for observed ingestion 3 days/week with maximum 2-day supply for home administration; after 2 years, clinic visits may be reduced to 2/wk with 3-day drug supplies; after 3 years, visits may be reduced to weekly with a 6-day supply.

Pain: 2.5–10 mg q 3–4 h not to exceed 80 mg/day.

Pharmacology

Bioavailability: >90% absorbed.

T1/2: 25 hours. Duration of action with repeated administration is 24–48 hours.

Elimination: Metabolized by liver. Parent compound excreted in urine with increased rate in alkaline urine; metabolites excreted in urine and gut.

Side Effects

Acute toxicity: CNS depression—stupor or coma, respiratory depression, flaccid muscles, cold skin, bradycardia hypotension. Treatment: Respiratory support, with or without gastric lavage (even hours after ingestion due to pylorospasm) and naloxone (but respiratory depression may last longer than naloxone and naloxone may precipitate acute withdrawal syndrome).

Chronic toxicity: Tolerance/physical dependence with abstinence syndrome following withdrawal—onset at 3–4 days after last dose with weakness, anxiety, anorexia, insomnia, abdominal pain, headache, sweating, and hot-cold flashes. Treatment: Detoxification.

Pregnancy: Category C. Avoid during first 3 months and use sparingly in small doses during last 6 months.

Drug interactions: Potentiate effects of other CNS depressants including alcohol and marijuana. Methadone levels are reduced with rifampin or rifabutin.

METRONIDAZOLE

Generic; Trade names: Flagyl (Searle); Femazole, Metizol, MetroGel, Metryl, Neo-Tric, Novonidazole, Protostat, Trikacids.

Forms and Price

	Generic	Flagyl
250 mg tab	$0.04	$ 1.21
500 mg tab	$0.08	$ 2.20
500 mg vial (VI)	$8.95	$15.50

Class: Synthetic nitroimidazole-derivative.

Indications and Dose Regimens

Gingivitis: 250 mg po tid or 500 mg po bid.
Intraabdominal sepsis: 1.5–2g/day po or IV in 2–4 doses.
Amebiasis: 750 mg po tid × 5–10 days.
Bacterial vaginosis: 2 g × 1 or 500 mg po bid × 7 days.
Trichomoniasis: 2 g × 1 or 250 mg po tid × 7 days.
C. difficile colitis: 500 mg po bid or 250 mg po tid × 10–14 days.

Pharmacology

Bioavailability: >90%.
T1/2: 10.2 hours; serum levels with 500 mg doses: 10–30 µg/ml.
Elimination: Hepatic metabolism; metabolites excreted in urine.
Dose adjustment in renal failure: None.
Liver failure: Half-life prolonged; reduce daily dose in severe liver disease and monitor serum levels.
Side effects: Uncommon—GI intolerance, unpleasant taste, glossitis, furry tongue, headache, ataxia, urticaria, dark urine; rare—seizures; prolonged use—reversible peripheral neuropathy; disulfiram (Antabuse)—type reaction with alcohol.

Pregnancy: Category B. Fetotoxicity in animals. Contraindicated in first trimester—although 206 exposures during the first trimester showed no increase in birth defects; use during the last 6 months is not advised unless essential. For trichomoniasis CDC recommends 2 g × 1 after first trimester. Alternative agents are available for most other conditions.

Drug interactions: Increases levels of coumadin, lithium, and possibly astemizole and terfenadine (Seldane); the latter may cause ventricular arrhythmias and the combination should be avoided. Mild disulfiram-like reactions noted with alcohol (flushing, headache, nausea, vomiting, cramps, sweating). This is infrequent and unpredictable. Patients should be warned and manufacturer recommends that alcohol be avoided. Concurrent use with disulfiram may cause psychoses or confusion; disulfiram should be stopped 2 weeks prior to use of metronidazole.

Note: Metronidazole is virtually completely absorbed with oral administration and should be given IV only if patient can take nothing by mouth.

MYAMBUTOL

See Ethambutol.

MYCELEX

See Clotrimazole.

MYCOBUTIN

See Rifabutin.

MYCOSTATIN

See Nystatin.

NEBUTEM

See Pentamidine.

NEUPOGEN

See G-CSF.

NIZORAL

See Ketoconazole.

NORFLOXACIN

See Ciprofloxacin (Fluoroquinolone Summary).

NORTRIPTYLINE

Generic; Trade names: Aventyl (Lilly); Pamelor (Sandoz).
Forms and prices: 10 mg caps—$0.19; 25 mg caps—$0.39; 50 mg caps—$.73; 75 mg caps—$1.11; oral suspension 10 mg/5 ml (480 ml)—$0.47/10 mg.
Class: Tricyclic antidepressant.
Indications and dose regimens: (1) Depression: 10–25 mg hs initially; increase to 25 mg 3–4 × /day or 50–150 mg hs over 2–3 weeks depending on response, side effects and serum levels (objective is 70–125 ng/ml). (2) Peripheral neuropathy: 10 mg hs; increase dose by 10 mg q 5 days to maximum of 50 mg hs.

Pharmacology

Bioavailability: >90% absorbed.
T1/2: 13–79 hours, mean—31 hours.
Elimination: Metabolized and renally excreted.
Side effects: Anticholinergic effects (dry mouth, dizzy, blurred vision, constipation, urinary hesitancy), orthostatic hypotension (less compared to other tricyclics), sedation, sexual dysfunction (decreased libido), and weight gain.
Pregnancy: Category D. Animal studies are inconclusive and experience in pregnant women is inadequate. Avoid during first trimester and limit use when possible in the last two trimesters.
Drug interactions: The following drugs should not be given concurrently: adrenergic neuronal blocking agents, clonidine, other alpha-2 agonists, disulfiram, excessive alcohol, fenfluramine, cimetidine, and MAO inhibitors. Drugs that increase nortriptyline levels—cimetidine, quinidine, fluconazole.

NYSTATIN

Generic: Mycostatin (Apothecon, Bristol-Myers).
Forms and cost: Lozenges (200,000 units)—$.93/Mycostatin lozenge; Cream (100,000 μ/g) 15 g—$1.46, 30 g—$2.18 (generic), 15 g—$14.48 (Mycostatin); Ointment (100,000 μ/g) 15 g—$1.46, 30 g—$3.60 (generic), 15 g—$14.48 (Mycostatin); Suspension (100,000 μ/ml) 60 ml—$3.29, 480 ml—$20.64 (generic),

60 ml—$21.84 (Mycostatin); Oral tabs (500,000 units)—$.12/tab (generic), $.55/tab (Mycostatin); Vaginal tabs (100,000 units)—$.15/tab (generic), $.98/tab (Mycostatin).

Class: Polyene macrolide similar to amphotericin B.

Activity: Active versus *Candida albicans* at 3 μg/ml and other *Candida* species at higher concentrations.

Indications and Dose Regimens

Thrush—5 ml suspension to be gargled $5 \times$/day $\times 14$ days.

Vaginitis—100,000 unit tab intravaginally $1-2 \times$/day $\times 14$ days.

Note: Some studies suggest topical treatment with imidazoles (clotrimazole, miconazole) may be superior.

Pharmacokinetics

Bioavailability: Poorly absorbed and not detectable in blood with oral administration. Therapeutic levels persist in saliva for 2 hours after oral dissolution of two lozenges.

Side effects: Infrequent, dose-related GI intolerance (transient nausea, vomiting, diarrhea).

OFLOXACIN

See Ciprofloxacin (Fluoroquinolone Summary).

PAMELOR

See Nortriptyline.

PAROMOMYCIN

Trade name: Humatin (Parke Davis).

Forms: 250 mg caps.

Price: $1.88/250 mg cap.

Class: Aminoglycoside (for oral use).

Indication: Cryptosporidiosis.

Dose: 500–750 mg po qid $\times 21$ days.

Efficacy: Anecdotal reports show clinical response in 42 of 43 patients, but there are no controlled studies and many unreported clinical failures (*Clin Infect Dis* 1992; 15:726).

Pharmacology

Bioavailability: Not absorbed; most of oral dose is excreted unchanged in stool; lesions of the GI tract may facilitate absorption and serum levels may increase in presence of renal failure.

Side effects: GI intolerance (anorexia, nausea, vomiting, epigastric pain), steatorrhea and malabsorption; rare complications include rash, headache, vertigo. There could be ototoxicity and nephrotoxicity with systemic absorption as with other aminoglycosides.

PENETREX

See Ciprofloxacin (Fluoroquinolone Summary).

PENTAM

See Pentamidine.

PENTAMIDINE

Trade name: Pentam for IV use and NebuPent for inhalation (Fujisawa).
Forms: 300 mg vial.
Price: $98.75/300 mg vial; PCP prophylaxis—$98.75/mo, PCP treatment—$2,100.
Patient assistance program: (708) 317-8636 or FAX letter of inquiry for contact (708) 317-5941.
Insurance reimbursement: (800) 366-6323.
Class: Aromatic diamidine-derivative antiprotozoal agent that is structurally related to stilbamidine.
Indications and dose regimen: (1) *P. carinii* pneumonia: 3–4 mg/kg IV × 21 days (TMP-SMX preferred). (2) *P. carinii* prophylaxis: 300 mg/month delivered by a Respirgard II Nebulizer using 300 mg dose diluted in 6 ml sterile water delivered at 6 L/min from a 50 psi compressed air source until the reservoir is dry. (TMP-SMX preferred due to superior efficacy in preventing PCP, efficacy in preventing other infections, reduced cost, and greater convenience.)

Pharmacology

Bioavailability: Not absorbed orally, with aerosol—5% reaches alveolar spaces via Respirgard II Nebulizer, 16% with Fisoneb nebulizer. Blood levels with monthly aerosol delivery are below detectable limits.
T1/2: Parenteral–6 hours.

Elimination: Primarily nonrenal, but may accumulate in renal failure.

Dose modification with renal failure: Cr Cl >50 ml/mm—4 mg/kg q 24 h; 10–50 ml/min—4 mg/kg q 24–36 h; <10 ml/min—4 mg/kg q 48 h.

Side Effects

Aerosolized pentamidine: Risk of TB to patients and health-care workers. Cough and wheezing—30% (prevented with β_2-agonist; sufficiently severe to require discontinuation of treatment in 5%) (*N Engl J Med* 1990; 323:769). Other reactions include laryngitis, chest pain, and dyspnea. The role of aerosolized pentamidine in promoting extrapulmonary *P. carinii* infection and pneumothorax is unclear.

Systemic pentamidine: *Nephrotoxicity* in 25%, usually gradual increase in creatinine in second week of treatment, but may cause acute renal failure. Risk is increased with dehydration and concurrent use of nephrotoxic drugs. *Hypotension* including death, most often with rapid infusions; drug should be infused over >60 min. *Hypoglycemia* with blood glucose <25 mg/dl in 5–10% usually after 5–7 days of treatment and sometimes several days after treatment is stopped. Hypoglycemia may last days or weeks and is treated with IV glucose with or without oral diazoxide. *Hyperglycemia* and insulin-dependent diabetes mellitus may occur with or without prior hypoglycemia. *Leukopenia and thrombocytopenia* are infrequent. *GI intolerance* with nausea, vomiting, abdominal pain, anorexia, and/or bad taste is common. *Local reactions* include sterile abscesses at IM injection sites (no longer advocated), and pain, erythema, tenderness, and induration (chemical phlebitis) at IV infusion sites. Other reactions include *hepatitis*, hypocalcemia (sometimes severe), *fever, rash, urticaria, toxic epidermal neurolysis, neurologic confusion, dizziness* (without hypotension), and anaphylaxis.

Monitoring

Aerosolized pentamidine: This is considered safe for the patient, but poses risk of TB to health-care workers and other patients. Patient should be evaluated for TB (PPD, x-ray, sputum exam). Suspected or confirmed TB should be treated prior to aerosol treatments. There needs to be adequate air exchanges with exhaust to outside and appropriate use of particulate air filters. Some suggest pregnant health-care workers should avoid environmental exposure to pentamidine until risks to fetus are better defined.

Parenteral administration: Adverse effects are common and may be lethal. Due to the risk of hypotension, the drug should be given in supine position, the patient should be hydrated, pentamidine should be delivered over ≥60 minutes, and BP should be monitored during treatment and after until stable. Regular laboratory monitoring (daily or every other day) should include creatinine, potassium, and glucose; other tests for periodic monitoring include CBC, LFTs, and calcium.

Pregnancy: Category C. Spontaneous abortion reported in patient receiving aerosolized pentamidine; causal relationship is unclear. Current recommendation is to avoid use of aerosolized pentamidine in pregnant women and in those planning to become pregnant.

Drug interactions: Avoid concurrent use of parenteral pentamidine with nephrotoxic drugs—aminoglycosides, amphotericin B, and foscarnet.

PROCRIT

See Erythropoietin.

PYRAZINAMIDE

Generic.
Forms and price: 500 mg—$1.12 (usually $4.12/day).
Class: Derivative of niacinamide.
Indication and regimen: Tuberculosis.
Daily regimen: 20–35 mg/kg in 3–4 daily doses up to 2 g/day; up to 60 mg/kg/day for drug resistant TB.
Twice weekly regimen: 50–70 mg/kg up to 4 g/day.
Thrice weekly regimen: 50–70 mg/kg up to 3 g/day.

Pharmacology

Bioavailability: Well absorbed.
T1/2: 9–10 hours.
CSF levels: Equal to plasma levels.
Elimination: Hydrolyzed in liver; 4–14% of parent compound and 70% of metabolite excreted in urine.
Renal failure: Usual dose unless creatinine clearance <10 ml/min—12–20 mg/kg/day.
Hepatic failure: Contraindicated.
Side effects: Hepatotoxicity in up to 15% receiving >3g/day—transient hepatitis with increase in transaminase, jaundice, and a syndrome of fever, anorexia, and hepatomegaly; rarely acute yellow atrophy. Monitor LFTs. Hyperuricemia is common, but gout is rare. Nongouty polyarthralgia in up to 40%; hyperuricemia usually responds to uricosuric agents. Use with caution in patients with history of gout. Rare—rash, fever, acne, dysuria, skin discoloration, urticaria, pruritis, GI intolerance, thrombocytopenia, sideroblastic anemia.
Pregnancy: Category C. Not tested in animals or in patients. Conclusion is that risk of teratogenicity has not been tested, so INH, rifampin, and ethambutol are preferred. Pyrazinamide is advocated for pregnant women if resistant *M. tuberculosis* is suspected or established.

PYRIMETHAMINE

Trade name: Daraprim (Burroughs Wellcome).
Forms and cost: 25 mg tabs at $.37/tab.
Class: Aminopyrimidine-derivative antimalarial agent that is structurally related to trimethoprim.
Indications and dose regimens: Toxoplasmosis: *Treatment*—Pyrimethamine, 50–100 mg/day po *plus* sulfonamide (sulfadiazine, sulfamethoxazole, or trisulfapyrimidine) 4–8 g po/d × ≥6 weeks *plus* folinic acid, 10 mg/day po *or* pyrimethamine, 50–100 mg/day po *plus* clindamycin, 600 mg q 6–8 h IV or 300–450 mg q 6 h po *plus* folinic acid, 10 mg/day po. *Prophylaxis*—Pyrimethamine, 25 mg po 2 × /wk *plus* dapsone 50 mg/day *plus* folinic acid, 25 mg/wk.

Pharmacology

Bioavailability: Well absorbed.
T1/2: 54–148 hours (average—111 hours).
Elimination: Parent compound and metabolites excreted in urine.
Dose modification in renal failure: None.
Side effects: *Reversible marrow suppression* due to depletion of folic acid stores with dose-related megaloblastic anemia, leukopenia, thrombocytopenia, and agranulocytosis; prevented or treated with folinic acid (leucovorin): 5–15 mg/day po, IM or IV × 3 days.
GI intolerance: Improved by reducing dose or giving drug with meals.
Neurologic: Dose-related ataxia, tremors, or seizures.
Hypersensitivity: Most common with pyrimethamine plus sulfadoxine (Fansidar).
Pregnancy: Category C; teratogenic in animals.
Drug interactions: Lorazepam—hepatotoxicity.

RETROVIR

See Zidovudine.

RIFABUTIN

Trade name: Mycobutin (Adria Labs).
Forms: 150 mg caps.
Class: Semisynthetic derivative of rifampin B that is derived from *Streptomyces mediterranei*.
Cost: $3.54/150 mg cap ($7.08/day).
Patient assistance program: (800) 795-9759. Patient must have no insurance coverage, income criteria (<$25,000/yr for single person + $5000 for each additional person in household), and cannot have TB or active *M. avium* infection.

Activity: Active vs. most strains of *M. avium* and rifampin-sensitive *M. tuberculosis*; cross-resistance between rifampin and rifabutin is common with *M. tuberculosis* and *M. avium*.

Indication and dose regimen: *M. avium* prophylaxis in HIV-infected patients with CD4 count <100/mm³. Dose: 300 mg/day q d; this is a CDC recommendation (*MMWR* 1993; 42:RR-9). Patients with GI intolerance: 150 mg po bid with food.

Efficacy: Placebo-controlled trials (Adria 023 and 027) with 1,146 AIDS patients with CD4 <200/mm³ treated an average of 270 days showed *M. avium* infections developed in 102 placebo recipients vs. 48 rifabutin recipients ($p < .001$) (*N Engl J Med* 1993; 329:828). Relative merit compared with clarithromycin is now being studied.

Pharmacology

Bioavailability: 12–20%.
T1/2: 30–60 hours.
Elimination: Primarily renal and biliary excretion of metabolites.
Dose modification in renal failure: None.
Side effects: Common—brown-orange discoloration of secretions: urine (30%), tears, saliva, sweat, stool, and skin. Infrequent—rash (4%), GI intolerance (3%), neutropenia (2%). Rare side effects—flu-like illness, hepatitis, hemolysis, headache, thrombocytopenia, myositis. Possible cause of uveitis, which presents as red and painful eye, blurring of vision, photophobia, or floaters. Possibly dose related (600 mg/d) and responsive to topical corticosteroids plus mydriatics.

Drug interactions: Rifabutin reduces activity of protease inhibitors anticoagulants (coumadin), barbiturates, benzodiazepines, β-adrenergic blockers, chloramphenicol, clofibrate, *oral contraceptives*, corticosteroids, cyclosporine, diazepam, *dapsone*, digitalis, doxycycline, haloperidol, hypoglycemics, ketoconazole, *methadone*, phenytoin, quinidine, theophylline, trimethoprim, and verapamil.

Comments

1. There is concern that widespread use of rifabutin will promote rifampin resistance of *M. tuberculosis*.
2. Rifampin and rifabutin are related drugs, but *in vitro* activity and clinical trials show that rifabutin is preferred for *M. avium* and rifampin is preferred for *M. tuberculosis*.
3. Clarithromycin is the preferred agent for treatment of disseminated *M. avium* infection; relative merits of clarithromycin and rifabutin for *M. avium* prophylaxis are currently being studied.
4. It is assumed that drug interactions are similar for rifabutin and rifampin although the studies to date are far more substantial for rifampin.

5. Uveitis is a possible side effect recently described and rquires immediate discontinuation of drug and ophthalmology consult.

RIFAMPIN

Trade name: Rifadin (Merrill-Dow) and Rimactane (CIBA); Combination with INH: Rifamate.
Forms: 150 and 300 mg caps; caps with 150 mg INH and 600 mg vials for IV use.
Price: $2.10/300 mg cap; $79.38/600 mg vial.
Active vs.: *M. tuberculosis*, *M. kansasii*, *S. aureus*, *H. influenzae*, Legionella, and many anaerobes.
Indications: (1) Tuberculosis (with INH, PZA and SM, or ETH): Dose = 600 mg/day; DOT = 600 mg 2–3 × /wk; prophylaxis (alone or in combination with PZA or ETH) = 600 mg/day. (2) Other infections: *S. aureus* (with vancomycin, fluoroquinolones, or penicillinase resistant penicillin): 300 mg po bid.

Pharmacology

Bioavailability: 90–95%, less with food.
T1/2: 1.5–5 hours, average—2 hours.
Elimination: Excreted in urine (33%) and metabolized.
Dose modification in renal failure: None.
Side effects: Common—orange-brown discoloration of urine, stool, tears (contact lens), sweat, skin. Infrequent—GI intolerance; hepatitis (no increase in risk when given with INH); jaundice (usually reversible with dose reduction or continued use); hypersensitivity, especially pruritis with or without rash (3%); flu-like illness with intermittent use—dyspnea, wheezing, purpura, leukopenia. Rare side effects—thrombocytopenia, leukopenia, hemolytic anemia, increased uric acid, and BUN. Frequency of side effects that require discontinuation of drug: 3% rifampin.
Pregnancy: Category C. Dose-dependent congenital malformations in animals. Isolated cases of fetal abnormalities noted in patients, but frequency is unknown. May cause postnatal hemorrhage in mother and infant if given in last few weeks of pregnancy. Must use with caution.
Drug interactions: Rifampin reduces activity of anticoagulants (coumadin), barbiturates, benzodiazepines, β-adrenergic blockers, chloramphenicol, clofibrate, *oral contraceptives*, corticosteroids, cyclosporine, diazepam, *dapsone*, digitalis, doxycycline, haloperidol, hypoglycemics, ketoconazole, *methadone*, phenytoin, quinidine, theophylline, trimethoprim, and verapamil.

ROFERON

See Interferon.

SEPTRA

See Trimethoprim-Sulfamethoxazole.

SPORANOX

See Itraconazole.

STAVUDINE

See D4T.

STREPTOMYCIN

Generic: Available from Pfizer at no charge. Order information—(800) 254-4445; FAX order request—(800) 251-4445. Comparative wholesale price for aminoglycosides (usual daily dose, 70 kg patient); streptomycin—free; gentamicin—$5.20 (400 mg); capreomycin—$20.86 (1 g); tobramycin—$36.80 (400 mg); amikacin—$128.97 (1 g).
Form: Ampules with 1 g/2.5 ml.
Class: Aminoglycosides.
Indication: Tuberculosis.
Dose: Daily regimen—15 mg/kg IM up to 1 g/day; DOT regimen—25–30 mg/kg IM up to 1.5 g for twice-weekly treatment and up to 1.0 g for thrice-weekly treatment. IM injections should be made in the upper outer quadrant of the buttock or midlateral thigh; deltoid muscle may be used if well developed. Injection sites should be alternated.

Pharmacology

Bioavailability: Not absorbed with po administration.
T1/2: 5–6 hours.
Peak levels (1 g dose)—25–30 mcg/ml. *CNS levels*: Low.
Elimination: Renal (30–80% recovered in urine).
Dose modification in renal failure: Cr cl >50 ml/min—15 mg/kg/day; 10–50 mg/kg—15 mg/kg q 24–72 hr; <10 ml/min—15 mg/kg q 72–96 hr.
Side effects: Ototoxicity especially nausea, vomiting, and vertigo—dose and duration related; hearing loss is less common and may be irreversible. Patients should be warned that tinnitus, roaring noises, or sense of fullness in ears indicates the drug should be discontinued. Caloric stimulation tests and audiometric tests are advised with long courses, with selected high-risk patients (elderly, renal failure) and with complaints suggesting ototoxicity. Vestibular dysfunction is usually reversible

within 2–3 months if the drug is promptly discontinued. Other less common forms of neurotoxicity include peripheral neuritis, arachnoiditis, encephalopathy, and respiratory paralysis. Renal failure is uncommon except with persons >65 years, prior renal failure, and/or concurrent nephrotoxic drugs. Paresthesias—perioral and hands in 15% (not important). Streptomycin contains a sulfite that may cause allergic-type reactions including anaphylaxis, rash, urticaria, and eosinophilia. Serious reactions are rare and are more common in asthmatic patients.

Drug interactions: Increased nephrotoxicity and ototoxicity with other drugs that have these side effects, especially other aminoglycosides. Ototoxicity is potentiated by coadministration of ethacrynic acid, furosemide, mannitol, and possibly other diuretics.

Pregnancy: Category D. This and other aminoglycosides have been implicated in irreversible congenital deafness. Streptomycin is the only major antituberculosis drug with established toxicity to the fetus.

SULFADIAZINE

Generic: Now available from Eon Labs (718) 276-8600.
Form: 500 mg tabs.
Class: Synthetic derivatives of sulfanilamide, which inhibits folic acid synthesis.

Indications and Doses

Toxoplasmosis: Initial treatment, 1–2 g po qid × ≥6 weeks; maintenance, 500 mg –1 g po qid indefinitely.
Nocardia: 1 g po qid × ≥6 months.
UTIs: 500 mg–1 g po qid × 3–14 days.

Pharmacology

Bioavailability: >70%.
T1/2: 17 hours.
Elimination: Hepatic acetylation and renal excretion of parent compound + metabolites.
CNS penetraion: 40–80% of serum levels.
Serum levels for systemic infections: 100–150 mcg/ml.
Dose modifications in renal failure: Cr cl >50 ml/min—0.5–1.5 g q 4–6 hr; 10–50 ml/min—0.5–1.5 g q 8–12 h (half dose); <10 ml/min—0.5–1.5 g q 12–24 hr (one-third dose).
Side effects: Hypersensitivity with rash, drug fever, serum-sickness, urticaria; crystalluria reduced with adequate urine volume (≥1,500 ml/day) and alkaline

urine-use with care in renal failure; marrow suppression—anemia, thrombocy-topenia, leukopenia, hemolytic anemia due to G6PD deficiency.

Drug interactions: Decreased effect of cyclosporine, digoxin; increased effect of coumadin, oral hypoglycemics, methotrexate (?), and phenytoin.

Pregnancy: Category C. Compete with bilirubin for albumin to cause kernic-terus—avoid near term or in nursing mothers.

3TC (LAMIVUDINE)

Forms: 150 mg tabs.

Class: Nucleoside analogues.

Availability: Treatment IND (no charge).

Enrollment criteria: Physician registration—(800) 248-9757, FDA form 1572, In-stitutional Review Board approval, patient registration, signed informed consent.

Patient eligibility criteria: CD4 count $<300/mm^3$ (two samples ≥ 30 days apart). Progression while receiving alternative FDA-approved antiretroviral therapy or in-tolerance/toxicity to these drugs (AZT, ddI, ddC, d4T); practice safe sex; informed consent; willing to attend clinic monthly for hematologic monitoring.

Dose: Participants in Treatment IND are randomized to receive 150 or 300 mg po bid. Most patients take AZT concurrently (see below).

Efficacy: Four comparative trials were reported at the 2nd National Conference on Human Retroviruses and Related Infections (ASM, February, Washington, DC, abstracts LB 31-34); compared efficacy of AZT, 3TC, and AZT + 3TC. Participants had CD4 counts of $100-500/mm^3$ with or without prior AZT therapy. Results at 24–52 weeks in all four trials showed increases in CD4 cell counts among recipients of AZT plus 3TC by $50-75/mm^3$ compared with baseline and decreased viral burden by about one log. Results with AZT or 3TC alone were inferior for both parameters. One hypothesis is that the mutation that confers resistance to 3TC at codon 184 reinstates susceptibility to AZT.

Pharmacokinetics

Oral bioavailability: 86%.

T1/2 (serum): 3 hours.

T1/2 intracellular: 12 hours.

CNS penetration: 10%.

Elimination: Renal.

Dose adjustment in renal failure: Not known.

Toxicity: Experience in 4,000 patients receiving 3TC on the Treatment IND or in studies has shown remarkably little toxicity. Infrequent complications include GI intolerance, neutropenia, rare cases of peripheral neuropathy, and rare cases of pancreatitis.

TRAZODONE

Trade name: Desyrel (Mead Johnson) and generic.

Forms and Price

	Generic	Desyrel
50 mg tab	$0.09	$1.19
100 mg tab	$0.13	$2.08
150 mg tab	$0.53	$1.79
300 mg tab	–	$3.19

Class: Nontricyclic antidepressant.

Indications and dose regimens: Depression, especially when associated with anxiety or insomnia; 150 mg/day in two doses; if insomnia or daytime sedation, give as single dose at hs. Increase dose 50 mg every 3–4 days up to maximum dose of 400 mg/day for outpatients and 600 mg/day for hospitalized patients.

Pharmacology

Bioavailability: >90%, improved if taken with meals.

T1/2: 6 hours.

Elimination: Hepatic metabolism, then renal excretion.

Side effects: Adverse effects are dose and duration related, are usually seen with doses >300 mg/day and may decrease with continued use, dose reduction, or schedule change. Major side effects—sedation in 15–20%; orthostatic hypotension (5%); nervousness; fatigue; dizziness; nausea and vomiting. Rare—anticholinergic effects (dry mouth, blurred vision, constipation, urinary retention); priapism (1/6,000), agitation; cardiovascular and anticholinergic side effects are less frequent and less severe compared with tricyclics.

Pregnancy: Category B.

Drug interactions: Increased levels of phenytoin and digoxin; alcohol and other CNS depressants potentiate sedative side effects; increased trazodone levels with fluoxetine; may potentiate effects of antihypertensive agents.

TRIAZOLAM

Trade name: Halcion (Upjohn).

Forms and price: 0.125 mg tab—$.68; 0.25 mg tab—$.74.

Class: Benzodiazapine, controlled substance category IV.

Indications and dose regimens: Insomnia: 0.125–0.5 mg (usually 0.25 mg) hs for 7–10 days.

Note: Current FDA guidelines state triazolam should be prescribed for short-term use (7–10 days), the prescribed dose should not exceed a one-month supply and use for >2–3 weeks requires reevaluation of patient.

Pharmacology

Bioavailability: >90%.

T1/2: 1.5–5 hours.

Elimination: Metabolized by liver to inactive metabolites that are renally excreted.

Side effects: See Benzodiazepines. Usual side effects of benzodiazepines. Most common are drowsiness, incoordination, dizziness, and amnesia. Anecdotal reports of delirium, confusion, paranoia, and hallucinations.

Pregnancy: Category X.

TRIMETHOPRIM

Generic.

Forms and price: 100 mg tab—$0.17; 200 mg tab—$0.28 (see Trimethoprim-Sulfamethoxazole).

Indications and dose regimen: (1) PCP (with sulfamethoxazole as TMP-SMX or with dapsone): 5 mg/kg po tid or qid (usually 300 mg tid or qid)×21 days. (2) UTIs: 100 mg po bid or 200 mg × 1/day × 3–14 days.

Pharmacology

Bioavailability: >90% absorbed.

T1/2: 9–11 hours.

Excretion: Renal.

Dose modification with renal failure: Cr cl >50 ml/min—full dose; 10–50 ml/min—half dose.

Side effects: Usually well tolerated; most common—pruritis and skin rash; GI intolerance; marrow suppression—anemia, neutropenia, thrombocytopenia; antifolate effects—prevent with folinic acid; recent reports of reversible hyperkalemia in 20–50% of AIDS patients given high doses (*Ann Intern Med* 1994; 119:291,296; *N Engl J Med* 1993; 238:703).

Drug interactions: Increased activity of phenytoin (monitor levels) and procainamide; levels of both dapsone and trimethoprim are increased when given concurrently.

Pregnancy: Category C. Teratogenic in rats with high doses; limited experience in patients shows no association with congenital abnormalities.

TRIMETHOPRIM-SULFAMETHOXAZOLE

Generic.
Trade name: Septra (Burroughs Wellcome); Bactrim (Roche).

Forms and Cost

	Single strength (80/400 mg)[a]	Double strength (160/800 mg)	IV preparation (16 mg/ml, 80 mg/ml)
Generic	$0.07	$0.07	10 ml, $3.53
Bactrim	$0.72	$1.19	10 ml, $15.25
Septra	$0.70	$1.14	10 ml, $7.24

[a]80 mg trimethoprim plus 400 mg sulfamethoxazole.

Indications and Regimens

PCP prophylaxis: 1 DS/day or 3 DS/wk, or 1 SS/day.
PCP treatment: 5 mg/kg (trimethoprim) po or IV q 6–8 hours × 21 days.
Toxoplasmosis prophylaxis: 1 DS/day.
Isospora: 5 mg/kg (trimethoprim) po bid, usually 2 DS po bid or 1 DS tid × 2–4 weeks; may need maintenance with 1–2 DS/day.
Salmonellosis: 5–10 mg/kg (trimethoprim) po/day × 2–4 weeks.
Nocardia: 4–6 DS/day × ≥6 mo.
Urinary tract infections: 1–2 DS/day × 3–14 days.
Prophylaxis for cystitis: ½ SS tab daily.

Pharmacology

Bioavailability: >90% absorbed with oral administration (both drugs).
T1/2: Trimethoprim, 8–15 hr; sulfamethoxazole 7–12 hr.
Elimination: Renal, $T_{1/2}$ in renal failure increases to 24 hr for trimethoprim and 22–50 hr for sulfamethoxazole.
Renal failure: Cr cl >50 ml/min—usual dose; 10–50 ml/min—half dose; <10 ml/min—avoid (some suggest further reduction in dose may be used).
Side effects: Noted in 10% of patients without HIV infection and about 50% of patients with HIV. Most common: nausea, vomiting, pruritus, rash, fever, and increased transaminase. Many HIV infected patients may be treated through side effects (GI intolerance and rash) if symptoms are not disabling or with dose reduction.

Role of desensitization is unclear. Mechanism of most sulfonamide reactions is unclear and cause of increased susceptibility with HIV is also unclear.

Rash: Most common is erythematous, maculopapular, morbilliform, and/or pruritic rash, usually 7–14 days after treatment is started. Less common are erythema multiforme, epidermal necrolysis, exfoliative dermatitis, Stevens-Johnson syndrome, urticaria, Schonlein-Henoch purpura. *GI intolerance* is common with nausea, vomiting, anorexia, and abdominal pain; rare side effects include *C. difficile* diarrhea/colitis and pancreatitis. *Hematologic side effects* include leukopenia, neutropenia, anemia, and/or thrombocytopenia. Rate is increased in patients with HIV infection and with folate depletion. Some respond to folinic acid (5–15 mg/day), but this is not routinely recommended. *Neurologic* toxicity may include ataxia, apathy, and ankle clonus that responds promptly with drug discontinuation. *Hepatitis* with cholestatic jaundice and hepatic necrosis has been described. *Hyperkalemia* in 20–50% of patients given trimethoprim in doses of >15 mg/kg/d (*N Engl J Med* 1993; 328:703).

Pregnancy: Category C. Teratogenic in animals. No congenital abnormalities noted in 35 children born to women who received TMP-SMX in first trimester. Use with caution due to effect on folic acid and avoid at term due to kernicterus associated with sulfonamides.

Drug interactions: Increased levels of oral anticoagulants, phenytoin, and procainamide. Risk of megaloblastic anemia with methotrexate.

TRIMETREXATE

Trade name: Neutrexin (U.S. Bioscience).
Forms and cost: 25 mg vials at $49/vial.
Patient assistance: (800) 887-2467.
Class: Synthetic folate-antagonist.
Dose: 45 mg/m^2 IV once daily over 60–90 min × 21 days combined with leucovorin: 20 mg/m^2 IV q 6 h (80 mg/m^2/day) or 20 mg/m^2 po q 6 h × 24 days.
Indication: Alternative treatment for moderate-to-severe *P. carinii* pneumonia in patients who are intolerant of TMP-SMX or who are refractory to TMP-SMX.
Efficacy: ACTG trial comparing trimetrexate with TMP-SMX among 220 patients with moderate or severe PCP (defined as A-a gradient >30 mm Hg) showed a mortality rate of 27% among those given trimetrexate compared with 16% in those given TMP-SMX.

Pharmacology

Bioavailability: Not bioavailable with oral administration.
T1/2: 11 hours.
Excretion: Renal excretion and hepatic metabolism.
Dose modification in renal failure or hepatic failure: No data.
Side effects: *Trimetrexate must be used with leucovorin to avoid potentially se-*

rious complications including bone marrow suppression, oral, or gastrointestinal ulceration, renal dysfunction, and hepatic toxicity.

Dose Modification for Hematologic Toxicity

PMNs	Platelets	Trimetrexate	Leucovorin
>1000/mm^3	>75,000/mm^3	45 mg/m^2/d	20 mg/m^2 q 6 h
750–1000/mm^3	50,000–75,000/mm^3	45 mg/m^2/d	40 mg/m^2 q 6 h
500–750/mm^3	25,000–50,000/mm^3	22 mg/m^2/d	40 mg/m^2 q 6 h
<500/mm^3	<25,000/mm^3	Day 1–9: Discontinue Day 10–21: Interrupt up to 96 hours	40 mg/m^2 q 6 h

Renal impairment (discontinue with creatinine >2.5 mg/dl); *hypotension*; *pancreatitis*; *dysglycemia* with hypoglycemia or hyperglycemia.

Pregnancy: Category D, teratogenic effects.

Drug interactions: Erythromycin, rifampin, rifabutin, ketoconazole, and fluconazole.

VANCOMYCIN

Trade name: Vancocin, Vancor, Vancoled Generic.

Forms and Price

Oral	10 day (*C. difficile*)
500 mg vial $7.80	$110
125 mg parvule $4.73	$189

Parenteral: 2 g/IV: $43.60/day.

Class: Tricyclic glycopeptide antibiotic.

Activity: Nearly all gram-positive bacteria including all *S. aureus*; 8% of hospital strains of *Enterococcus facecium* are resistant.

Indications and Regimens

Deep infections involving MRSA and *S. epidermidis*; infections involving other gram-positive bacteria in penicillin-allergic patients: 1 g IV q 12 h infused (±rifampin or gentamicin).

C. difficile colitis: 125 mg po qid × 10–14 days.

Pharmacology

Bioavailability: Not absorbed with po admin, but may accumulate in serum with inflamed gut plus renal failure.

T1/2: 4–6 hours.

Elimination: Renal.

Dose modification in renal failure: Cr cl >50 ml/mm—15 mg/kg IV q 12 h; 10–50 ml/min—15 mg/kg q 3–10 days; <10 ml/min—15 mg/kg q 10 days.

Side effects:

1. *Red man syndrome*: hypotension and flushing with or without dyspnea, urticaria, pruritis, and/or wheezing ascribed to histamine release from mast cells, which is directly related to rate of infusion. This usually begins shortly after infusion starts and may require antihistamine, corticosteroids, or IV fluids; some patients benefit from pretreatment with antihistamine.
2. *Otic and nephrotoxicity*: Infrequent and most likely with renal failure, high doses, long courses and concurrent use of nephrotoxic or ototoxic drugs. Many authorities feel that current supplies of vancomycin are not nephrotoxic if used alone, but vancomycin appears to promote nephrotoxicity of other nephrotoxic drugs such as aminoglycosides. Relationship to serum levels is unclear and use of serum levels to monitor toxicity is unclear.
3. Thrombophlebitis and pain at infusion site.
4. Hypersensitivity reactions are rare; most reactions are the result of histamine release due to rapid infusion.

VIBRAMYCIN

See Doxycycline.

VIDEX

See Didanosine.

XANAX

See Alprazolam.

ZALCITABINE

See Dideoxycytideine.

ZERIT

See D4T.

ZIDOVUDINE (AZT)

Trade name: Retrovir (Burroughs Wellcome).
Forms and price: 100 mg tabs—$1.55/tab; $9.30/day, $3,395/year; IV vials—10 mg/ml, 20 ml (200 mg)—$16.74.
Patient assistance program: (800) 722-9294. Eligibility based on lack of third-party drug coverage, monthly income criteria using Medicaid guidelines and asset information; forms are reviewed on an individual case basis.
Class: Nucleoside analogue.

Indications and Regimen

Condition	Regimen
CD4 $<500/mm^3$, symptomatic[a]	200 mg po tid (daily dose 600 mg)
CD4 $<200/mm^3$, asymptomatic[a]	200 mg po tid (daily dose 600 mg)
CD4 200–500/mm³, asymptomatic[a]	Consider use (above dose)
HIV-associated ITP	200 mg po 3–5 × /day (daily dose 600–1200 mg) (response may be dose related; see *AIDS* 1993; 7:209)
HIV-associated dementia	200 mg po 5–6 × /day (daily dose 1000–1200 mg)
Toxicity (minimum effective dose)	100 mg po tid (daily dose 300 mg)
Combination treatment	Most use standard dose (600 mg/day)
IV formulation	1 mg/kg q 4 h

[a]Based on NIAID/CDC Expert Panel recommendations: *JAMA* 1993; 270:2583.

Pharmacology

Bioavailability: 60%.
CSF levels: 60% serum levels.
T1/2: 1.1 hour; *intracellular* $T_{1/2}$: 3 hours.
Elimination: Metabolized by liver to glucuronide (GAZT) that is renally excreted.
Dose modification in renal failure: No specific guidelines, but some use half dose with creatinine clearance <10 m/min.

Side Effects

1. *Subjective*: GI intolerance, insomnia, myalgias, asthenia, malaise, and/or headaches noted in 76% of health-care workers taking 1,000 mg/day and sufficiently severe so that 31% discontinued use (*Ann Intern Med* 1993; 118:913). Patients

often note these complaints, but standard dose is less (600 mg/day) and most improve with continued treatment and/or with reduced dose.

2. *Marrow suppression*, which is stage and dose dependent:

	Asympt. HIV	AIDS	Management
Anemia (Hgb <8 g/dl)	2%	29%	Reduce dose or discontinue.Substitute ddI or ddC. Initiate EPO and/or transfusions.
Neutropenia (ANC <750/mm^3)	1%	37%	Reduce dose or discontinue. Substitute ddI or ddC. Initiate G-CSF.

3. *Myopathy*: Infrequent complication related to advanced disease and cumulative dose, usually AZT treatment >1 year. Clinical features are extremity weakness, muscle tenderness, atrophy, increased LDH, and increased CPK, with return to normal at 2–4 weeks after discontinuing AZT. May not be easily distinguished from HIV-associated myopathy.

4. *Macrocytosis*: Noted within 4 weeks of starting AZT in virtually all patients and serves as an indicator of compliance.

5. Hepatitis with reversible increases in transaminase levels, sometimes within 2–3 weeks of starting treatment.

6. Lactic acidosis and fulminant hepatic failure in rare patients, especially obese women; etiologic role of AZT is unclear.

7. Fingernail discoloration with dark bluish discoloration at base of nail noted at 2–6 weeks.

8. Carcinogenicity: Long-term treatment with high doses in mice caused vaginal neoplasms; relevance to humans is not known.

Pregnancy: Category C. Not teratogenic in animals. Administration to pregnant women showed no teratogenic effect and no adverse outcomes.

Drug interaction: Additive or synergistic versus HIV with ddI, ddC, alpha interferon, and foscarnet; acyclovir is neutral; antagonism with ribavirin. Marrow suppression precludes concurrent use with ganciclovir. Early studies suggested acetaminophen increased risk of AZT-induced granulocytopenia, possibly by competitive inhibition of glucuronidation, but most clinicians feel intermittent use of acetaminophen is safe.

ZITHROMAX

See Azithromycin.

ZOVIRAX

See Acyclovir.

A Clinical Guide to AIDS and HIV,
edited by Gary P. Wormser.
Lippincott-Raven Publishers, Philadelphia © 1996.

12

Pharmacotherapy of Pain in AIDS

William Breitbart

Department of Psychiatry, Cornell University Medical College; and Memorial Sloan-Kettering Cancer Center; Psychiatry Service, Memorial Hospital, New York, New York 10021

Pain management is an integral part of the total care of patients with HIV infection. Pain in individuals with HIV infection or AIDS is highly prevalent, diverse and varied in syndromal presentation, associated with significant psychological and functional morbidity, and alarmingly undertreated. Health care professionals working with HIV-infected patients must be aware of the prevalence and types of pain encountered, and make pain control a focus of care. This chapter outlines the major issues relevant to the management of pain in AIDS, and provides guidelines and principles for treating pain in the AIDS patient.

PREVALENCE OF PAIN IN HIV INFECTION

The prevalence of pain in HIV infected individuals varies depending on the stage of disease, care setting, and study methodology. Estimates of the prevalence of pain in HIV-infected individuals range from 30% to 80% with prevalence rates increasing as the disease progresses. Thirty-eight percent of ambulatory HIV-infected patients reported significant pain in a prospective study of pain prevalence over a 2-week period. Fifty percent of patients with AIDS reported pain, while only 25% of those with earliest stages of HIV infection had pain. Patients had an average of two or more pains at one time. Patients with AIDS reported average pain intensities that were comparable to, if not more severe, than published reports of pain intensity in cancer patients. A recent review of ambulatory HIV-infected men demonstrated that 28% of those who were asymptomatic seropositive versus 80% of those with AIDS reported one or more painful symptoms over a 6-month period. A study of pain in hospitalized patients with AIDS revealed that over 50% of patients required treatment for pain, with pain being the presenting complaint in 30% (second only to fever). In one study 53% of patients with far-advanced AIDS cared for in a hospice setting had pain. Investigators in a French national study demonstrated that patients with AIDS being cared for by hospice at home had prevalence rates and intensity ratings for pain that were comparable to and even exceeded those of cancer patients.

PAIN SYNDROMES IN HIV/AIDS

Pain syndromes encountered in AIDS are diverse in nature and etiology. The most common pain syndromes reported in studies to date include painful sensory peripheral neuropathy, pain due to extensive Kaposi's sarcoma, headache, pharyngeal and abdominal pain, arthralgias and myalgias, as well as painful dermatologic conditions. Pain syndromes seen in HIV disease (Table 1), are often categorized into three types: (1) those directly related to HIV infection or consequences of immunosuppression, (2) those due to AIDS therapies, and (3) those unrelated to AIDS or AIDS therapies. In studies to date, approximately 50% of pain syndromes encountered are directly related to HIV infection or consequences of immunosuppression, 30% are due to therapies for HIV- or AIDS-related conditions as well as diagnostic procedures, and the remaining 20% are unrelated to HIV or its therapies.

Pain syndromes of a neuropathic nature occur in up to 40% of AIDS patients with pain. While several types of peripheral neuropathy have been described, the most common painful neuropathy encountered is the predominantly sensory neuropathy (PSN) of AIDS, affecting up to 30% of people with HIV infection. The PSN of AIDS is postulated to be a direct or indirect result of HIV infection of the peripheral nervous system and is characterized by a sensation of burning, numbness, or pins and needles in the feet and hands. Other potentially painful neuropathies encountered in HIV-infected patients, however, can be caused by a variety of medical conditions, toxins, and HIV-related therapies, as listed in Table 2. It is important to note that several antiretroviral drugs such as didanosine (ddl) and zalcitabine (ddC), chemotherapy agents used to treat Kaposi's sarcoma (vincristine), as well as a num-

TABLE 1. *Pain syndromes in AIDS patients*

Pain related to HIV/AIDS
  HIV neuropathy
  HIV myelopathy
  Kaposi's sarcoma
  Opportunistic infections (intestines, skin)
  Organomegaly
  Arthritis/vasculitis
  Myopathy/myositis
Pain related to HIV/AIDS therapy
  Antiretrovirals, antivirals
  Antimycobacterials, PCP prophylaxis
  Chemotherapy (vincristine)
  Radiation
  Surgery
  Procedures (bronchoscopy, biopsies)
Pain unrelated to AIDS
  Spinal disk disease
  Diabetic neuropathy

PCP, *Pneumocystis carinii* pneumonia.

TABLE 2. *Neuropathies encountered in HIV-infected patients*

Predominantly sensory neuropathy (PSN) of AIDS
Immune-mediated
    Inflammatory demyelinating polyneuropathies (IDPs)
        Acute (Guillain-Barré syndrome)
        Chronic
    Infectious
        Cytomegalovirus polyradiculopathy
        Cytomegalovirus multiple mononeuropathy
        Herpes zoster
        Mycobacterial
Toxic/nutritional
    Alcohol, vitamin deficiencies (B_6, B_{12})
    Antiretrovirals: ddI (didanosine), ddC (zalcitabine), D4T (stavudine)
    Antivirals: foscarnet
    PCP prophylaxis: dapsone
    Antibacterial: metronitazole
    Antimycobacterials: INH (isoniazad), rifampin, ethionamide
    Antineoplastics: vincristine, vinblastin
    Other medical conditions
        Diabetic neuropathy
        Postherpetic neuralgia

PCP, *Pneumocystis carinii* pneumonia.

ber of medications used in the treatment of *Pneumocystis carinii* pneumonia (PCP), mycobacterial infection, and other HIV-associated infections can cause painful neuropathy. HIV virus can attack the spinal cord as well and cause painful myelopathy. In addition, plexopathies and radiculopathies have been reported in AIDS patients with pain complaints.

While pains of a neuropathic nature are an important clinical problem that has attracted a great deal of attention, pains of somatic and visceral etiologies make up the bulk of the causes of pain in AIDS. Somatic, visceral, and neuropathic pains often occur concurrently, and the neuropathic pain is not always the predominant pain. Pains of somatic and visceral etiologies commonly encountered in AIDS patients include Kaposi's sarcoma–related pain; headache; gastrointestinal pains (e.g., abdominal, esophageal, oral) and diarrhea due to opportunistic infections such as cryptosporidiosis; painful rheumatologic manifestations of HIV infection including various forms of arthritis (painful articular syndrome, septic arthritis, psoriatic arthritis, Reiter's syndrome, reactive arthritis) vasculitis, Sjögren's syndrome, polymyositis, zidovudine (AZT) myopathy, and dermatomyositis.

Children with HIV infection also experience pain (see Chapter 4). HIV-related conditions in children that are observed to cause pain include meningitis and sinusitis (headaches), otitis media, shingles, cellulitis and abscesses, severe *Candida* dermatitis, dental caries, intestinal infections such as *Mycobacterium avium* complex (MAC) and cryptosporidium, hepatosplenomegaly, oral and esophageal candidiasis, and spasticity associated with encephalopathy that causes painful muscle spasms.

THE IMPACT OF PAIN ON QUALITY OF LIFE

Pain appears to have a profound impact on levels of emotional distress and disability. In a pilot study of the impact of pain on ambulatory HIV-infected patients, depression was significantly correlated with the presence of pain. In addition to being significantly more distressed and depressed, those with pain were twice as likely to have suicidal ideation (40%) as those without pain (20%). HIV-infected patients with pain were more functionally impaired. Such functional interference was highly correlated to levels of pain intensity and depression. Those who felt that pain represented a threat to their health reported more intense pain than those who did not see pain as a threat. Patients with pain were more likely to be unemployed or disabled, and reported less social support. One group has also reported an association between the frequency of multiple pains, increased disability, and higher levels of depression.

Psychological variables such as the amount of control people believe they have over pain, emotional associations and memories of pain, fears of death, depression, anxiety, and hopelessness all contribute to the experience of pain in people with AIDS and can increase suffering. Our group recently reported that negative thoughts related to pain were associated with greater pain intensity, psychological distress, and disability in ambulatory patients with AIDS.

UNDERTREATMENT OF PAIN IN AIDS

While still preliminary in nature, reports of dramatic undertreatment of pain in AIDS patients are appearing in the literature. These studies suggest that opioid analgesics are underutilized in the treatment of pain in AIDS. Our group has reported that, in our cohort of AIDS patients, only 6% of individuals reporting pain in the severe range (8–10 on a numerical rating scale of pain intensity) received a strong opioid, such as morphine, as recommended in the WHO Analgesic Ladder. Utilizing the Pain Management Index (PMI), a measure of adequacy of analgesic therapy derived from the Brief Pain Inventory's record of pain intensity and strength of analgesia prescribed, only 15% of our sample received adequate analgesic therapy. This degree of undermedication of pain in AIDS (85%) far exceeds published reports of undermedication of pain in cancer populations of 40%. As with cancer, we have found that factors that influence undertreatment of pain in AIDS include gender (women are more often undertreated), education, substance abuse history, and a variety of patient-related barriers. While opioid analgesics are underutilized, it is also clear that adjuvant analgesic agents such as the antidepressants are also dramatically underutilized. Only 6% of subjects in our sample of AIDS patients reporting pain received an adjuvant analgesic drug (i.e., an antidepressant). This class of analgesic agents is an essential part of the WHO Analgesic Ladder.

MANAGEMENT OF PAIN IN AIDS

Overview

Federal guidelines developed by the Agency for Health Care Policy and Research (AHCPR) for the management of cancer pain also address the issue of management of pain in AIDS, and state: "The principles of pain assessment and treatment in the patient with HIV positive/AIDS are not fundamentally different from those in the patient with cancer and should be followed for patients with HIV positive/AIDS." In contrast to pain in cancer, pain in HIV infection is more likely to have an underlying treatable cause.

Optimal management of pain in AIDS is multimodal and requires pharmacologic, psychotherapeutic, cognitive-behavioral, anesthetic, neurosurgical, and rehabilitative approaches. A multidimensional model of AIDS pain that recognizes the interaction of cognitive, emotional, socioenvironmental, and nociceptive aspects of pain suggests a model for multimodal intervention. This chapter focuses on the pharmacologic aspects of pain management in the AIDS patient.

Assessment Issues

The initial step in pain management is a comprehensive assessment of pain symptoms. The health professional must have a working knowledge of the etiology and treatment of pain in AIDS. This would include an understanding of the different types of AIDS pain syndromes discussed above, as well as a familiarity with the parameters of appropriate pharmacologic treatment. A close collaboration of the entire health care team is optimal when attempting to manage pain adequately in the AIDS patient.

A careful history and physical examination may disclose an identifiable syndrome (e.g., herpes zoster bacterial infection, or neuropathy) that can be treated in a standard fashion. A standard pain history may provide valuable clues to the nature of the underlying process, and indeed, may disclose other treatable disorders. A description of the qualitative features of the pain, its time course, and any maneuvers that increase or decrease pain intensity should be obtained. Pain intensity (current, average, at best, at worst) should be assessed to determine the need for weak versus potent analgesics, and as a means to evaluate serially the effectiveness of ongoing treatment. Pain descriptors (e.g., burning, shooting, dull, or sharp) will help determine the mechanism of pain (somatic, nociceptive, visceral nociceptive, or neuropathic), and may suggest the likelihood of response to various classes of traditional and adjuvant analgesics [nonsteroidal antiinflammatory drugs (NSAIDs) opioids, antidepressants, anticonvulsants, oral local anesthetics, corticosteroids, etc.]. Additionally, detailed medical, neurologic, and psychosocial assessments (including a history of substance use or abuse) must be conducted. Where possible, family members or partners should be interviewed. During the assessment phase, pain should be aggressively treated while pain complaints and psychosocial issues are subject to an ongoing process of reevaluation.

An important concept is that pain assessment is continuous and needs to be repeated over the course of time. There are essentially four aspects of the pain experience in AIDS that require ongoing evaluation: (1) pain intensity, (2) pain relief, (3) pain-related functional interference (e.g., mood state, general and specific activities), and (4) monitoring of intervention effects (analgesic drug side effects, abuse). The Memorial Pain Assessment Card (MPAC) is a helpful clinical tool that allows patients to report their pain experience. The MPAC consists of visual analogue scales that measure pain intensity, pain relief, and mood. Patients can complete the MPAC in less than 30 seconds. The patient's report of pain intensity, pain relief, and present mood state provides the essential information required to help guide pain management. The Brief Pain Inventory is another pain assessment tool that has useful clinical and research applications.

Pharmacotherapies for Pain in AIDS

The World Health Organization has devised guidelines for analgesic management of cancer pain. These guidelines, also known widely as the "WHO Analgesic Ladder" are well validated for cancer patients. This approach advocates selection of analgesics based on severity of pain. For mild to moderate severity pain, nonopioid analgesics such as NSAIDs and acetaminophen are recommended. For pain that is persistent and moderate to severe in intensity, opioid analgesics of increasing potency (such as morphine) should be utilized. Adjuvant agents, such as laxatives and psychostimulants, are useful in preventing as well as treating opioid side effects such as constipation and sedation, respectively. Adjuvant analgesic drugs, such as the antidepressant analgesics, are suggested for use, along with opioids and NSAIDs, in all stages of the analgesic ladder (mild, moderate, or severe pain).

This WHO approach, while not yet validated in AIDS, has been recommended by the AHCPR, and clinical authorities in the field of pain management and AIDS (Fig. 1). Clinical reports describing the successful application of the principles of the WHO Analgesic Ladder to the management of pain in AIDS, with particular emphasis on the use of opioids, have also recently appeared in the literature.

Authorities have described the indications for and use of three classes of analgesic drugs that have applications in the management of AIDS patients with pain: (1) nonopioid analgesics (such as acetaminophen, aspirin, and other NSAIDs), (2) opioid analgesics (of which morphine is the standard), and (3) adjuvant analgesics (such as antidepressants and anticonvulsants).

Nonopioid Analgesics

The nonopioid analgesics are prescribed principally for mild to moderate pain or to augment the analgesic effects of opioid analgesics in the treatment of severe pain.

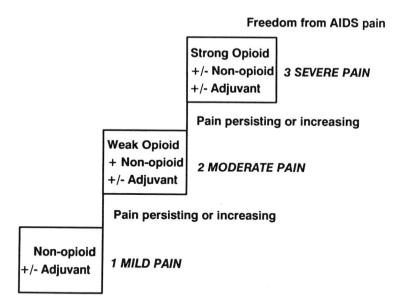

FIG. 1. WHO Analgesic Ladder for the management of pain in HIV-infected patients. (Adapted from *Cancer Pain Relief*, WHO, 1986.)

Commonly utilized nonopioid analgesics (as well as the "weaker" opioids) are described in Table 3. The analgesic effects of NSAIDs result from their inhibition of cyclooxygenase and the subsequent reduction in prostaglandin biosynthesis in the tissues. Concurrent use of NSAIDs or acetaminophen and opioids provides more analgesia than does either of the drug classes alone. In contrast to opioids, NSAIDs have a ceiling effect for analgesia, do not produce tolerance or dependence, have antipyretic effects, and have a different spectrum of adverse effects.

The physiochemical properties of the NSAIDs, mechanisms of action, pharmacokinetics, and pharmacodynamics influence the analgesic response. Selection of the NSAID should take into account the etiology and severity of the pain, concurrent medical conditions that entail relative contraindications (e.g., bleeding diathesis), associated symptoms, and favorable experience by the patient as well as physician. From a practical point of view, a NSAID should be titrated to effect as well as to side effects. There is also variability in patient response to both relief and adverse reactions, so if the results are not favorable an alternative NSAID should be tried.

The major adverse effects associated with NSAIDs include gastric ulceration, renal failure, hepatic dysfunction, and bleeding. Use of NSAIDs has been associated with a variety of gastrointestinal toxicities including minor dyspepsia and heartburn as well as major gastric erosion, peptic ulcer formation, and gastrointestinal hemorrhage. The nonacetylated salicylates, such as salsalate, sodium salicylate, and choline magnesium salicylate, theoretically have fewer gastrointestinal (GI) side effects and might be considered in cases where GI distress is an issue. Pro-

TABLE 3. *Oral analgesics for mild to moderate pain in AIDS*

Analgesic (by class)	Starting dose (mg)	Duration (hours)	Plasma half-life (hours)	Comments
Nonsteroidal				
Aspirin	650	4–6	4–6	The standard for comparison among nonopioid analgesics
Ibuprofen	400–600	4–8	3–4	Like aspirin, can inhibit platelet function
Choline magnesium trisalicylte	700–1500	8–12	8–12	Essentially no hematologic or gastrointestinal side effects
Weaker opioids				
Codeine	32–65	3–4	3–4	Metabolized to morphine, often used to suppress cough in patients at risk of pulmonary bleed
Oxycodone	5–10	3–4	3–4	Available as a single agent and in combination with aspirin or acetaminophen
Proxyphene	65–130	4–6	3–4	Toxic metabolite, norpropoxy, accumulates with repeated dosing

phylaxis for NSAID-associated GI symptoms include H2 antagonist drugs (cimetidine 300 mg tid–qid or ranitidine 150 mg bid), misoprostal 200 mg qid, omeprazole 20 mg qd, or an antacid. Patients should be informed of these symptoms, issued guaiac minds with reagent, and taught to check their stool weekly for occult blood.

NSAIDs also may affect kidney function. Prostaglandins are involved in the autoregulation of renal blood flow, glomerular filtration, and the tubular transport of water and ions. NSAIDs can cause a decrease in glomerular filtration, acute and chronic renal failure, interstitial nephritis, papillary necrosis, and hyperkalemia. In patients with renal impairment, NSAIDs should be used with caution since many of these drugs (e.g., ketoprofen, feroprofen, naproxen, and carpofen) are highly dependent on renal function for clearance. The risk of NSAID-induced renal dysfunction is greatest in patients with advanced age, preexisting renal impairment, hypovolemia, concomitant therapy with other nephrotic drugs, and heart failure. Prostaglandins modulate vascular tone and their inhibition by the NSAIDs can cause hypertension as well as interference with the pharmacologic control of hypertension. Caution should be used in patients receiving β-adrenergic antagonists, diuretics, or angiotensin-converting enzyme inhibitors. Several studies have suggested that there is substantial biliary excretion of several NSAIDs including indomethacin and sulindac. In patients with hepatic dysfunction these drugs should be used with caution. NSAIDs, with the exception of the nonacetylated salicylates (e.g., sodium salicylate, choline magnesium trisalicylate), produce inhibition of platelet aggregation (usually reversible, but irreversible with aspirin). NSAIDs should be used with extreme caution, or avoided, in patients who are thrombocytopenic or who have a clotting impairment.

The use of NSAIDs in patients with AIDS must be accompanied by heightened awareness of toxicity and adverse effects. NSAIDs are highly protein bound and the free fraction of available drug is increased in AIDS patients who are cachectic, wasted, and hypoalbuminic, often resulting in toxicities and adverse effects. Patients with AIDS are frequently hypovolemic, on concurrent nephrotoxic drugs, and experiencing HIV nephropathy, and so are at increased risk for renal toxicity related to NSAIDs. Finally, the antipyretic effects of the NSAIDs may interfere with early detection of infection in patients with AIDS.

Opioid Analgesics

Opioid analgesics are the mainstay of pharmacotherapy of moderate to severe intensity pain in the patient with HIV infection (Table 4). Principles that are helpful in guiding the appropriate use of opioid analgesics for pain include the following: (1) choose an appropriate drug; (2) start with the lowest dose possible; (3) titrate dose; (4) use "as needed" doses selectively; (5) use an appropriate route of administration; (6) be aware of equivalent analgesic doses; (7) use a combination of opioid, nonopioid, and adjuvant drugs; (8) be aware of tolerance; and (9) understand physical and psychological dependence.

In choosing the appropriate opioid analgesic for cancer pain one authority highlights the following important considerations: (1) opioid class, (2) "weak" versus "strong" opioids, (3) pharmacokinetic characteristics, (4) duration of analgesic effect, (5) favorable prior response, and (6) opioid side effects. Opioid analgesics are divided into two classes, the agonists and the agonist-antagonists, based on their affinity for opioid receptors. Morphine and the other opioid analgesics listed in Table 4 are agonist drugs. Pentazocine, butorphanol, and nalbuphine are examples of opioid analgesics with mixed agonist-antagonist properties. These drugs can reverse opioid effects and precipitate an opioid withdrawal syndrome in patients who are opioid tolerant or dependent. They are of limited use in the management of chronic pain in AIDS. Oxycodone, hydrocodone, and codeine are the so-called weaker opioid analgesics and are indicated for use in step 2 of the WHO ladder for mild to moderate intensity pain. They are often prescribed/available in combination with either aspirin or acetaminophen. Oxycodone (Roxicodone) and codeine are available as single agents without aspirin or acetaminophen. More severe pain is best managed with morphine or another of the stronger opioid analgesics, such as hydromorphone, methadone, levorphanol, or fentanyl.

A basic understanding of the pharmacokinetics of the opioid analgesics is important for the AIDS care provider. Opioid analgesics with long half-lives, such as methadone, and levorphanol require approximately 5 days to achieve a steady state. Despite their long half-lives, the duration of analgesia that they provide is considerably shorter (i.e., most patients will require administration of the drug every 4 to 6 hours). As both methadone and levorphanol tend to accumulate with early initial dosing, delayed effects of toxicity can develop (primarily sedation and more rarely respiratory depression).

TABLE 4. Narcotic analgesics for moderate to severe pain in AIDS

Analgesic	Route	Equianalgesic dose (mg)	Analgesic onset (hours)	Analgesic duration (hours)	Plasma half-life (hours)	Comments
Morphine	po	30–60	1–1½	4–6	2–4	Standard of comparison for the narcotic analgesics; now available in long-acting sc oral sustained release preparations
	im, iv	10	½–1	4–6	3–4	
Hydromorphone	po	7.5	½–1	3–4	2–3	Short half-life, ideal for elderly patients; comes in rectal suppository and injectable forms
	im, iv	1.5	¼–½	3–4	2–3	
Methadone	po	20	½–1	4–6	15–30	Long half-life; tends to accumulate with initial dosing, requires careful titration; good oral potency
	im, iv	10	½–1	ND	15–30	
Levorphanol	po	4	1–1½	4–6	12–16	Long half-life; requires careful dose titration in first week; note that analgesic duration is only 4 hours
	im	2	½–1	4–5	12–16	
Meperidine	po	300	1–1½	4–6	3–4	Active toxic metabolite, normeperidine, tends to accumulate (plasma half-life is 12–16 hours), especially with renal impairment and in elderly patients, causing delirium, myoclonus, and seizures
	im	75	½–1	4–5	3–4	
Fentanyl	td	0.1	12–18	48–72	20–22	Transdermal patch is convenient, bypassing GI absorption; long duration of analgesia, slow onset of analgesia until depot is formed; not suitable for rapid titration
	iv	0.1	ND	ND	–	

po, per oral; td, transdermal; im, intramuscular; iv, intravenous; sl, sublingual; sc, subcutaneous; ND, no data available.

The duration of analgesic effects of opioid analgesics varies considerably as outlined in Tables 3 and 4. Oxycodone will often provide only 3 hours of relief, and it must be prescribed on an every 3 hour around-the-clock basis (not as needed). Methadone and levorphanol may provide up to 6 hours of analgesia. There is individual variation in the metabolism of opioid analgesics, and there can be significant differences between individuals in drug absorption and disposition. These differences lead to a need for alterations in dosing, route of administration, and scheduling for maximum analgesia in individual patients. While parenteral administration (intravenous, intramuscular, subcutaneous) will yield a faster onset of pain relief, the duration of analgesia is shorter unless a continuous infusion of opioid is instituted. The use of continuous subcutaneous or intravenous infusions of opioids, with or without patient-controlled analgesia (PCA) devices, has become commonplace in caring for AIDS patients with escalating pain, and in hospice and home settings during late stages of disease.

The oral route is often the preferred route of administration of opioid analgesics, from the perspectives of convenience and cost. Immediate-release oral morphine or hydromorphone preparations require that the drug be taken every 3 to 4 hours. Longer-acting, sustained-release oral morphine preparations (MS Contin, Oramorph SR) are now available that provide up to 8 to 12 hours of analgesia, minimizing the number of daily doses required for the control of persistent pain. Rescue doses of short-acting, immediate-release opioids are often necessary to supplement the use of sustained-release morphine, particularly during periods of titration or pain escalation. The transdermal fentanyl patch system (Duragesic) also has applications in the management of severe pain in AIDS. Each transdermal fentanyl patch contains a 48- to 72-hour supply of fentanyl, which is absorbed from a depot in the skin. Levels in the plasma rise slowly over 12 to 18 hours after patch placement. So, with the initial placement of a patch, alternative opioid analgesia, either oral, rectal or parenteral, must be provided until adequate levels of fentanyl are attained. The elimination half-life of this dosage form of fentanyl is long (21 hours), implying that significant levels of fentanyl will remain in plasma for about 24 hours after the removal of a transdermal patch. The transdermal system is not optimal for rapid dose titration of acutely exacerbated pain; however, a variety of dosage forms are available. As with sustained-release morphine preparations, all patients should be provided with oral or parenteral, rapidly acting, short-duration opioids to manage breakthrough pain. The transdermal system is convenient, and eliminates the reminders of pain associated with repeated oral dosing of analgesics. In AIDS patients, it should be noted that the absorption of transdermal fentanyl can be increased with fever, resulting in higher plasma levels and shorter duration of analgesia from the patch.

It is important to note that opioids can be administered through a variety of routes: oral, rectal, transdermal, intravenous, subcutaneous, intraspinal, and even intraventricularly. The advantages and disadvantages as well as indications for use of these various routes is beyond the scope of this chapter; however, interested readers are directed to the Agency for Health Care Policy and Research Clinical

Practice Guideline: Management of Cancer Pain available free of charge through 1-800-4-CANCER.

Adequate treatment of pain in AIDS also requires consideration of the equianalgesic doses of opioid drugs, which are generally calculated using morphine as a standard (Table 4). Cross-tolerance is not complete among these drugs. Therefore, one half to two thirds of the equianalgesic dose of the new drug should be given as the starting dose when switching from one opioid to another. For example, if a patient receiving 20 mg of parenteral morphine is to be switched to hydromorphone, the equianalgesic dose of parenteral hydromorphone would be 3.0 mg. Thus, the starting dose of parenteral hydromorphone should be approximately 1.5 mg to 2 mg. There is also considerable variability in the parenteral to oral ratios among opioid analgesics. Both levorphanol and methadone have 1:2 intramuscular/oral ratios, whereas morphine has a 1:6 and hydromorphone a 1:5 intramuscular/oral ratio. Failure to appreciate these dosage differences in route of administration can lead to inadequate pain control.

Regular ("standing") scheduling of the opioid analgesics is the foundation of adequate pain control. It is preferable to prevent the return of pain as opposed to treating pain as it recurs. "As-needed" orders for chronic cancer often create a struggle between patient, family, and staff that is easily avoided by regular administration of opioid analgesics. The typical prescribing of methadone is a notable exception. It is often initially prescribed on an as-needed basis to determine the patient's total daily requirement and to minimize toxicity (due to its long half-life).

Opioid Side Effects

While the opioids are extremely effective analgesics, their side effects are common and can be minimized if anticipated in advance. Sedation is a common side effect, especially during the initiation of treatment. Sedation usually resolves after the patient has been maintained on a steady dosage. Persistent sedation can be alleviated with a psychostimulant, such as dextroamphetamine, pemoline, or methylphenidate. All are prescribed in divided doses in early morning and at noon. Additionally, psychostimulants can improve depressed mood and enhance analgesia. Delirium, of an either agitated or somnolent variety, can also occur while on opioid analgesics, and is usually accompanied by attentional deficits, disorientation, and perceptual disturbances (visual hallucinations and more commonly illusions). Myoclonus and asterixis are often early signs of neurotoxicity that accompany the course of opioid induced delirium. Meperidine (Demerol) when administered chronically in patients with renal impairment can lead to a delirium due to accumulation of the neuroexcitatory metabolite normeperidine.

Opioid-induced delirium can be alleviated through the implementation of three possible strategies: (1) lowering the dose of the opioid drug presently in use, (2) changing to a different opioid, or (3) treating the delirium with low doses of high-potency neuroleptics such as haloperidol. The third strategy is especially useful for agitation and clears the sensorium. For agitated states intravenous haloperidol in doses starting at between 1 and 2 mg is useful, with rapid escalation of dose if no effect is noted. Gastrointestinal side effects of opioid analgesics are common. The most prevalent are nausea, vomiting, and constipation. Concomitant therapy with prochlorperazine for nausea is sometimes effective. Since all opioid analgesics are not tolerated in the same manner, switching to another narcotic can be helpful if an antiemetic regimen fails to control nausea. Constipation caused by narcotic effects on gut receptors is a problem frequently encountered and it tends to be responsive to the regular use of senna derivatives. A careful review of medications is imperative, since anticholinergic drugs such as the tricyclic antidepressants can worsen opioid-induced constipation and can cause bowel obstruction. Respiratory depression is a worrisome but rare side effect of the opioid analgesics. Respiratory difficulties can almost always be avoided if two general principles are adhered to: (1) start opioid analgesics in low doses in opioid-naive patients, and (2) be cognizant of relative potencies when switching opioid analgesics, routes of administration, or both.

Adjuvant Analgesics

Adjuvant analgesics are the third class of medications frequently prescribed for the treatment of chronic pain and have important applications in the management of pain in AIDS (Table 5). Adjuvant analgesic drugs are used to enhance the analgesic efficacy of opioids, treat concurrent symptoms that exacerbate pain, and provide independent analgesia. They may be used in all stages of the analgesic ladder. Commonly used adjuvant drugs include antidepressants, neuroleptics, psycho-stimulants, anticonvulsants, corticosteroids, and oral anesthetics.

Antidepressants

Current literature supports the use of antidepressants as adjuvant analgesic agents in the management of a wide variety of chronic pain syndromes including cancer pain, postherpetic neuralgia, diabetic neuropathy, fibromyalgia, headache, and low back pain. The antidepressants are analgesic through a number of mechanisms that include antidepressant activity, potentiation or enhancement of opioid analgesia, and direct analgesic effects. The leading hypothesis suggests that both serotonergic and noradrenergic properties of the antidepressants are probably important and that variations among individuals in pain (as to the status of their own neurotransmitter systems) is an important variable. Other possible mechanisms of antidepressant analgesic activity that have been proposed including adrenergic and serotonin receptor effects, adenosinergic effects, antihistaminic effects, and direct neuronal effects such as inhibition of paroxysmal neuronal discharge and decreasing sensitivity of adrenergic receptors on injured nerve sprouts.

There is substantial evidence that the tricyclic antidepressants, in particular, are analgesic and useful in the management of chronic neuropathic and nonneuropathic

TABLE 5. *Psychotropic adjuvant analgesic drugs for AIDS pain*

Generic name	Trade name	Approximate daily dosage (mg)	Route
Tricyclic antidepressants			
Amitriptyline	Elavil	10–150	PO, IM
Nortriptyline	Pamelor, Aventyl	10–150	PO
Imipramine	Tofranil	12.5–150	PO, IM
Desipramine	Norpramin	10–150	PO
Clomipramine	Anafranil	10–150	PO
Doxepin	Sinequan	12–150	PO, IM
Heterocyclic and noncyclic antidepressants			
Trazadone	Desyrel	125–300	PO
Maprotiline	Ludiomil	50–300	PO
Serotonin reuptake inhibitors			
Fluoxetine	Prozac	20–60	PO
Paroxetine	Paxil	10–40	PO
Sertraline	Zoloft	50–200	PO
Amine precursor			
L-Tryptophan		500–3,000	PO
Psychostimulants			
Methylphenidate	Ritalin	2.5–20 bid	PO
Dextroamphetamine	Dexedrine	2.5–20 bid	PO
Pemoline	Cylert	3.75–75 bid	PO
Phenothiazines			
Fluphenazine	Prolixin	1–3	PO, IM
Methotrimeprazine	Levoprome	10–20 q6h	IM, IV
Butrophenones			
Haloperidol	Haldol	1–3PO	IM, IV
Pimozide	Orap	2–6 bid	PO
Antihistamines			
Hydroxyzine	Vistaril	50 q 4–6h	PO
Dexamethasone	Decadron	4–16	PO, IV
Benzodiazepines			
Alprazolam	Xanax	0.25–2.0 tid	PO
Clonazepam	Klonopin	0.5–4 bid	PO

PO, per oral; IM, intramuscular; PR, parenteral; IV, intravenous; q6h, every 6 hours.

pain syndromes. Amitriptyline is the tricyclic antidepressant most studied and has been proved effective as an analgesic in a large number of clinical trials, addressing a wide variety of chronic pain syndromes, including neuropathy, cancer pain, fibromyalgia, and others. Other tricyclics that have been shown to have efficacy as analgesics include imipramine, desipramine, nortriptyline, clomipramine, and doxepin.

The heterocyclic and noncyclic antidepressant drugs such as trazadone, mianserin, maprotiline, and the newer serotonin specific reuptake inhibitors (SSRIs), fluoxetine and paroxetine, may also be useful as adjuvant analgesics for chronic pain syndromes. Fluoxetine, a potent antidepressant with specific serotonin reuptake inhibition activity, has been shown to have analgesic properties in experimental animal pain models, but failed to show analgesic effects in a clinical trial for neuropathy. Several case reports suggest fluoxetine may be a useful adjuvant analgesic in the management of headache and fibrositis. Paroxetine, a newer SSRI, is the first antidepressant of this class shown to be a highly effective analgesic in a controlled trial for the treatment of diabetic neuropathy.

Given the diversity of clinical syndromes in which the antidepressants have been demonstrated to be analgesic, trials of these drugs can be justified in the treatment of virtually every type of chronic pain. The established benefit of several of the antidepressants in patients with neuropathic pains, however, suggests that these drugs may be particularly useful in populations, such as cancer and AIDS patients, where an underlying neuropathic component to the pain often exists. While studies of the analgesic efficacy of these drugs in HIV-related painful neuropathies have not yet been conducted, they are widely applied clinically using the models of diabetic and postherpetic neuropathies.

While antidepressant drugs are analgesic in both neuropathic and nonneuropathic pain models, their clinical use is most commonly in combination with opioid drugs, particularly for moderate to severe pain. Antidepressant adjuvant analgesics have their most broad application as "co-analgesics," potentiating the analgesic effects of opioid drugs. The "opioid-sparing" effects of antidepressant analgesics have been demonstrated in a number of trials, especially in cancer populations with neuropathic as well as nonneuropathic pain syndromes. A placebo controlled study demonstrated that imipramine was a potent co-analgesic when used along with morphine in the treatment of cancer-related pain, allowing for a reduction in morphine consumption of greater than 25%. Similar co-analgesic and opioid sparing effects were demonstrated for amitriptyline and other antidepressants in two multicenter clinical trials for cancer pain.

The dose and time course of onset of analgesia for antidepressants when used as analgesics appear to be similar to their use as antidepressants. While some investigators have argued that a low-dose regimen of amitriptyline (10 to 30 mg) is equally analgesic to a high-dose regimen (75 to 150 mg), others have demonstrated only modest analgesic results from low-dose amitriptyline. Some authorities have felt that there was a "therapeutic window" (20 to 100 mg) for the analgesic effects of amitriptyline. More recently, there is compelling evidence that the therapeutic analgesic effects of amitriptyline are correlated with serum levels, as are the antidepressant effects, and that analgesic treatment failure is due to low serum levels. A high-dose regimen of 150 mg (or higher) of amitriptyline is suggested. The proper analgesic dose for paroxetine is likely in the 40- to 60-mg range, with the major analgesic trial utilizing a fixed dose of 40 mg. There is anecdotal evidence to suggest that the debilitated medically ill (cancer or AIDS patients) often respond (re: depression or pain) to lower doses of antidepressants than are usually required in the physically healthy, probably because of impaired metabolism of these drugs. As to the time course of onset of analgesia, a biphasic process appears to occur. There are immediate or early analgesic effects that occur within hours or days, which are probably mediated through inhibition of synaptic reuptake of catecholamines. In addition, there are later, longer analgesic effects that peak over a 2- to 4-week period that are probably due to receptor effects of the antidepressants.

PSYCHOSTIMULANTS

Psychostimulants such as dextroamphetamine, methylphenidate, and pemoline may be useful antidepressants in patients with HIV infection or AIDS who are cognitively impaired. Psychostimulants also enhance the analgesic effects of the opioid drugs, and are useful in diminishing their sedating properties. Investigators have demonstrated that a regimen of 10 mg methylphenidate with breakfast and 5 mg with lunch significantly decreased sedation and potentiated the effect of narcotics in patients with cancer pain. Methylphenidate has also been demonstrated to improve functioning on a number of neuropsychological tests, including tests of memory, speed, and concentration, in patients receiving continuous infusions of opioids for cancer pain. Dextroamphetamine has been reported to have additive analgesic effects when used with morphine in postoperative pain. In relatively low doses, psychostimulants stimulate appetite, promote a sense of well-being, and improve feelings of weakness and fatigue in cancer patients.

Pemoline is a unique alternative psychostimulant that is chemically unrelated to amphetamine, but may have similar usefulness as an antidepressant and adjuvant analgesic in AIDS patients. Advantages of pemoline as a psychostimulant in AIDS pain include the lack of abuse potential, the lack of federal regulation and requirement for special triplicate prescriptions, the final sympathomimetic effects, and the fact that it comes in a chewable tablet form that can be absorbed through the buccal mucosa, and thus can be used by AIDS patients who have difficulty swallowing. Clinically, pemoline is as effective as methylphenidate or dextroamphetamine in the treatment of depressive symptoms and in countering the sedating effects of opioid analgesics. There are no studies of pemoline's capacity to potentiate the analgesic properties of opioids. Pemoline should be used with caution in patients with liver impairment, and liver function tests should be monitored periodically with longer-term treatment.

Neuroleptics

Neuroleptic drugs such as methotrimeprazine, fluphenazine, haloperidol, and pimozide may play a role as adjuvant analgesics in AIDS patients with pain. Their use, however, must be weighed against what appears to be an increased sensitivity to the extrapyramidal side effects of these drugs in AIDS patients with neurologic complications. Anxiolytics such as alprazolam and clonazepram may also be useful as adjuvant analgesics, particularly in the management of neuropathic pains.

PAIN MANAGEMENT AND SUBSTANCE ABUSE IN AIDS

Individuals who inject drugs are among the AIDS exposure categories with the highest rate of increase over the past 5 years, especially in large urban centers. Pain management in the substance abusing AIDS patient is perhaps the most challenging of clinical goals. Fears of addiction and concerns regarding drug abuse affect both patient compliance and physician management of pain and use of narcotic analgesics, often leading to under treatment of pain. Studies of patterns of chronic narcotic analgesic use in patients with cancer, burns, and postoperative pain have demonstrated that although tolerance and physical dependence commonly occur, addiction, that is, psychological dependence, and drug abuse are rare and almost never occur in individuals who do not have histories of drug abuse.

More problematic, however, is managing pain in the growing segment of HIV-infected patients who are actively abusing drugs. The use of opiates for pain control raises several issues: how to treat pain in people who have a high tolerance to narcotic analgesics; how to mitigate this population's drug-seeking and potentially manipulative behavior; how to deal with patients who may offer unreliable medical histories or who may not comply with treatment recommendations; and how to counter the risk of patients spreading HIV while high and disinhibited. In addition, clinicians must rely on a patient's subjective report, which is often the only indication of the presence and intensity of pain, as well as the degree of pain relief, achieved by an intervention. Physicians who believe they are being manipulated by drug-seeking patients often hesitate to use appropriately high doses of narcotic analgesics to control pain. Most clinicians experienced in working with this population of patients recommend that practitioners set clear and direct limits. While this is an important aspect of the care of IV drug users with HIV infection, it is by no means the whole answer. As much as possible, clinicians should attempt to eliminate the issue of drug abuse as an obstacle to pain management by dealing directly with the problems of opiate withdrawal and drug treatment. Clinicians should err on the side of believing patients when they complain of pain, and should utilize knowledge of specific HIV-related pain syndromes to corroborate the report of a patient perceived as being unreliable.

Experience reported in the cancer pain literature suggests that it is possible to manage pain adequately in substance abusers with life-threatening illness, and to do so safely and responsibly, utilizing opioid analgesics and several sound principles of pain management outlined in Table 6. Perhaps of greatest concern to clinicians is the possibility that they are being lied to by a substance-abusing AIDS patient complaining of pain. The fear is that the clinician is being "duped" into prescribing narcotic analgesics that will then be abused or sold. Clinicians do not want to contribute to or help sustain addiction. This leads to an immediate defensiveness on the part of the clinician and an impulse to avoid prescribing opioids and even to avoid full assessment of a pain complaint. Unfortunately, the existence or severity of pain cannot be objectively proven. The clinician must accept and respect the report of pain in spite of the possibility of being duped and proceed in the evaluation, assessment, and management of pain.

The clinician must be familiar with and understand the current terminology relevant to substance abuse and addiction. It is important to distinguish between the terms *tolerance*, *physical dependence*, and *addiction* or *abuse* (psychological dependence). Tolerance is a pharmacologic property of opioid drugs defined by the

TABLE 6. *Guidelines for pain management in substance abusers with AIDS*

Accept and respect the report of acute pain in spite of the possibility of being duped
Prevent or minimize withdrawal symptoms
Define the pain syndrome (comprehensive pain assessment) and provide treatment for both
 the underlying disorder and the pain complaint
Utilize the WHO "Analgesic Ladder" schema to select appropriate pharmacologic approach
Apply appropriate pharmacologic principles when using opioids
Provide nonopioid and nonpharmacologic therapies as indicated
Recognize specific drug abuse behaviors
Set realistic goals for pain therapy
The care of the substance abusing AIDS patient with pain requires a team effort
Evaluate and treat other distressing physical and psychological symptoms that may contrib-
 ute to pain and suffering
Constant assessment and reevaluation of the effects of pain interventions must take place in
 order to optimize care

Adapted from McCaffery M, Vourakis C: Assessment and relief of pain in chemically dependent patients. *Orthopedic Nursing* 1992;11:13–27, and Portenoy RE, Payne R: Acute and chronic pain. In: Lowenson JH, Ruiz P, Millman RB, eds.: Comprehensive textbook of Substance
Abuse. Baltimore: Williams and Wilkins, 1992; 691–721.

need for increasing doses to maintain an (analgesic) effect. Physical dependence is
characterized by the onset of signs and symptoms of withdrawal if narcotic analgesics are abruptly stopped or a narcotic antagonist is administered. Tolerance usually
occurs in association with physical dependence. Addiction or abuse is a psychological and behavioral syndrome in which there is drug craving, compulsive use (despite physical, psychological, or social harm to the user), other aberrant drug-re-
lated behaviors, and relapse after abstinence. The term *pseudo-addiction* has been
coined to describe the patient who exhibits behavior that clinicians associate with
addiction, such as requests for higher doses of opioid, but in fact is due to uncontrolled pain and inadequate pain management.

The clinician must also distinguish between the "former" addict who has been
drug free for years, the addict in a methadone maintenance program, and the addict
who is actively abusing illicit and/or prescription drugs. Actively using addicts and
those on methadone maintenance with pain must be assumed to have some tolerance
to opioids and may require higher starting and maintenance doses of opioids. Preventing withdrawal is an essential first step in managing pain in this population. In
addition, "active" addicts with AIDS will understandably require more in the way of
psychosocial support and services to deal adequately with the distress of their pain
and illness. Former addicts may pose the challenge of refusing opioids for pain
because of the fear of relapse. Such patients can be assured that opioids, when
prescribed and monitored responsibly, may be an essential part of pain management, and use of the drug for pain is quite different than its use when they were
abusing similar drugs.

Some authorities emphasize the importance of conducting a comprehensive pain
assessment in order to define the pain syndrome. Specific pain syndromes often
respond best to specific interventions (i.e., neuropathic pains respond well to anti-

depressants or anticonvulsants). Adequate assessment of the cause of pain is essential in all AIDS patients, and particularly in the substance abuser. It is critical that adequate analgesia be provided while diagnostic studies are under way. Often therapy of the underlying disorder causing pain is effective in improving the condition and its accompanying symptoms, such as pain; headache from CNS toxoplasmosis responds well to primary treatments and steroids.

When deciding on an appropriate pharmacologic intervention in the substance abuser, it is also advisable to follow the Analgesic Ladder. For mild to moderate pain, NSAIDs are indicated. The NSAIDs are continued with adjuvant analgesics (antidepressants, anticonvulsants, neuroleptics) if a specific indication exists. Patients with moderate to severe pain, or those who do not achieve relief on NSAIDs are treated with a "weak" opioid, often in combination with NSAIDs and adjuvant drugs if indicated. Finally, patients who have severe pain or do not get adequate relief from these agents are prescribed a "strong" opioid, with or without NSAIDs or adjuvants.

It has been pointed out that it is critical to apply appropriate pharmacologic principles for opioid use. One should avoid using agonist-antagonist opioid drugs. The use of prn dosing often leads to excessive drug-centered interactions with staff that are not productive. While patients should not necessarily be given the specific drug or route they want, every effort should be made to give patients more of a sense of control and a sense of collaboration with the clinician. Often a patient's report of beneficial or adverse effects of a specific agent is useful to the clinician.

Management of pain in substance-abusing AIDS patients requires a team approach. Early involvement of pain specialists, psychiatric clinicians, and substance abuse specialists is necessary. Nonpharmacologic pain interventions should be appropriately applied, not as a substitute for opioids but as an important adjunct. Realistic goals for treatment must be set, and problems related to inappropriate behavior around the handling of prescriptions and interactions with staff should be anticipated. Hospital staff should be made aware that such difficult patients evoke feelings that if acted on could interfere with providing good care. Clear limit setting is helpful for both the patient and treating staff. Sometimes written rules about what behaviors are expected and what behaviors are not tolerated, and their consequences, should be provided. The use of urine toxicology monitoring, restrictions of visitors, and strict limits on the amount of drug per prescription can all be very useful. It is important to remember that rehabilitation or detoxification from opioids is not appropriate during an acute medical crisis and should not be attempted at that time. Once more stable medical conditions exist, referral to a drug rehabilitation program may be very useful. Constant assessment and reevaluation of the effects of pain interventions must also take place in order to optimize care. Special attention should be given to points in treatment where routes of administration are changed or where opioids are being tapered. It must be made clear to patients what drugs and or regimen will be used to control pain when opioids are tapered or withdrawn, and what options are available if the nonopioid regimen is ineffective.

Finally, it is important to recognize that substance abusers with AIDS are quite likely to have comorbid psychiatric symptoms as well as multiple other physical symptoms that can all contribute to increased pain and suffering. Adequate attention must be paid to these physical and psychological symptoms if pain management is to be optimized.

SUMMARY

Pain in AIDS is a clinically significant problem contributing greatly to psychological and functional morbidity. Pain can be adequately treated and so must be a focus of care in the AIDS patient. Substance abusers with pain and AIDS are a particularly challenging problem that needs special attention.

ACKNOWLEDGMENTS

This work has been supported by NIH grant 45664 and the Open Society Institute, Project on Death in America Faculty Scholars Program.

SUGGESTED READING

Agency for Health Care Policy and Research, Public Health Service, U.S. Department of Health and Human Services. *Management of cancer pain: clinical practice guideline*, number 9. (AHCOR Publication No. 94-0592). Rockville, MD, 1994.

Anand A, Carmosino L, Glatt AE. Evaluation of recalcitrant pain in HIV-infected hospitalized patients. *J AIDS* 1994;7:52–56.

Barone SE, Gunold BS, Nealson TF, et al. Abdominal pain in patients with acquired immune deficiency syndrome. *Ann Surg* 1986;204:619–623.

Breitbart W, Patt RB. Pain management in the patient with AIDS. *Hematol Oncol Ann* 1994;2(6):391–399.

Carr DB, Dubois M, Luu M, Shepard KV. Pharmacotherapy of pain in HIV/AIDS. In: Carr DB, ed. *Pain in HIV/AIDS: Proceedings of a workshop convened by France–U.S.A. Pain Association*. Washington, D.C.: France-U.S.A. Pain Association, 1994;18–28.

Cornblath DR, McArthur JC. Predominantly sensory neuropathy in patients with AIDS and AIDS-related complex. *Neurology* 1988;38:794–796.

Gaut P, Wong PK, Meyer RD. Pyomyositis in a patient with the acquired immunodeficiency syndrome. *Arch Intern Med* 1988;148:1608–1610.

Kaye BR. Rheumatologic manifestations of infection with human immunodeficiency virus (HIV). *Ann Intern Med* 1989;111:158–167.

Lebovits AK, Lefkowitz M, McCarthy D, et al. The prevalence and management of pain in patients with AIDS. A review of 134 cases. *Clin J Pain* 1989;5:245–248.

Lipton RB, Feraru ER, Weiss G, Chhabria M, Harris C, Aronow H, Newman LC, Solomon S. Headache in HIV-1-related disorders. *Headache* 1991;31:518–522.

McCormack JP, Li R, Zarowny D, Singer J. Inadequate treatment of pain in ambulatory HIV patients. *Clin J Pain* 1993;9:279–283.

O'Neill WM, Sherrard JS. Pain in human immunodeficiency virus disease: a review. *Pain* 1993;54:3–14.

Schofferman J, Brody R. Pain in far advanced AIDS. In: Foley KM, et al., eds. *Advances in Pain Research and Therapy*, vol 16. New York: Raven Press, 1990;379–386.

Simpson DM, Wolfe DE. Neuromuscular complication of HIV infection and its treatment. *AIDS* 1991;5:917–926.

Singer EJ, Zorilla C, Fehy-Chandon B, et al. Painful symptoms reported for ambulatory HIV-infected men in a longitudinal study. *Pain* 1993;54:15–19.

A Clinical Guide to AIDS and HIV,
edited by Gary P. Wormser.
Lippincott-Raven Publishers, Philadelphia © 1996.

13

Alternative Therapies

Donald I. Abrams

AIDS Program, San Francisco General Hospital, University of California at San Francisco, San Francisco, California 94110

Despite a decade of progress in understanding the molecular virology and pathophysiology of the human immunodeficiency virus (HIV), acquired immunodeficiency syndrome (AIDS), the disease caused by infection with this novel retrovirus, remains incurable. Many patients who were initially encouraged by the prospects of early intervention with antiretroviral agents have lost confidence in available orthodox treatments offered by their medical providers. The continued lack of effective therapies has sparked a return to the alternative treatment movement begun prior to the availability of prescription therapies for HIV infection. By now the alternative therapies movement has grown to the point that most health care providers treating patients with HIV infection regardless of their risk group are likely to have interacted with patients who have utilized alternative therapies.

The alternative therapy movement is not unique to HIV-infected patients. These therapies have been studied extensively in patients with malignant diseases; increased use of unorthodox treatments is related to disillusionment with standard medical practice. A *Time*/CNN poll reported in 1991 that 30% of 500 people questioned in a telephone survey had tried some form of unconventional therapy, one half within the year before the survey. Among those who responded that they had never sought help from a practitioner of alternative medicine, 62% stated that they would consider seeking such assistance if conventional medicine failed to help them. Of those who had sought help from a practitioner of alternative medicine, 84% responded that they would go back to an alternative doctor.

The prevalence, costs, and patterns of use of unconventional medicine in the United States was studied by investigators who conducted telephone interviews with 1,539 adults in 1990. Of those surveyed, 34% reported using one or more unconventional therapies in the past year. The two most frequently reported unconventional modalities of therapy reported, exercise (26%) and prayer (25%), were excluded from the overall 34% result. Of the numerous unconventional techniques, relaxation (13%), chiropractic (10%), massage (7%), imagery (4%), and spiritual healing (4%) were all more frequently cited than any interventions requiring ingestion of a substance. Weight loss programs, lifestyle diets, herbal medicine, and megavitamin therapy were reported by only 2% to 4% of respondents. The greatest use of unconventional therapies was reported by nonblack persons, aged 25 to 49 years, with higher income and educational levels. Of the 34% who used unconventional therapies for serious medical conditions, 83% also sought treatment from a medical doctor. However, nearly three quarters of these individuals did not inform their doctor. Based on these findings, the authors estimate that annual visits to providers of unconventional therapy number 425 million, a figure that exceeds the number of visits to all primary care physicians, at an approximate cost of $13.7 billion. Concluding that the frequency and use of unconventional therapy is higher than previously reported, the authors urged physicians to inquire about their patients' use of unconventional therapy whenever they obtain a medical history.

Greater use of alternative therapies is noted among patients with diseases for which treatment is limited. It is therefore not surprising that people with HIV infection have become frequent users of alternative therapy. The earliest studies of the use of alternative therapies by patients with HIV infection in the United States suggested that 20% to 30% of this population have sought such interventions. Subsequent surveys have reported even higher proportions. Preliminary reports of studies from London, Amsterdam, and Basel, Switzerland, found that 40% to 50% of patients who were interviewed while attending AIDS outpatient clinics were using one or more alternative remedies or treatments. Vitamins were the most commonly ingested treatment. In general, patients believed that their alternative regimens were safe, although not likely to be curative. The main reasons cited for using alternative therapies were to strengthen the body and immune system and to delay progression of disease. Failure or lack of confidence in traditional medical treatments was not the primary reason for seeking alternative interventions in these European surveys reported in 1992. However, in the Swiss study, subjects using a visual analogue scale estimated their benefits to be higher from alternative than traditional medicine, with fewer adverse effects.

AN ALTERNATIVE THERAPY TIME LINE

The history of alternative therapy use among persons infected with HIV is intricately associated with the availability and perceived efficacy of orthodox antiretroviral interventions. At the beginning of the AIDS epidemic, before the etiologic agent had been identified, alternative therapies included high-dose intravenous or oral vitamin C and topical application of the sensitizer dinitrochlorobenzene (see below). Immunomodulators and antivirals, such as isoprinosine and ribavirin, respectively, were available through over-the-counter purchases from foreign markets, at the same time that they were undergoing more formal evaluation in U.S. research centers. Alternative use and acquisition of therapies filled the gap created by the absence of a standard treatment during the first 5 years of the epidemic.

Zidovudine (AZT) was approved in 1987 for use in patients with symptomatic HIV disease and $<200/mm^3$ CD4 cells. For the first time, orthodox treatment was available by prescription to patients. Following this breakthrough, interest in alternative therapies slowed for a short time. However, a surge occurred in the alternative therapy movement from 1987 to 1989 when it became clear that newer and possibly better antiviral agents would not soon be released. In 1989, results of large clinical trials demonstrated that AZT prevented progression to advanced HIV disease in patients treated earlier in the course of infection. This led to the approval of the drug for patients with $<500/mm^3$ CD4 cells, significantly increasing the number of individuals able to obtain a licensed agent by prescription from their provider. At the same time the expanded access program for didavosine (ddI) was initiated, allowing access to this drug for patients who had progressive disease while receiving AZT. The strength of the alternative therapies movement and the fact that treatment activists would likely gain unmonitored access to ddI even in the absence of the "parallel track," were probably the primary factors that encouraged the initiation of such expanded access programs for faster delivery of drugs still in early stages of conventional clinical trials.

In 1991, just 3 years after it entered phase I clinical trials in humans, ddI was approved by the Food and Drug Administration (FDA) as the second antiretroviral agent for patients with HIV infection. Despite the availability of these antiretroviral therapies by prescription, many HIV-infected individuals continued to use alternative treatments. Some employed these alternatives as complements to their prescribed antiretrovirals. However, as experience with nucleoside analogues has increased over the years, the perceived benefits of these agents has become less evident. Many patients have opted for a strictly alternative pathway. In one group of 232 HIV-infected men with AIDS or CD4 lymphocyte counts $<500/mm^3$, all eligible for treatment under existing guidelines, one third had never taken AZT. Of those who took AZT 46% used it in combination with nonconventional therapies. AZT users were more likely to have AIDS and lower CD4 counts, not be treated in a clinic, and have private insurance. Those who used complementary therapy in conjunction with their AZT were reported to be sicker, but otherwise to be similar to those who used AZT alone.

In 1993 the alternative therapy movement picked up momentum following the preliminary report of the results of the large collaborative Concorde trial, which evaluated early versus deferred AZT therapy in patients with asymptomatic HIV infection. The study suggested that although a definite CD4 cell benefit was apparent throughout the trial in the early treatment group, the previously reported decrease in progression of disease was short-lived and did not extend through the entire 3 years of follow-up. Similarly, although the study was not powered with death as an endpoint, no survival benefit was seen for those intervening early with AZT. In fact, there were more deaths in the early treatment group compared with the deferred cohort; although disturbing, this was not statistically significant. Further dissemination of Concorde results at the 1993 International Conference on AIDS in Berlin, coupled with discouraging news from combination therapy studies and trials of other agents for which there had been high expectations, fueled the disenchantment over currently available treatments. Further disillusionment greeted the perceived ambiguity of the recommendations from the State-of-the-Art Conference on antiretroviral therapy for adult HIV-infected patients. In the absence of any breakthrough developments, the next few years should again see a resurgence of interest in and use of alternative therapies in patients with HIV infection. Primary providers should become cognizant of potential alternative therapies and understand the side effects and potential drug interactions of these agents.

CURRENTLY USED ALTERNATIVE THERAPIES

A number of the alternative treatments have had varying degrees of popularity over the last decade. The rationale behind the use of these agents and results from various trials of early popular alternative therapies have been reviewed elsewhere. Some of the earlier "favorites" are again being used to an appreciable extent within the community (Table 1); others are becoming more widely touted as complementary treatments (Table 2). These agents and their rationale for use and potential toxicities should be familiar to providers who treat AIDS and HIV-infected patients. With increasing frequency, agents initially chosen as alternatives have begun to enter orthodox clinical trials through university centers or the government-sponsored AIDS Clinical Trial Group (ACTG) or the Community Programs for Clinical Research on AIDS (CPCRA) of the National Institutes of Allergy and Infectious Diseases (NIAID).

Vitamin C and Antioxidants

Vitamin C was one of the first interventions proposed as a potential alternative therapy. Rationale for use of vitamin C was based on anecdotal observations of broad antiviral activity and *in vitro* activity against a human retrovirus. The recom-

TABLE 1. *Alternative therapies still in current use*

Agent	Nature of agent	Suggested activity	Potential side effects
Antioxidants	Vitamin C Beta-carotene	Antiviral Free radical scavengers	Gastrointestinal distress
Dinitrocholobenzene	Organic compound used in photographic processing	Enhanced cellular immunity	Contact dermatitis
Compound Q (GLQ223)	Chinese cucumber extract	Antiviral	Influenza symptoms, myalgias, throat pain, central nervous system effects
Oral alpha interferon	Human cytokine on a wafer	Immunomodulator	Rare influenza symptoms

TABLE 2. *Alternative therapies with increased current use*

Agent	Nature of agent	Suggested activity	Potential side effects
NAC	Cysteine precursor, mucolytic, acetaminophen antidote	Antiviral via TNF inhibition	None reported
Pentoxyfylline	Approved vasodilator	Antiviral via TNF inhibition	Fever, gastrointestinal distress, fatigue
Chinese herbs	Traditional herbal mixture	Symptom palliative	Generally none seen, but numerous possible
Tumeric	Circumin, food spice	Antiviral via LTR inhibition	Ulcers seen in rats

TNF, tumor necrosis factor; LTR, long terminal repeat.

mended doses were high (up to 50 g/day) and were administered by either oral routes or intravenous infusion. Patients were advised to escalate their vitamin C intake to "bowel tolerance"—to ingest as much ascorbate as possible without developing completely intolerable diarrhea. Enthusiasm for further pursuit of this agent waned in the community, however, as many of the advocates of ascorbate therapy died secondary to progression of their AIDS-related illness.

In the ensuing years a resurgence of interest in the potential therapeutic utility of antioxidants in general and vitamin C in particular has led researchers to once again explore the potentially beneficial effects of this drug. At an NIH sponsored conference in 1990 the biologic and clinical actions of vitamin C were reviewed. Vitamin C was reported to be the first line of defense against free-radical damage. It is postulated that oxidative stress may be toxic to lymphocytes, thus potentiating the destructive effect of HIV in infected patients.

In addition to vitamin C's potential role in preservation of immune function, recent reports support the notion of *in vitro* antiretroviral activity. At the Linus Pauling Institute of Science and Medicine, investigators demonstrated that continuous exposure of HIV-infected cells to noncytotoxic ascorbate concentrations resulted in significant inhibition of viral replication in both chronically and acutely infected cell lines. A subsequent study from this same group of researchers suggested that another benefit of vitamin C is its ability to raise intracellular glutathione levels *in vitro*, which leads to synergistic *in vitro* anti-HIV activity when combined with *N*-acetylcysteine (see below).

This research, coupled with the general wave of enthusiasm generated by results of large studies of vitamin/antioxidant therapies in non–HIV-related conditions, has spawned a new wave of ascorbate activists, reminiscent of the vitamin C proponents in the early 80s. Current proponents of vitamin C treatment for HIV infection are convinced, more so than previously, that because vitamins are not patentable, and because they pose a threat to the pharmaceutical industry and the medical profession, they will never be seriously studied in clinical trials.

The impetus to study beta-carotene in conjunction with vitamin C is in response to preliminary studies involving this carotenoid with provitamin A activity. Vitamin A deficiency is associated with increased frequency and severity of infections, and beta-carotene has been reported to have an immunostimulating effect. Based on this finding, a 21-patient double-blind, placebo-controlled crossover trial of beta-carotene in HIV-infected patients was conducted. Participants received either beta-carotene 180 mg daily or placebo for 4 weeks, after which they received the alternate intervention for the next 4 weeks. Treatment with beta-carotene resulted in a statistically significant rise in total white blood cell count and percent change in CD4 count and CD4:CD8 ratios. However, although the absolute CD4 count rose on beta-carotene and fell during placebo, the change was not statistically significant. The investigators concluded that further studies are needed to determine whether beta-carotene has an adjunctive role in the treatment of HIV-infected persons. In an attempt to address this issue, the CPCRA has been developing a pilot study to evaluate the tolerability and anti-HIV activity of high-dose vitamin C with or without beta-carotene to be conducted through its community-based clinical trials network.

DNCB

Another of the early AIDS alternative treatments currently enjoying a comeback, particularly in the San Francisco Bay area, is the chemical 1-chloro-2,4-dinitrobenzene (DNCB). DNCB is an organic compound used to process color photography. It has a medical application as a topical sensitizer and is used as an agent for anergy testing. It also has been successful in the treatment of common warts and alopecia areata. While experimenting with the compound as a potential therapy for patients with AIDS-related Kaposi's sarcoma, a community dermatologist in San Francisco reported observing an increase in the CD4 lymphocyte number in patients repeatedly painted with sensitizing quantities of DNCB in a 1% concentration dissolved in acetone. Word of the improvement in immune function caused by the compound spread throughout the community. Because DNCB was a widely available chemical, one group began purchasing the compound in kilogram quantities from photographic supply houses and producing the treatment solution in bulk. It was subsequently distributed to individuals interested in DNCB's potential immunomodulating effect and its activity against Kaposi's sarcoma. A network of similar buyers' groups took shape, thereby creating an infrastructure for drug distribution of alternative treatments on a national level. Enthusiasm for DNCB eventually waned when it became apparent that it had no efficacy against lesions of Kaposi's sarcoma and many of the early users died of progressive HIV infection. However, the "guerilla clinics" of alternative treatments that evolved became the forerunners of the current "buyers' clubs" that continue in the current for-profit distribution of potentially therapeutic agents for patients with HIV infection.

A group of proponents, however, has continued to support weekly application of

DNCB to the skin of HIV-infected patients. Not convinced that HIV is solely responsible for the pathogenesis of AIDS and more supportive of an underlying autoimmune mechanism, staunch DNCB advocates seemed vindicated by news that HIV infects Langerhans cells of the skin. Because the principal antigen-presenting cell for contact sensitization is the Langerhans cell, a possible mechanism for DNCB as a treatment for HIV infection now seemed plausible. It was postulated that the cell-mediated immune response that results from topical application of DNCB may allow the immune system to rid itself of HIV-infected Langerhans cells. As replacement Langerhans cells may ultimately become infected as well, treatment with DNCB must be continued indefinitely.

This author, in collaboration with DNCB activists and university researchers, wrote a protocol to study the effects of DNCB application on viral infection of Langerhans cells, which was denied funding. Small trials with immunologic and clinical endpoints have been conducted by the remaining DNCB enthusiasts. One trial reported on the results of weekly DNCB application in a cohort of 24 HIV-infected gay men with a mean CD4 cell count of $353/mm^3$ at study entry. Of the 24 subjects, 14 patients were not taking any antiretroviral therapy. The mean duration of follow-up was 12 months, at which time CD4 cell counts showed a significant decrease to a mean of $251/mm^3$. The CD8 count also declined during the course of therapy. A significant increase in natural killer cells from 99 to $162/mm^3$ was observed. Two participating patients developed Kaposi's sarcoma. The authors "conclude that prolonged use of topical DNCB is associated with a stable clinical course in most patients, despite a significant decrease in CD4 T-cells. Lack of disease progression is associated with a stable CD8 CD38 count, and may be related to a persistent increase in natural killer cells . . . probably due to DNCB-induced delayed type hypersensitivity that may be beneficial in HIV disease."

Because it is not patentable, is easily synthesized, and is very inexpensive, DNCB advocates claim that the compound poses a threat to the medical and pharmaceutical industries. A vocal advocacy group in the San Francisco gay community with access to local press has been stepping up the DNCB hype, capitalizing on recent disappointments with nucleoside analogues. DNCB has been catapulted to the number one bestseller at the Healing Alternatives Buyer's Club in San Francisco. While DNCB application is nontoxic, except for its expected contact dermatitis reaction, the incongruity between the vehemence of DNCB's supporters and the available objective results is certainly perplexing, but not at all unique to this alternative therapy.

Oral Alpha Interferon

Similar to the DNCB phenomenon described in factions of the gay community is the debate over the interpretation of data from trials of low-dose oral alpha interferon between its supporters in the African-American community and the "AIDS medical establishment." Alpha interferon has generally been used as a parenteral agent because it was believed that oral administration would destroy the active moieties. Thus, a report of possible efficacy of low-dose oral natural human alpha interferon (KEMRON) in a study conducted in HIV-infected patients in Kenya came as a surprise to the AIDS treatment world. Investigators used an extremely low-dose preparation (2 units/kg/day) that was held in the mouth for sustained mucosal absorption. Reseachers evaluated 40 patients over 6 weeks of treatment; after 6 weeks, researchers reported that all symptomatic patients experienced dramatic relief of constitutional symptoms, weight gain, and remarkable CD4 cell count increases. In an attempt to reproduce these findings, the World Health Organization (WHO) assisted in the development of a multicenter 28-day trial testing the same interferon preparation used in the Kenyan study. Multiple logistic problems, however, resulted in a paucity of data that could be evaluated from this 108-patient trial. Subsequently a number of trials in the United States were initiated to confirm the initial KEMRON findings. Unfortunately, access to the specific preparation used in the first study was difficult; other interferon preparations were used, but this made the resulting data unacceptable to KEMRON supporters. None of the studies demonstrated significant increases in CD4-positive lymphocyte numbers, although stabilization of counts compared with those of placebo-treated patients was suggested. Except for a few instances of influenza-like symptoms, no significant adverse reactions are said to result from oral administration of low-dose alpha interferon.

The largest single trial of low-dose oral interferon-α (INF-α) published to date was conducted by the Community Research Initiative of Toronto (CRIT). Investigators studied 149 HIV-infected patients in a randomized, double-blind trial of placebo versus low-dose (50 U) versus high-dose (100 U) oral INF-α. Patients were assessed after 4 and 8 weeks for adverse events and measurements of disease status, including weight, performance status, CD4 cell counts, and β_2-microglobulin levels. Mean CD4 cell counts decreased in all groups during the 8-week trial. Disease status, weight, performance score, and β_2-microglobulin levels remained unchanged. The investigators concluded "that while oral interferon-alpha does not seem to cause adverse effects, it does not appear to provide short-term benefits to the Toronto CRIT population of patients with HIV infection." In qualifying their conclusion with regard to the population studied, the authors recognize the major criticism of the oral interferon enthusiasts: all but one of the 149 patients enrolled were men and only three were nonwhite. With growing concerns that response to any therapeutic intervention may be affected by gender and racial differences, supporters in the African-American community were not about to accept the Toronto results as a death knell to low-dose oral INF-α therapy.

Advocates of INF-α claim that CD4 counts and impact on disease progression are not appropriate endpoints for measuring oral interferon's benefits and that the quality of life improvements described in the original KEMRON trial deserve validation. A recently reported trial from the Mt. Sinai School of Medicine support this claim. During an initial 6-week double-blind phase, symptomatic patients with CD4 counts between 100 and 350/mm^3 were randomized to placebo or interferon alfa-n3 150 U daily. No differences were seen in CD4 cell count changes, weight, incidence of fever, or prevalence of thrush. However, prevalence of common symptoms such as anorexia and fatigue showed greater improvement in the interferon (11.8%) group than in the placebo (5.6%) ($p = .02$). No adverse experiences were attributed to the oral interferon therapy.

Because of continued pressure from members of the African-American community, the division of AIDS of the NIAID agreed to develop in collaboration with the National Medical Association what is hoped will be the definitive study of the impact of a number of different preparations of low-dose oral INF-α on quality of life in a demographically diverse patient population.

It remains uncertain whether conclusively negative results from a study of any particular alternative therapy will ever be enough to dissuade that treatment's advocates. More than likely someone will always be able to find fault with the preparation of the agent studied, the population enrolled, or some aspect of trial design. This appears to be a continuing theme throughout the history of the alternative therapies movement and one that seems destined to maintain many agents in wide use for years to come.

Cysteine Precursors

Cysteine, an essential amino acid, is used in the biosynthesis of the peptide glutathione. HIV-infected patients have decreased intracellular glutathione. N-acetyl-cysteine (NAC), the N-acetyl derivative of cysteine, is available in aerosolized form as a mucolytic treatment for bronchitis in Europe. It is administered systemically in the United States for management of acetaminophen overdose (Mucomyst). It is believed that cysteine precursors may indirectly inhibit HIV replication by raising intracellular glutathione levels. In *in vitro* studies, cysteine and NAC were shown to raise intracellular glutathione and inhibit HIV-1 replication in persistently infected cell lines, which may occur by blocking the effects of tumor necrosis factor (TNF) in HIV-infected cells. TNF levels are elevated in people with HIV infection and may be associated with accelerated HIV replication. In a recent review of the multifactorial nature of the pathogenesis of HIV disease, it is suggested that TNF-α acts as a cytokine that may contribute to symptomatology, especially HIV-related wasting, as well as upregulation of HIV infection, and urges researchers to seek out agents that may block TNF-α for clinical trials. In addition to NAC, a number of agents popular as alternative therapies have TNF blockade as their presumed mechanism of action (see below). Because it is readily available from foreign markets, has a well-understood biochemical profile, and except for occasional dyspepsia and diarrhea, lacks significant toxicity, NAC ranks as one of the biggest selling items in buyers' clubs nationwide.

The NIAID conducted a small study to evaluate the safety, pharmacokinetics, and antiviral activity of both intravenous and orally administered NAC. Eligible patients with HIV infection and fewer than 500/mm^3 CD4 lymphocytes received 6 weeks of escalating intravenous NAC three times per week. This was followed by 6 weeks of oral administration of doses ranging from 600 to 4,800 mg daily. Of the 23 patients enrolled with a mean CD4 count of 209/mm^3, 22 were receiving concurrent antiretroviral therapy; the maximum tolerated dose was 100 mg/kg. First-order pharmacokinetics were observed following intravenous treatment, with a half-life of 30 minutes. Following oral administration, however, plasma free NAC was barely detectable (22 μM). Although this implies that there was little or no oral bio-availability, NAC advocates countered that the short half-life indicates the compound's rapid conversion into cysteine, and subsequently glutathione, following ingestion. Similarly, advocates claim that NAC could not be the effective mucolytic or antidote to acetaminophen that it is, if it were not absorbed. The NIAID study showed no significant changes in CD4 cell counts, p24 antigen levels, HIV plasma viremia, or plasma cysteine levels. Still, NAC advocates were not phased and suggested that the true endpoint is the intracellular glutathione level, which is currently being investigated in a Stanford-based clinical trial. Of concern, however, is a recent report of an *in vitro* study demonstrating that NAC and glutathione enhanced the replication of HIV-1 in macrophages up to 160%, leading the investigators to conclude that "other oxygen radical scavengers than NAC should be considered as therapeutic agents in AIDS."

Pentoxifylline

Pentoxifylline (Trental), a trisubstituted derivative of xanthine, is approved for the treatment of patients with intermittent claudication and peripheral vascular disease. A reduction of HIV replication *in vitro* has been reported in acutely infected peripheral blood mononuclear and T cells treated with pentoxifylline. It is believed that this agent indirectly inhibits HIV, possibly through suppression of TNF. Pentoxifylline may upregulate adenosine 3:5'-cyclic monophosphate (cAMP), which downregulates TNF. TNF increases HIV infection in chronically infected T cells; its repression may lead to reduced viral replication.

Although the treatment activist community remains frustrated by the lack of definitive trial data on NAC, pentoxifylline was more rapidly evaluated in an ACTG study. Investigators have reported the results of ACTG 160, wherein two cohorts of AIDS patients on concurrent nucleoside analogue therapies were studied. Of 28 patients studied, 17 patients with a mean CD4 cell count of 32/mm^3 received 400 mg of pentoxifylline three times a day; 11 received twice that dose. Laboratory parameters followed include HIV load by cocultivation, TNF messenger RNA (mRNA) levels in peripheral blood mononuclear cells, and serum triglycerides as a surrogate marker for cytokine activation. None of the patients at either dose developed opportunistic infections during the 12 months of follow-up. The only side effect was fever, which was documented in one patient at each dose level. Anecdotal observations from those using pentoxifylline as an alternative therapy outside of controlled clinical trials suggest that fatigue and gastrointestinal distress are also associated adverse experiences. At the 400 mg tid dose level, triglyceride levels declined by 67 mg/dl; TNF mRNA levels declined in 10 of 16 evaluable patients; and HIV load decreased in four patients, rose in one patient, and remained stable in 10 patients. In the group receiving 800 mg three times daily, serum triglycerides declined in two of three patients with baseline levels above 300 mg/dl; TNF mRNA levels fell in half the patients; and HIV load as measured by cocultivation decreased in four patients, rose in one patient, and remained stable in six patients. Although equivocal, the results of this small early trial suggest that further trials of pentoxifylline may be warranted.

A recent report demonstrated that pentoxifylline significantly enhanced the *in vitro* antiretroviral effect of ddI as measured by detection of HIV-1 reverse transcriptase RNA in infected peripheral blood mononuclear cells. It had previously been observed that TNF blocks the antiretroviral activity of the nucleoside analogue reverse transcriptase inhibitors.

Chinese Herbs and Acupuncture

A significant number of HIV-infected individuals seek alternative therapies from sources other than Western health care providers. In the San Francisco Bay area, where many traditional Chinese therapies are still practiced by the large local Asian community, patients in various stages of HIV infection have taken advantage of the abundance of providers as an alternative to Western medicine. These therapies are generally sought, not for their antiretroviral or immunomodulatory actions, but as treatment for certain clinical or systemic manifestations of HIV disease, including wasting, nausea, sleep disturbances, and pain syndromes. Anecdotal reports of the effectiveness of these interventions in patients who have failed previous attempts at Western treatments are abundant. Recognition of the widespread use of these interventions is evidenced by the inclusion of the following statement regarding concomitant medications in an ACTG protocol comparing combinations of nucleoside analogue antiretroviral agents: "Alternative therapies such as vitamins, acupuncture, herbal therapies, and visualization techniques will be permitted. Participants should, however, report the use of these therapies; alternative therapies will be recorded but not keyed."

In an effort to obtain pilot information on the efficacy of Chinese herbal therapies in patients with symptomatic HIV infection, 30 HIV-infected patients were enrolled in a collaborative trial conducted by the AIDS Clinic at the San Francisco General Hospital using treatments prepared by a doctor of oriental medicine from the Quan Yin Healing Arts Center. The herbal formulation was a 31-herb combination based on two herbal formulas, Enhance and Clear Heat, which have been used extensively in the treatment of HIV-infected patients. The herbs in the combination were selected for their purported antiviral and immunomodulatory properties. All enrolled patients had CD4 cell counts between 200 and 500/mm^3 and no prior AIDS-defining diagnosis. All patients reported experiencing at least two HIV-related symptoms to be eligible for the trial. In this randomized, double-blind, placebo-controlled pilot study, participants took 28 pills per day for 12 weeks. Outcome variables evaluated included changes from baseline in overall well-being, physical and social functioning, and symptoms. Changes in weight, CD4 count, hemoglobin, and depression and adherence to the regimen were also measured. Compliance was excellent and the only adverse reaction was the development of diarrhea in one placebo recipient, which required discontinuation of therapy. No significant changes were seen in any of the major outcome variables. Median life satisfaction change was greater in the herbal group. After presentation of these results at an international AIDS conference, a practitioner from China commented that it is not possible to evaluate Chinese herbal interventions using placebo-controlled studies and that no one should expect isolated herbal capsule preparations to work in the absence of the entire herb and outside of the context of a regimen that includes acupuncture and meditation.

Perhaps the same caution will apply to the interpretation of a CPCRA-sponsored multicenter trial of acupuncture for the treatment of HIV-related peripheral neuropathy. Cognizant of the wide use of acupuncture for this painful condition, which is often refractory to other analgesic interventions, the CPCRA designed a factorial trial of a standard acupuncture regimen or amitriptylene compared with placebo. The target enrollment is 260 patients. Patients are randomized to one of four treatment arms for 14 weeks. The protocol defines study medication as follows: "Amitriptyline 75 mg/day or placebo, in combination with standardized acupuncture with Spleen 9,7,6 (Lower Three Kings) or alternate points acupuncture (Lower Three Jesters). Standardized additional points may be used with the Lower Three Kings depending on patient symptoms."

Although this seems quite progressive for a government sponsored protocol, the patient community is less than enthusiastic. Many patients are aware of the side effects associated with amitriptylene and are therefore not interested in possibly being randomized to an active amitriptylene arm. Those who may be particularly attracted to the study because of the opportunity to receive acupuncture treatments are discouraged by the 50% chance that needles will be inserted in sham points for 14 weeks. Although the exact efficacy of amitriptylene for the indication of HIV-related neuropathy has never been formally studied, the known benefit of this drug for other neuropathic syndromes has been extrapolated by many providers who are uncomfortable with the prospect of offering a quarter of the randomized patients both placebo and alternate acupuncture points for 14 weeks. The study has recently been modified to include two substudies: one comparing amitriptylene to placebo and the other a randomization to standard versus alternate points acupuncture.

Cucumbers and Melons

Compound Q (GLQ223), a purified extract from the root tuber of a Chinese cucumber (*Trichosanthes kirilowii*), has been demonstrated in *in vitro* studies to kill HIV-infected macrophages and block replication of virus in T-helper lymphocytes. In China the root itself has been used as an abortifacient for centuries and more recently it has been used to treat choriocarcinomas. As phase I trials of compound Q were commencing in the United States, treatment activists were obtaining trichosanthin, a similar product, from a manufacturer in Shanghai. Sufficient quantities of compound Q were exported from Shanghai to establish a treatment network in four U.S. cities, where patients were given vials of the substance to bring to their collaborating physicians. The provider was asked to inject the patient with the substance, thereby forgoing the need for the physician to obtain regulatory approval to participate in this "treatment experience." Extensive information was collected by the collaborating physicians to accumulate a database on the toxicity and efficacy of the agent. This community network had already treated 35 patients with a fixed dose, at the same time that the phase I protocol began evaluation of its first four patients, who were receiving one twentieth of the community-regimen dose.

News of the underground treatment network was exposed by the national media when one of the study participants died. Accompanying this reported fatality were reports of additional individuals sustaining significant adverse effects sustained by patients using compound Q. The FDA then intervened, asking that the underground cease its unsanctioned AIDS drug trial. Despite their unsuccessful results, the treatment activists maintained that with this treatment experience they had successfully challenged the usual and slower channels of academic medicine, the government's clinical trials program, and the FDA. After further negotiations, the FDA granted a treatment IND (investigational new drug) to the community network group. Orthodox trial centers and the community-based network continued parallel trials of compound Q. Despite nearly 4 years of both conventional and underground trials, very little is actually reported about the clinical efficacy of the agent. Combination studies of compound Q and AZT have also now been completed.

Unlike some of the previously mentioned alternative therapies, compound Q has demonstrated the potential for serious toxicity. Many patients experience influenza-like symptoms, which continue for days after the intravenous injections. Elevated creatine phosphokinase levels may accompany the myalgias. Throat pain is common. Central nervous system (CNS) toxicities, including stupor and coma, have been reported in some patients. Patients with evidence of preexistent HIV-related CNS disease are more likely to experience the untoward CNS effects. These symptoms generally respond to acetaminophen.

Mamordica charantia (bitter melon) is a relative of *Trichosanthes kirilowii* in the cucurbitacea family. The bitter bumpy fruit of the vine-like climbing plant is used as a medicinal folk remedy by Asians, particularly Filipinos. In this folk arena, bitter melon has reported utility against colds, influenza, dysentery, and inflammatory conditions of the skin and eyes. The plant contains several seed lectins that inhibit *in vitro* protein synthesis, but cannot enter cells. Investigators have noted similar activities in an aqueous extract from the bitter melon fruit that have cytotoxic effects against a variety of malignant cells *in vitro* and in animal tumors. MAP 30 (momordica anti-HIV protein) has now been isolated and purified from the seeds and fruit of the bitter melon. Investigators have demonstrated that MAP 30 exhibits a dose-dependent inhibition of cell-free HIV infection and replication. Syncytium formation was inhibited in acutely infected CD4 positive indicator cells, suggesting that MAP 30 affects initial HIV infection and cell-to-cell transmission. Viral p24 antigen expression and reverse transcriptase activity were also inhibited, indicating that MAP 30 affects virion production and replication. Because no cytotoxic or cytostatic effects were observed under assay conditions, the investigators suggested that MAP 30 may be a useful therapeutic agent against HIV infection.

Bitter melon has been described as "a kinder, gentler compound Q" in the underground literature, which has led to the first observational evaluations of bitter melon in the alternative treatment communities. Therapy with bitter melon to date is being championed by members of the gay Asian-Pacific community along the West Coast. The bitter melon extract is made from vines and leaves and administered as an enema to bypass the unpleasant bitter taste of the resultant tea. Most of the enthusiasm for the treatment has been generated by the fruit's pioneer recipient, who reports dramatic increases in his CD4 count and a halt in all the typical downward trends of HIV disease. Despite the vague endorsement, bitter melon enemas are being increasingly utilized, and providers should be aware that, except for diarrhea secondary to the retention, the only other reported side effect is insomnia due to increased energy if taken too late in the day.

Curcumin

Alternative treatment activists are extremely adept at keeping up with basic science literature that may suggest any potential therapeutic intervention with a glimmer of hope for arresting HIV. Harvard researchers have described three inhibitors of HIV-1 long terminal repeat (LTR)-directed gene expression and viral replication. The LTR governs activation of latent provirus. The activity of the LTR is determined by a complex interaction of positive and negative transcriptional regulators binding to specific sequences within the LTR. For example, tumor necrosis factor is felt to be a potent LTR activator. Compounds that block activation or suppress activity of the HIV-1 LTR could be useful for extending the viral latency period or inhibition of the persistent progressive infection. Curcumin, the major active component of the spice tumeric, has been demonstrated by these investigators to block HIV LTR activity. It was effective in both acute and chronically infected cells. This information generated enthusiasm to call for the initiation of clinical trials investigating the antiretroviral activity of tumeric. Already tumeric has surpassed Chinese herbs as the second leading seller at the San Francisco buyers' club, outsold only by DNCB.

Search Alliance, a Los Angeles "community-based fast-track AIDS research" organization has conducted an "accelerated pilot study to assess the potential clinical benefits of curcumin." Nineteen volunteers received 2.5 g of encapsulated curcumin in three daily divided doses over a period of 20 weeks. Baseline CD4 lymphocyte counts were in the 50 to 400/mm^3 range; one half of the participants were HIV p24 antigen positive at entry. Four patients developed opportunistic infections during the study and were withdrawn from the trial. Two patients withdrew because of complaints of upset stomach and nausea, the only adverse effects observed with the relatively large dose of curcumin used. Two additional patients withdrew for nonmedical reasons, which left 11 of the original 19 patients evaluable (58%).

This pilot study used HIV p24 antigen levels and polymerase chain reaction (PCR) techniques for measuring viral load. In the 11 evaluable patients, PCR testing of viral load demonstrated a decline of 2.2 logs between weeks 4 and 12 of curcumin treatment. By week 20, baseline levels were returning. Curcumin did not cause a significant sustained reduction in p24 antigen. CD8 lymphocyte counts were noted to rise slightly. No clinical improvements were observed or reported by the participants. Although no bioavailability studies were conducted, Search Alliance investigators were concerned that curcumin may not be well absorbed by the gastrointestinal tract. They concluded that "the initial results of this pilot study indicate that curcumin looks less promising as an antiretroviral agent. Curcumin appears to behave like other new agents (i.e., protease inhibitors), with low bioavailability, transient viral load reduction, and rapid viral resistance emergence."

ACQUISITION OF ALTERNATIVE THERAPIES

Although many individuals procure their alternative therapies on their own, an increasing number are using the services of the buyers' club. A cottage industry has developed based on import and resale of desirable alternative treatments. Initially established as centers for sale of vitamins and herbal remedies to patients interested in restoring immune function, the buyers' clubs have now moved into the business of providing patients with a veritable menu of desired alternative regimens and orthodox agents acquired through alternative means. Following a controversy regarding improper doses of ddC being distributed, the FDA conducted an investigation of buyers' clubs activities. They determined that four general classes of agents were available: (1) Unapproved versions of products approved and available in the United States, such as foreign pentamidine; such drugs are usually sold at lower cost. (2) Agents that have been approved elsewhere, such as isoprinosine or KEMRON. (3) Agents, such as compound Q, that are available in the United States but are as yet unapproved. (4) Products that are produced "underground," such as peptide T and nonpharmaceutically manufactured ddC. Recently the FDA has been making an effort to keep abreast of which agents require buyers' club distribution so that they may more quickly shepherd them into clinical trials or expanded access, thus limiting the underground organizations' need to exist. It has been found that numerous health care providers have taken advantage of the ease of acquisition of agents through the buyers' club mechanism rather than do the copious amounts of paperwork and monitoring required to obtain similar agents through expanded access programs. Despite the fact that the drugs available through expanded access programs are free of charge to patients, many prefer the ease of obtaining the drugs through the buyers' club.

Individuals with HIV infection and their providers obtain information about which alternative treatments are currently being used through a number of regular publications. As an infrastructure for distribution of alternative therapies was established and the number of treatments from which to choose increased, a need for information dissemination arose. Organizations and publications devoted entirely to spreading up-to-date information on available underground treatments began to appear in 1987. Project Inform, a community-based group of AIDS activists, was one of the first organizations established to provide such information. Using a 24-hour hotline and a monthly newsletter, Project Inform quickly became one of the major clearinghouses for the alternative treatment movement.

AIDS Treatment News, a biweekly update of AIDS treatment information, was first published in 1987. With a current circulation of 5,000, the newsletter informs readers of both alternative and experimental treatments. *Treatment Issues, the Gay Men's Health Crisis Newsletter of Experimental AIDS Therapies*, also appeared in 1987. It cautions subscribers that "describing an experimental therapy should not be misconstrued as recommending it. All new treatments should be conducted under a physician's care." It is ironic, however, that despite increased availability of these sophisticated publications geared at the consumer population, providing physicians are frequently ignorant of a particular new agent about which their patients inquire. Focused at the health care provider in addition to the consumer is the *AIDS/HIV Treatment Directory*. This quarterly directory published by the American Foundation for AIDS Research (AMFAR) reviews both orthodox and unorthodox agents that are currently in both early and later stages of clinical development.

Despite widespread enthusiasm for the increased number of licensed and approved conventional therapies, the future introduction of additional alternative treatments can be expected. Practitioners caring for patients with HIV-infection have a number of options with regard to the use of alternative treatments in their patient populations (Table 3). Some providers may remain unaware of the use of alternatives, and some may choose to ignore that their patients are using unprescribed agents. Often patients fear that they cannot be forthcoming with their providers, concerned about possible condemnation for not being fully content or confident

TABLE 3. *Providers'*
attitudes toward
alternative therapies in
their HIV patient
population

Remain unaware
Ignore
Condemn
Acknowledge
Monitor
Encourage
Refer

with the medications prescribed by the primary care physician. Condemning a patient's use of alternative treatment regimens without trying to understand what motivates the individual to seek these options is counterproductive in establishing and maintaining trust in the patient-doctor relationship.

Physicians should acknowledge the possibility that their patients are using alternative therapies. In taking the medical history physicians should stress in a nonjudgmental manner the need to understand all medications and substances their patients are ingesting so they can best be able to evaluate the patient's clinical condition and determine what, in fact, may be the adverse effects of potential treatments. In some situations providers enter into a partnership with the patient and choose to assist in monitoring their use of alternative treatments. Some providers have taken an even more active stance in their approach to the use of alternative treatments by their patients. Often discouraged by the slow pace of drug development for HIV disease and enthusiastic about early *in vitro* reports of activity, some providers have encouraged the use of unorthodox, unproved treatments by their patients, especially for patients with advanced disease whose life span may not permit them to survive until actual clinical trials of an agent commence or to benefit from the result of such studies. These providers may encourage patients to seek alternative therapies and in fact refer them to a buyers' club to obtain the agents.

CONCLUSION

The impact of the alternative therapy movement can already be appreciated (Table 4). Drug approval is accelerating. The FDA has already responded to the alternative treatment movement in a number of ways over the past decade. Allowing personal drug use importation, codifying the parallel track-expanded access program, coexisting with the buyers' club industry, and conducting timely reviews for accelerated approval are all demonstrations that the regulatory agency is not responding in a vacuum. Further evidence that the Public Health Service is listening carefully to the public is seen in the establishment of the Alternative Medicine Office at the National Institute of Health.

It is hoped that more effective therapies for HIV infection and its manifestations will emerge in the upcoming decade. The alternative therapies movement has encouraged strides in modernizing and accelerating the drug approval process that will benefit patients with AIDS and HIV infection as well as those with other serious and

TABLE 4. *Impact of the alternative therapy movement*

Importation for personal use allowed
Buyers' club industry established
Parallel track and expanded access mechanisms created
Protocols for patients with prior drug exposure designed
Accelerated approval modified by FDA
Office of Alternative Medicine established

life-threatening diseases. Unfortunately, in the absence of a cure the need for alternatives persists. John James, the editor of *AIDS Treatment News* and an effective treatment activist, poignantly summarizes the quandary. "In the past years, the only way the AIDS community could move a drug forward in the face of institutional neglect was to develop it as an 'alternative' treatment, i.e., let it go into widespread use, in the hope that if there were any substantial value it would be noticed, and if not, the substance would be retired through the usual 'drug of the month' process. Maybe we can do better today."

Providers caring for patients with HIV infection should make every attempt to inform themselves about complementary therapies that may be in use in their community. Establishing trust and open communication will allow the health professionals to enter a caring partnership with their patients, including those who may be empowering themselves by using alternative treatments.

SUGGESTED READING

Abrams D. Dealing with alternative therapies for HIV. In: Sande M, Volberding P, eds. *The medical management of AIDS*, 4th ed. Philadelphia: WB Saunders, 1995; 183–207.

Abrams D, Cotton D, Mayer K, eds. *AIDS/HIV treatment directory*. New York: Am Found AIDS Res (AmFAR).

Byers VS, Levin AS, Waites LA, et al. A phase I/II study of trichosanthin treatment of HIV disease. *AIDS* 1990;4:1189–1196.

Coodley GO, Nelson HD, Loveless MO, et al. Beta-carotene in HIV infection. *J AIDS* 1993;6:272–276.

Dwyer JT, Salvato-Schille AM, Coulston A, et al. The use of unconventional remedies among HIV-positive men living in California. *JANAC* 1995;6:17–28.

Eisenberg DM, Kessler RC, Foster C, et al. Unconventional medicine in the United States: prevalence, costs and patterns of use. *N Engl J Med* 1993;328:246–252.

Greenblatt RM, Hollander H, McMaster JR, et al. Polypharmacy among patients attending an AIDS clinic: utilization of prescribed unorthodox, and investigational treatments. *J AIDS* 1991;4:136–143.

Harakeh S, Jariwalla RJ, Pauling L. Suppression of human immunodeficiency virus replication by ascorbate in chronically and acutely infected cells. *Proc Natl Acad Sci USA* 1990;87:7245–7249.

Hulton MR, Levin DL, Freedman LS. Randomized placebo-controlled, double-blind study of low-dose oral interferon-alpha in HIV-1 antibody positive patients. *J AIDS* 1992;5:1084–1090.

James JS. New kind of HIV antiviral: food spice, cancer drug show activity. *AIDS Treatment News* No. 174, May 7, 1993.

James JS. Curcumin update: could food spice be low-cost antiviral? *AIDS Treatment News* No. 176, June 4, 1993.

Li CJ, Zhang LJ, Dezube BJ, et al. Three inhibitors of type 1 human immunodeficiency virus long terminal repeat-directed gene expression and virus replication. *Proc Natl Acad Sci USA* 1993; 90:1839–1842.

Mihm S, Ennen J, Pessara U, et al. Inhibition of HIV-1 replication and NF-nB activity by cysteine and cysteine derivatives. *AIDS* 1991;5:497–503.

P.I. Perspective. (Quarterly) Project Inform. National hotline 1-800-822-7422; California hotline, 1-800-334-7422.

Stricker RB, Elswood BF. Topical dinitrochlorobenzene in HIV disease. *J Am Acad Dermatol* 1993; 28:796–797.

Treatment Issues. *The GMHC newsletter of experimental AIDS therapies*. New York: Gay Mens Health Crisis.

A Clinical Guide to AIDS and HIV,
edited by Gary P. Wormser.
Lippincott-Raven Publishers, Philadelphia © 1996.

14

Nursing Perspectives in Care of Persons with HIV Infection

Richard L. Sowell, *Arlene J. Lowenstein, and †Troy Spicer

*Department of Administrative and Clinical Nursing, University of South Carolina,
Columbia, South Carolina 29208; *Department of Nursing Administration,
School of Nursing, Medical College of Georgia, Augusta, Georgia 30912-4230;
†Early Intervention Program, AID Atlanta Inc., Atlanta, Georgia 30309-2955*

HIV infection and the resultant AIDS, first thought to be a disease of urban homosexual males, is now growing at a rapid pace among other populations. HIV infection is increasingly associated with drug use and heterosexual transmission, and is occurring in both urban and rural communities. Providing quality care to such a diverse population with HIV infection provides a complex and challenging task.

THE NURSING RESPONSIBILITY MODEL

HIV infection is a care-intensive disease across the continuum of the illness and involves client contact with many health care and social service disciplines. Nurses have a major role in providing care for HIV-infected patients and are also involved in many activities other than direct patient care, as illustrated in the model of nursing responsibility (Fig. 1). An overview of the model is presented here.

Nursing involvement actually begins before diagnosis, through the provision of health education about prevention strategies and wellness care in the community. From the point of the original HIV-antibody testing through to the end stage of AIDS, nurses provide client assessment and direct patient care, counseling support, health education, and bereavement support for families and friends. Care problems are both complex and unique for each patient, as differing constellations of symptoms are exhibited as the disease progresses. Nursing care is provided in homes and ambulatory care settings, as well as in hospitals and in all types of urban and rural communities.

Nurses must take responsibility in coordination of interdisciplinary resources to link the HIV-infected individual to appropriate services, including primary and acute care facilities and social and community support services that may be needed

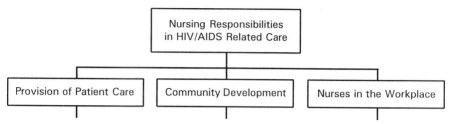

ACCESS TO CARE
- Availability of Services
  - early intervention
  - acute health care
  - supportive care
- Financial Considerations
- Redirection of Stigma & Discrimination
- Case Management
  - legal & ethical issues
  - financial issues
  - housing
  - transportation
- Emotional Support
- Spiritual Support

ADEQUACY OF CARE
- Interdisciplinary Approach
  - comprehensive care
  - discharge planning
- Patients Rights
  - confidentiality
  - informed consent
  - right to self-determination
- Patient Advocacy
  - patient, family, and staff education
  - continued support
- Infection Control
- Assessment and Care in All Settings, Ambulatory, Acute & Home
- Health Education
- Bereavement Support
- Quality Assurance/ Improvement
- Interdisciplinary Coordination
- Therapeutic Environment

ALTERNATIVE CARE SYSTEMS
- Hospice
- Home Care
- Non hospital institutional care
- Support groups
- Community services

COMMUNITY EDUCATION
- Health Education
- HIV/AIDS Education
- Community
  - prevention/risk behavior
  - health promotion
  - facilitate supportive community climate

POLITICAL AWARENESS
- Legislative
  - health care regulations
  - social policy
  - advocacy

NURSING MANAGEMENT
- HIV/AIDS Program Planning
- Standards & Policies
- Employee Protection

ORGANIZATIONAL EMPLOYEES
- Protection
  - infection control procedures
  - staff education
- Employee Rights
  - safe working environment
  - employee support
  - freedom from unreasonable fear
- Employee Responsibilities
  - job requirements
  - disciplinary/grievance process

EMPLOYEE WITH AIDS/HIV
- CDC Guidelines
- HIV Testing
  - confidentiality
  - counseling
  - cost
- State and Federal Antidiscrimination Laws
- Workman Compensation Laws
- Employee Assistance

NURSING EDUCATION
- Updated Information
- Student Support

RESEARCH
- Clinical
- Care Coordination

during the course of illness. Nurses are in a position to provide education about the importance of recognizing both families of biologic origin and families of choice, including significant others and partners, as participants in care and decision making when that is the client's choice. Financial, housing, nutrition, and transportation problems frequently grow worse as the disease progresses. Clients need to be linked to services that will help them make decisions in these areas as well as in the treatment plan. Nurses must understand and navigate the legal and ethical issues that relate to the necessary linkages and services for their clients. In many locations, nurses take full responsibility as case managers, or work within interdisciplinary case management systems that are based on client need for type of services.

Nurses are well positioned for involvement in community advocacy, encouraging those communities with inadequate services to develop programs and linkages, and political awareness to develop financial resources to carry out programs. Nurses are also a prime resource for providing information to the community at large and to other health care professionals, to reduce fear and discriminatory behaviors toward persons with HIV infection.

As the numbers of HIV-infected persons continues to grow, nursing administrators will need to encourage their staff to develop and implement HIV/AIDS patient care program planning in the community and in hospitals, in both urban and rural settings. Nursing care standards and quality improvement programs should be developed and monitored for effectiveness. Nursing administrators, as part of the senior management team, need to be involved in ensuring a safe workplace through development and implementation of appropriate orientation, workplace safety programs, and supportive human resource policies.

Nurse educators must take responsibility for their own education about HIV infection so that their students can benefit from accurate, up-to-date information and a supportive rather than judgmental attitude toward HIV-infected clients. Students and beginning practitioners will work with diverse populations of persons with HIV infection, diagnosed and undiagnosed, and they must learn to confront their own fears and attitudinal barriers. Nurse educators must also provide guidance and emotional support for students as they learn to understand, elicit, and negotiate their own as well as their clients' multicultural health beliefs. Students need support as they deal with occupational hazards and become aware of the necessity of self-protection through the use of universal precautions and personal safe health care practices. HIV-related research is needed to provide the research base for future nursing practice. Nurses in academic settings have the responsibility to develop and facilitate research programs and studies that will add to the current knowledge base.

MAJOR CONCEPTS ACROSS THE CONTINUUM OF ILLNESS

When structuring care of persons with HIV infection, there are underlying concepts that providers must consider throughout the illness, regardless of stage. These concepts may be emphasized more strongly at certain points or developed differently during the course of illness, but they shape the assessment and structuring of care.

Holistic nursing practice concepts can provide a framework for care. The focus of holistic practices, according to one group, is "aimed not at ameliorating symptoms but at improving client's ability to live, to be well, to live a high quality of life, and to focus their lives in meaningful and useful direction." They view the essence of nursing practice as helping clients to develop and fully use their sense of self as they cope with whatever changes they are finding in their physical, psychological, spiritual, and social worlds. This client-nurse relationship must also be expanded to families, both families of origin and families of choice.

The chronic disease model of Corbin and Strauss holds that persons with any chronic disease must "work hard" to manage their illness. There are whole sets of decisions to be made and tasks to be carried out by the individual, or parents in the case of children. These decisions and tasks may be carried out by the client alone or in conjunction with others. Each person fashions his/her own unique response to the illness and to health care provider recommendations for treatment. Some examples of required tasks by the affected individual and/or their families are: to become informed about the disease and its progression; to meet personal resistance to staying in treatment; to prepare for pain management; and to encounter issues of needing to be cared for, coping with body concept changes and body deterioration, and "making friends with the notion of dying."

Relationships with supportive practitioners can allow the person and family members to incorporate and expand their sense of self while engaging in the myriad of decisions that will be required as they work to manage their illness. Client and family involvement in decision making needs to occur over the illness continuum and is essential to the death-relating tasks and dissolution of the relationship in the end stage. Investigators have found that clients with HIV infection who participated in illness management activities improved their quality of life. Others have also found that bereavement partners of gay men who died from AIDS were better able to work through the loss when they and their partners were involved in those activities. Nurses are in a pivotal position to foster client and family participation in decision making and to assist in gathering information on which to base those decisions.

Besides the provision of care, nurses also work to prevent further transmission of HIV in the community at large and within health care settings. Prevention of transmission can be fostered through the practice of universal precautions and by the provision of health education and information not only to clients and their families but also in broader-based communities.

Many HIV-infected clients have a history of health behaviors that place them at risk for poor health outcomes. These behaviors may be related to cultural norms within their ethnic background or chosen lifestyle. These behaviors and attitudes may be difficult, if not impossible, to change. According to one study the more symptoms persons with AIDS reported, the greater the change toward unhealthy behaviors.

The Mersey Harm Reduction model was developed to deal with the harmful consequences of the growing substance abusing population in the Mersey area of Liverpool, England. However, this model can also be applied to other populations with protracted illness. The first principle is that total avoidance of unhealthy behaviors should not be the only objective of services to this population, since that would exclude a substantial proportion of people who are committed to their current lifestyle. For example, many clients are well aware that HIV can be transmitted through sexual activity, but they will not or cannot practice abstinence or even protected sexual activity. Nurses and other providers who are committed to changing unhealthy behaviors in their clients will face frustration and burnout when those clients ignore the information and education that they have worked hard to provide.

The second principle of the adapted Harm Reduction Model holds that behavior change should be conceptualized as the final goal in a series of harm-reduction objectives. Rather than anticipating total change in behavior, nurses and health care providers need to recognize that small changes may be easier for clients to adopt. When a series of health promoting behaviors are developed, the clients may choose to select those behaviors that they feel they can accomplish, while ignoring those they have no intention of changing. For example, clients who are not willing to abstain from sexual activity, may accept information about types of sexual activities that provide sexual gratifications, other than direct unprotected intercourse.

The third principle is to provide user-friendly services. Nurses should help establish a supportive rather than judgmental milieu; they should avoid overwhelming clients with excessive information and instead emphasize information and explanations that the clients feel they can handle. If trust can be established, clients will be more likely to maintain contact. Continuing contact provides an opportunity to provide reinforcement and support for behavior changes that have been accomplished. In addition, it will enable clients to obtain assistance for further behavior change and other problems as they arise.

The harm reduction concept is gaining growing acceptance as a realistic approach in the areas of care delivery, education, and prevention. Initial evidence of effectiveness has been encouraging. Harm reduction considers the user's wants along with the provider's wants, so that consensus and realistic goal setting can occur. Harm reduction is future oriented rather than concentrated on past practices. Information that can lead to positive behavior changes can be supplied without negative judgments about past practices. Outreach is required; social and health services need to be brought to people on their own turf and on their own terms. Services need to be user-friendly rather than judgmental and punishment based, and less-harmful options need to be made available and considered as acceptable in lieu of abstinence or total avoidance of harmful behaviors. Harm reduction considers providers as well as clients and is focused on future-oriented community health rather than institutional agendas. The harm reduction model provides a useful framework within which nurses can work effectively to integrate the complexity of issues associated with HIV infection. It can be successfully implemented with diverse populations and across the continuum of illness. Nurses can take leadership in interdisciplinary planning to introduce and support these concepts.

NURSING RESPONSIBILITIES IN PREVENTION AND TESTING

The various physical, social, and psychological consequences of HIV infection may result in severe stress for clients and their families. Many people are aware that their behavior and lifestyle decisions have put them into a high-risk category for HIV infection. Fear of stigmatization and/or discrimination and real or perceived lack of access to services may keep them from confirming their fears of infection. Diagnosis and medical intervention may be delayed until symptoms can no longer be ignored, and when they may be less effective.

The seemingly sudden advent of the HIV/AIDS epidemic had a profound impact on both health care professionals and the overall health care system. In the early 1980s, a generation of health care providers were faced with an incurable, life-threatening, infectious disease to which they were ill prepared to respond. The response of health care workers has mirrored that of society in general. This response has often been characterized by fear of contagion and avoidance of individuals infected with or thought to be at risk for AIDS.

Today, some 14 years into the AIDS epidemic, there has been rapid advancement in knowledge related to the causative agent of AIDS, modes of transmission of HIV and the course of the disease. Such information should provide a rational basis for the health care professional's response to the care of persons with this illness. However, to the contrary, research examining the attitudes and knowledge of health professionals (including nurses) regarding HIV infection indicates that fear, misinformation, and prejudice remain prevasive.

Nurses have been in the forefront of responding to the HIV/AIDS epidemic both in the provision of direct care and in organization of care delivery systems. Yet, many nurses lack knowledge and experience related to the care of patients with HIV infection. This lack of experience has resulted from nurses' avoiding care of these patients or working in communities with a low incidence of HIV infection.

The rapid increase of reported cases of AIDS in diverse segments of the population, as well as in all geographic regions, including rural areas, strongly suggest that all nurses will be involved. For nurses having limited experience with this disease, ongoing education is necessary to provide a knowledge base that supports quality nursing practice. However, education does not always change attitudes or behavior. Additionally, some clinically based health care providers continue to mistrust the experts and question exactly how much is really known about transmission of HIV in the patient care setting.

Fear of HIV infection by health care professionals can still result in refusal to provide care and in unnecessary isolation practices. The more likely scenario, however, is the exhibiting of behaviors by health care providers that make the HIV-infected person feel stigmatized or devalued. In a focus group study of HIV-infected women, it was reported that fear and insensitive behavior by health care providers were frequently encountered by these women when seeking care. The women reported that such behavior by providers affected their quality of care, and their willingness to seek health care services. Other studies of low-income and gay populations have shown similar results.

Nurse practitioners are providing an increasing amount of care for vulnerable populations and may be in a primary position to provide education and encourage appropriate testing and early intervention for populations at high risk for HIV infection. Other nurses who are involved in community activities, including school and community health education programs, should also be a major resource for information regarding available services. Nurses can provide a nonthreatening atmosphere in which questions can be raised, thus encouraging earlier diagnosis and treatment, and prevention of further transmission of the infection. School health programs provide an ideal opportunity to instruct and encourage children in developing good hygiene and age appropriate healthful behaviors. Risk-related sexual and drug practices may begin in adolescence, and this group needs to be a prime target for health education and risk-reducing programs. Studies of school-based AIDS education have been shown to have impact on risk-related behaviors. However, adolescents are not all alike, and effective health education and sex education programs must be tailored to their culture and lifestyle. Investigators found that different interventions were needed for sexually active and high-risk teenage populations than were effective with lower-risk groups.

Making the decision to undergo antibody testing requires the courage to face the possibility of HIV infection and the courage to take the chance that the provider will exhibit a professional, supportive attitude and maintain confidentiality. Regardless of whether the test results are positive or negative, posttest counseling is essential. Figure 2 models a comprehensive approach to HIV/AIDS education and prevention.

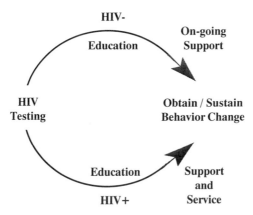

FIG. 2. Comprehensive approach to HIV/AIDs education and prevention. (© 1994, Richard Sowell, reproduced with permission.)

The person who tests negative may still be at risk for HIV infection and needs continuing health education and ongoing counseling or peer support for behavioral changes to reduce the likelihood of infection. Also, follow-up testing may be needed if the incubation period has not been long enough to reveal a positive test. Knowledge of the disease may be "street knowledge," learned from friends, filled with many untruths, half-truths, and inappropriate emotional overtones. This is an opportune time for nursing intervention to help correct some of those impressions.

Persons testing positive have had their worst fears confirmed. Counseling support is crucial at this point and must be delivered with sensitivity to the gender and cultural and ethnic background of the client. Clients need to know what the test results actually mean, and unless Western blotting was done, about the need for confirmation to avoid false positives. Persons who test positive will need to learn a whole new vocabulary as providers talk about T cells and CD4s. They must be linked to services that may be needed over the course of the illness. Even though the person testing positive may be asymptomatic, this is an appropriate time to begin case management activities. A case manager may assist the client to develop a plan of care. Case managers may provide education about the natural history of the disease and information on accessing health services so that early symptoms may be reported and treated appropriately. Case managers must assess the psychosocial, spiritual, and educational needs and prepare for linkages to services as needed in the future.

EARLY INTERVENTION

Increasingly, testing and counseling are being viewed as early intervention activities. Individuals identifying their HIV-positive status in the early stages of infection have the opportunity to implement behavior changes and health promotion activities that can potentially delay deterioration of immune status. Early identification allows a thorough medical and psychosocial assessment to define immediate and long-term needs in order to maximize the length and quality of life.

The goal of early intervention is to keep people well as long as possible. The tasks required in early intervention for both client and provider are many. Clients seeking early intervention may require treatment for many common illnesses not associated with HIV infection. The health assessment can identify additional infections and health care problems that need treatment. The nursing assessment should incorporate the health assessment into the psychosocial and spiritual context of the individual's life in devising they comprehensive client plan of care.

Education and information may be one of the greatest needs at this point to permit the client to take part in the shared decision making that will be necessary. Decisions such as when or if to start antiretroviral therapy, prophylaxis for opportunistic infections, and the appropriate course of management and treatment need to be jointly made by a well-informed client and provider. When decisions are made unilaterally by the provider, the client may not find them relevant or acceptable, decreasing chances of adherence to the prescribed treatment or regimen. It is important to acknowledge the use of alternative therapies by many individuals with HIV infection. When possible, incorporation of such therapies promotes adherence to the treatment plan, and allow providers to be knowledgeable about all the medications and approaches being used by clients.

To be effective, education needs to be ongoing and interactive. A trusting relationship needs to be developed between client and provider. The provider must acknowledge and respect the client's competence in making decisions about his or her own life. In addition, some clients with HIV infection are better informed about their condition and its treatment than many providers. We have found that when providers were not forthright with information, some clients interpreted this as a lack of knowledge by the provider, diminishing their willingness to adhere to treatment.

The nurse has a critical role to play in explaining a treatment program to the client. Medications currently in use to treat HIV infection and related opportunistic infections can have many unpleasant side effects. Clients must receive explanations about the reasons for taking the medications, potential side effects, and information that will allow them to make an informed choice as to whether the expected benefit outweighs the potential harm for side effects. Nurses can be particularly helpful in providing information that can assist the client and family as appropriate in managing those side effects, so that discomfort can be reduced to a tolerable level.

Certain studies indicate that good nutrition, exercise, and stress management may have positive impacts on the body's ability to fight infection and maintain or improve functioning. Nurses can provide health information in these and other health-promoting behaviors to both the client and family. Family members may better contribute to these health promotional behaviors when they are well informed. Such information may also benefit the family members directly by enhancing their own general health behaviors.

Whenever possible, a comprehensive plan of care that includes both medical and psychosocial issues needs to be developed early. Tables 1 and 2 list frequent nursing diagnoses and selected interventions across the stages of HIV infection. The plan will differ for each client, and nursing diagnoses and interventions other than the ones illustrated will also be needed.

Decisions such as advanced medical directives, medical power of attorney, and guardianship of children need to be considered before the potential neurologic and emotional complications associated with AIDS places legal decision making at risk. Many HIV-infected patients are not ready to deal with the prospect severe of illness, disability, or death when they do not yet feel sick. Because of their role in direct care and education with clients and their families, nurses are in a good position to develop a trusting relationship. This relationship will be necessary to assist clients in confronting these issues in a timely manner, when they may still be in denial or unprepared to consider such sensitive and distressing issues. However, one of the most important issues to be considered is how to balance the need to plan for future illness with the desire to maintain hope and a focus on living.

TABLE 1. *Physiologic challenges: selected nursing interventions*

Nursing diagnosis	Potential source/cause	Early interventions	Late interventions
Impaired gas exchange	*Pneumocystis carinii* pneumonia (PCP) Anemia Cytomegalovirus (CMV) pneumonia Pulmonary Kaposi's sarcoma	Educate populations at risk of benefits of early intervention and treatment Encourage and provide early HIV screening to identifiy at risk persons Monitor compliance with PCP prophylaxis Monitor hemoglobin and hematocrit	Monitor mental status Monitor vital signs, blood gases Position for comfort, elevate head of bed Educate regarding treatments and examinations Implement actions to reduce fear and anxiety Monitor effects of assisted ventilation
Diarrhea	Cryptosporidium Isospora Mycobacterium avium-intracellulare complex (MAC) Cytomegalovirus (CMV) Salmonella Giardia	Educate regarding dietary risks, e.g., raw chicken, eggs, meat Educate regarding good hygiene and handwashing Educate regarding refraining from risky oral-anal sexual practices	Monitor for weight loss, malnutrition Implement measures to ensure adequate hydration Educate regarding good hygiene and handwashing Diet counseling Educate regarding treatments and examinations
Potential for infection due to disruption of skin integrity	IV devices Herpes zoster Psoriasis Herpes simplex virus Immobility Poor nutritional status Diarrhea	Assess skin for lesions, pressure areas, turgor Monitor for signs and symptoms of secondary infection Monitor for disruptions of skin integrity Educate regarding good hygiene	Ensure good hygiene Use pressure-relieving devices Turn and position frequently Meticulous IV device care Infection control measures Work with physician to eliminate/treat underlying conditions
Pain	Peripheral neuropathy Tumor Reiter's syndrome Herpes zoster Herpes simplex	Monitor for pain; assess location, duration, type, etc. of pain Identify contributing and/or risk factors for pain Monitor and educate regarding drug therapy and reporting symptoms	Explore alternative techniques to cope with pain, e.g., relaxation, visualization, distraction Encourage client to verbalize pain Comfort measures such as egg-crate mattresses, positioning and supporting limbs

TABLE 1. *Continued.*

Nursing diagnosis	Potential source/cause	Early interventions	Late interventions
Altered nutrition	Anorexia Nausea/vomiting Malabsorption Cachexia Inflammation/lesions of GI tract Diarrhea	Educate and monitor regarding measures to promote lean body mass Educate and assess regarding sound nutritional practices Early detection and treatment of conditions such as inflammation/lesions of GI tract and diarrhea	Administer and monitor the effectiveness of analgesics Assess and monitor nutrition parameters (e.g., weight, serum albumin, food intake) Treat underlying conditions Dietary change as appropriate (high calorie–high protein, bland) Offer dietary supplements Implement and monitor parenteral nutrition and assess effectiveness and related complications or side effects; begin nursing measures to respond to complications

Psychological assessment needs to be done to identify levels of depression, anxiety, and suicide risk. Anxiety and depression are two of the most common emotional responses to a diagnosis of HIV infection. Such emotional responses can be linked to the uncertainty and stigma associated with this illness. For some people peer support groups can be an effective method to help cope with fear, anxiety and feelings of isolation. Nurses can provide information and linkages about available resources. Identification of problems with drug and alcohol use is also an important part of psychosocial assessment. Many people with poor social conditions have used drugs and alcohol as a means of coping and the option of substance abuse treatment needs to be made available. Behavior change related to substance abuse may require long-term solutions and incorporate principles of the harm-reduction model previously discussed.

Financial, housing, nutrition, and transportation problems frequently grow worse as the disease progresses. Problems in these areas may be preexisting or begin emerging after the diagnosis of HIV infection, especially if clients lose their jobs because their HIV status becomes known. The usual debilitating course of HIV infection mandates that issues of long-term housing, financing medical care and general financial management be regularly addressed in psychosocial care planning.

TABLE 2. *Psychosocial challenges: selected nursing interventions*

Nursing diagnosis	Potential source/cause	Early interventions	Late interventions
Knowledge deficits	New diagnosis Impaired or decreased learning ability Lack of awareness of need for education Development of new conditions	Increase awareness of need for education Assess level and readiness to learn Develop an individualized teaching plan Evaluate and revise education approaches Referral of client to other services such as peer or professional counseling services Include family/significant others in education process Provide sufficient, accurate, timely information (e.g., treatment options, informed consent, prevention of transmission, health promotion)	Refocus education of information from general to specific with regard to each client's infections and conditions Provide specific teaching regarding treatments and procedures Educate regarding realistic self-care goals; teach specific delegated nursing tasks such as IV maintenance Referral to resources/agencies providing supportive care
Social isolation	Stigmatizing disease Fear of contagion by others Alterations of body image Decreased ability to socialize Alterations in lifestyle due to chronic illness (related to fatigue, medications, and changes in physical appearance, hospitalizations) Avoidance and/or pity by family and friends of client	Establish open and therapeutic communication Referral to peer and professional counseling Assist client in inventorying sources of social support Assist client in identifying need and timing for disclosure of HIV status to significant others Referral of family and significant others to sources of social support across the potential circumstances of disease progression Identify HIV sensitive health and social services providers as potential referral sources	Develop a supportive, therapeutic environment in clinical setting Establish open communication across the continuum including talking and explaining procedures during nursing care, even with clients with limited ability to respond Appropriate but not excessive infection control measures Establish liberal visitation with incorporation of family and significant others in the plan Provision of safe space and opportunity for socialization for clients and significant others

TABLE 2. *Continued.*

Nursing diagnosis	Potential source/cause	Early interventions	Late interventions
			Use radio and television as source of stimulation
			Appropriate use of touch
Altered body image	Stigma of disease	Assess for early problems of altered body image, e.g., ruminating about imagined alterations, issues of contagion	Work with client to maximize functional abilities
	Past experiences with others with disease		Work with client to minimize physical manifestations
	Urinating		Refer to peer and professional counseling
	Skin lesions	Assess clients understanding and acceptance with physical manifestations of disease progression	Establish open, accepting communication with client
	Fatigue		
	Decreased mobility		
	Reaction to responses of others	Provide accurate information and assist client in establishing realistic plans to respond to physical changes in appearance	Establish and support a therapeutic caring clinical environment
		Assist client in exploring measures to control or disguise manifestations (e.g., skin lesions, eruptions)	Assist client and significant others in establishing an accepting and supportive home environment
		Referral to peer support and counseling	Identify and implement nursing measures to decrease effects of physical problems such as incontinence, nausea, vomiting, fatigue
		Provide information and education to family and significant others related to client's need for acceptance and emotional support in the face of physical manifestations of disease	
Anxiety	Stigmatizing disease	Provide accurate information	Facilitate return of control to patient
	Uncertainty	Open communication	Facilitate open communication
	Perceived lack of control		

TABLE 2. *Continued.*

Nursing diagnosis	Potential source/cause	Early interventions	Late interventions
	New diagnoses Fear of rejection/discrimination related to societal attitudes Fear of pain Fear of disfigurement Fear of death	Assist client in articulating source of anxiety Acknowledge the basis of anxiety Assist client in developing a plan to address anxieties Refer for peer and professional counseling Spiritual/pastoral support Informed consent regarding power of attorney, living will, advanced directions Support and educate regarding shared decision making	Provide accurate information regarding treatments and procedures Spiritual/pastoral support Implement nursing measures to control pain Maximize functional abilities Inclusion of family and significant others in plan of care Obtain informed consent regarding treatments and procedures Facilitate shared decision making
Altered role performance	Fatigue Physical debilities Pain Emotional Distress/fear Alteration in body image Lack of information	Assess client's emotional status, physical status, and knowledge level regarding transmission of virus and legal rights Educate and advocate for client regarding his rights Refer to peer and professional counseling Identify HIV-sensitive services and make appropriate referrals Job/career counseling as appropriate Family counseling Referral to community-based case management	Explore and assist negotiating of role expectations and obligations with client and family Identify and assist in obtaining entitlements Referral to community-based case management Maximize functional abilities Support maintenance of control

Practical concerns such as mobility and wheelchair access should be considered. Case management can provide a framework in which medical and psychosocial aspects can be integrated into a comprehensive care plan.

Case management models are found in both inpatient and community settings. Models in both settings have the overall objective of coordinating and linking clients to an appropriate level of service based on need. Nurses have the expertise needed to be effective case managers. Nurse care managers can be particularly beneficial to clients in early HIV infection when information and health promotion is a critical need and in later stages when physical assessment and symptom management become prime considerations. An interdisciplinary approach is critical and the case management role may be to link to available services and provide a conduit for appropriate information to reach service providers. In instances where services are not available, the nurse case manager, in collaboration with social service providers, can take the initiative to develop services or community networks that support the needed services. Where formal case management services have not been established, both hospital and community nurses need to provide health care networks that promote the continuity of services for people with HIV infection across the continuum of their illness.

ACUTE CARE

Persons with HIV infection can be hospitalized for a wide range of infections and symptoms related to immune suppression. For the individual patient, hospitalization can represent the initial acute disease or one in a series of debilitating opportunistic infections. Regardless of the person's stage of illness, a primary reason for admission to the hospital is the need for supportive nursing care.

An important objective for the professional nurse providing care to HIV-infected patients is to establish a therapeutic environment. The overall nursing goal is to maximize quality of life for the patient while responding to the individual's current manifestations of HIV disease. A challenge for nurses is to maintain functional ability even when the person is experiencing rapid disease progression.

Hospitalization may exacerbate emotional distress and be viewed by the individual and family members as representing a deterioration of health status. The HIV-infected patients often enter the hospital uncertain of the future, concerned about loss of functional ability and afraid that this will be the infection that they are unable to overcome. Universally, the health care professional having the most frequent contact with patients is the nurse. It is the nurse who is responsible for establishing open communications that acknowledge the fears and concerns of the patient. There is a valid need for health care workers to take appropriate precautions to prevent transmission of disease within the hospital setting. However, the practice of unnecessary or exaggerated precautions with the HIV-infected patient can limit patient-nurse interactions and increase the patient's sense of isolation, abandonment, and anger. There is a growing understanding that emotional stress can negatively affect an individual's physical status. For the patient entering the hospital in a state of immune suppression, unnecessary stress encountered within the health care setting may potentially further compromise the patient's ability to respond to treatment.

While respecting the patient's confidentiality, inclusion of family and significant others in the daily hospital routine can serve to decrease the sense of isolation. As part of the nursing function, nurses need to establish a flexible schedule with their patients and families that promotes a balance between the patient's need to rest and receive treatment and to interact with significant other individuals who provide ongoing emotional support. It is essential that the nursing plan of care be developed with the patient and that it integrates the medical treatment required into a holistic approach.

Nurses can appropriately serve as coordinators within the interdisciplinary therapeutic inpatient care team. An important nursing responsibility is to ensure that the hygiene, nutrition, emotional, and spiritual needs of a patient are adequately considered in the overall delivery of treatment and care. Additionally, nurses serve a central role in providing information/education to patients and family members. An understanding of treatment options, care procedures, and relevant infection control precautions by the patient and family can be facilitated by ongoing communication and education by the professional nursing staff.

Provision of Care

Persons with HIV infection are often admitted to the hospital in acute crisis or having the potential for their condition to deteriorate rapidly. This requires that nurses fully utilize their assessment skills in establishing baseline measurements from which future changes in condition can be evaluated. Nursing assessment should focus acutely on respiratory, neurologic, and gastrointestinal status because opportunistic infections affecting these systems can be life threatening.

The nurse as the direct care member of the treatment/care team should attend to frequent ongoing monitoring of the patient who is potentially unstable or in distress. The nurse needs to detect changes in the patient's condition as early as possible and be prepared to respond knowledgeably, as well as communicate the necessary information to the physician and other team members. Once an initial assessment of the patient is complete, the nursing process (assessment, planning, intervention, and evaluation/reassessment) provides a framework for providing comprehensive nursing care to the patient.

Special Problems

Frequently associated with the HIV-related gastrointestinal opportunistic infections (such as those caused by cryptosporidium, cytomegalovirus, or *Mycobacterium avium* complex) are alterations in hygiene and nutritional needs. Diarrhea, due to these and other causes, is a common condition encountered in HIV-infected patients. Episodes of diarrhea can be explosive and last for days or weeks. Profuse diarrhea can affect the individual's willingness to eat, affect electrolyte balance, and be associated with severe abdominal pain. Skin breakdown in the perianal area may result, providing a new avenue of infection. Diarrhea also adds to the psychological burden of the patient, with fear of loss of control and embarrassment. Monitoring response to antidiarrheal therapy and communications with the physician regarding the treatment plan are essential.

Debility and weight loss that typically accompany HIV infection over time also carry enormous psychological implications for the patient. The physical and emotional complications of HIV infection are quite complex and often interrelated. Maintaining or assisting the patient with this challenging illness and its special problems will test the nursing skills of even the most experienced nurse.

Alteration of Nutrition Status

In addition to diarrhea, prolonged fevers and poor nutritional intake contribute to generalized wasting in many individuals with HIV infection. Nutritional assessment for each patient and early intervention by the nurse are crucial in identifying and modifying the risk of this complication. Assessment should include a review of pertinent laboratory values, patient weights, diet recall, plus direct observation of nutritional intake. Once those patients at risk are identified, the nurse must institute early nutritional interventions such as frequent weights, dietary intake monitoring, offering foods of choice, and teaching patients dietary strategies. Consultation with a dietician or nutritionist may be helpful to individualize a dietary program. Appropriate strategies to avoid weight loss include assisting patients in selecting high calorie, high protein foods, avoidance of lactose in the intolerant, and offering frequent small meals. Nurses must also be alert to factors that contribute to poor dietary intake such as stomatitis, early filling, or a disagreeable taste in the mouth from medications, and then take the appropriate actions to ameliorate these conditions.

Early assessment of those at risk for weight loss and wasting, initiating appropriate interventions, and identification and communication of factors associated with poor dietary intake to other members of the health care team offer the patient the hope of avoiding enteral and parenteral interventions. Early nutritional intervention and preservation of normal dietary routines as much as possible are more palatable to patients than the inconvenient, expensive, and potentially harmful invasive interventions such as long-term intravenous lines and parenteral nutrition. Prompt recognition of correctable problems combined with appropriate nutritional interventions by the nurse can delay and possibily diminish the impact of intractable wasting.

Alteration of Mental Status

Alteration of mental status, including cognitive, motor, affective, and behavioral changes, is common in patients with HIV infection, especially those with advanced immune deficiency. An estimated 20% to 30% of persons with very late stage HIV infection will suffer profound cognitive and motor impairment. The difficulty experienced in performing a health assessment in any acutely ill patient is often made even more complicated by such severe alterations in mental status in HIV-infected individuals. This difficulty in assessment can complicate the formulation of an appropriate plan of intervention for the patient. Maintaining meaningful and effective patient-nurse communication is a challenge under such circumstances and can make evaluation of significant changes in physical and mental condition even more difficult.

Mental status alterations can also present the nurse with another dilemma. The nurse is often faced with making decisions related to preserving the mentally compromised patient's safety. Decisions to physically restrain or chemically sedate the patient are most often made by the nurse. The patient's need for safety must be weighed by the nurse against the patient's right of self-determination and need for self-care.

Dual Infection with Tuberculosis

The development of tuberculosis in the HIV-infected individual represents a serious situation with pressing implications for the nurse. First, it may be the nurse who is responsible for ensuring the initiation of respiratory precautions for any patient with HIV infection and suspicious pulmonary symptoms. Further, the nurse must vigilantly insist that appropriate respiratory precautions are maintained by staff and patient families. The importance of adherence to proper respiratory precautions goes beyond the nurse's responsibility to advocate for the patient and their families. Although HIV is rather difficult to transmit from patient to nurse, pulmonary tuberculosis represents a real occupational hazard for the nurse and others in health care. Therefore, the nurse is obligated to ensure that the workplace is made as safe as possible.

In addition to supplies and teaching regarding isolation, the patient and family must receive from the nurse timely and accurate information about treatments, procedures, and examinations. Establishing continuity with community agencies, particularly public health nurses and epidemiologists, is essential for follow-up upon discharge.

Discharge Planning

An ideal example of the importance of discharge planning is tuberculosis follow-up after hospital discharge. Due to the requirement for compliance with long-term treatment, effective discharge planning for a patient with tuberculosis has public health implications. As discharge planner, the nurse identifies potential needs of the patients as they return to the community and also identifies the resources in the community to meet those needs. Communication and feedback between hospital nurses and nurses and other health care providers in the community (hospice, the public health departments, and home health) are critical for continuity of care. Nurses should work to provide discharge planning and encourage that communication. Communication information systems need to be developed to permit hospital nurses to be kept up-to-date on community resources and allow for those necessary linkages outside of the hospital.

END STAGE

"I am not afraid of death, I am afraid of dying" is a major concern as the disease process takes its course. The psychological work of coping with the fear of disability is replaced by the specter of going through the process of dying. A major issue for persons in the final stage of the disease is the need to stay in control of their life and their death. There are several important issues to be addressed in this area. Considerations of quantity versus quality of life will require decisions about life support and advanced directives, aggressive treatment versus supportive care options, and institutional or home care.

Choices of where dying will take place need to be made. Patients and families have the task of deciding if dying at home is an option. Home care is not easy, given the physical, mental, and financial problems to be faced, but may be an option in those families with the necessary resources. Hospice support may be available at home or in an institution. Nurses have the responsibility to ensure that individuals and families understand their available options and support them in their choices.

Fear of pain may be a major component in facing the process of dying. Pain management takes on special importance in the end stage. Pain is common in people with AIDS. Common types of pain include abdominal, neuropathic, esophageal, head, and pain related to Kaposi's sarcoma. Pain may make it impossible to maintain quality of life. Negative attitudes about the need for pain relief have been documented among health care providers for their patients who were chemically dependent, and affected the treatment provided. This is especially important since substance abusers are the second most common risk group for HIV infection in the United States. Pain control needs to be highly individualized. The client has a right to define when pain exists and to expect adequate interventions to provide relief when possible.

Issues around family relationships often come to a head at this time. Special problems may arise for HIV-infected parents with regard to their ability to maintain a relationship with their children. This can be especially difficult for women who are traditionally caretakers within families. As parents approach the end stage of their illness, issues related to the care and well-being of children after their death must be faced. A growing number of children who are orphaned by parents with AIDS are requiring foster care. Many of these children are also HIV-infected. In 1991, 1,149 HIV-antibody positive children were already in the foster care system. Issues around families of choice and families of origin and how family members will be integrated into the final stage of life can create conflict. Responsibilities for making final decisions need to be clearly spelled out. Nurses need to support clients' decisions about who is most important to them and who will play integral roles in the final stages of life. Finally, surviving families cannot be forgotten once death has occurred; bereavement counseling may be needed to resolve issues of loss. Some family members or significant others will face their own death from AIDS, and may require support to deal not only with loss but also with their future prospects.

NURSING ADMINISTRATION

Nurse managers may be found in hospital or outpatient settings, and are responsible for establishing specific policies that outline clinical standards and procedures that ensure the quality of care received by patients with HIV infection. Clearly linked to standards of care is the need to establish personnel performance criteria. Consumerism in health care demands that quality care measures focus on patient care outcomes. This does not suggest that the "end result" outcome for HIV-infected patients will be cure, but rather that incremental process outcomes are achieved. Patient satisfaction with care can be an important outcome for patients with terminal disease. Nurse managers can support the nursing staff in delivering quality care by establishing consistent organizational policies and procedures that guide staff in making controversial decisions encountered in the care of HIV-infected patients. Issues such as self-determination, use of alternative therapies, or referral to sources that may offer specific medical treatments can produce controversial patient care situations in which nurse managers need to support the patient's rights, as well as those of the nursing staff.

Refusal by a nurse to care for an HIV-infected patient presents an important challenge for the nurse manager. Institutional-specific policies are needed to guide supervisory actions in such situations. Often, existing personnel and grievance procedures can be used if disciplinary measures are required. The optimal approach to responding to staff fear or concerns associated with the care of persons with HIV infection is the establishment of an ongoing in-service program focusing on updated information related to this disease. Education should then be reinforced by clearly articulated clinical guidelines that promote a safe working environment for all staff. The low risk of infection with HIV when following the Centers for Disease Control (CDC) guidelines for handling blood and other bodily fluids make understanding universal precautions and safe needle disposal practices crucial elements in any educational activity.

Approximately 80% of the significant exposures to HIV among health care workers involve needle sticks. Of those health care workers most likely to sustain a needle stick, nurses constitute 60% to 70%. However, even among nurses who have a good understanding of HIV related issues, implementation of universal precautions is not consistent.

Universal precautions guidelines need to be mandated as part of institutional policy. Employees unwilling to incorporate these precautions into routine practice need to expect corrective or disciplinary action. It is no longer acceptable to isolate or avoid the admission of persons with HIV infection because nurses or other hospital staff do not take advantage of available safety precautions when caring for patients.

HEALTH CARE WORKERS—CONCERNS AND EMPLOYEE ASSISTANCE

Persons with HIV infection require a large physical and emotional investment from nurses. Hospitalized patients are often young and exhibit a wide range of disfiguring signs. No direct care provider should be expected to withstand repeated encounters with this stress without support. Nurse managers need to work creatively to develop strategies that support their staff. While support efforts need to be individualized to specific agencies, the inclusion of psychologists and pastoral care workers in the interdisciplinary care team may be valuable to patients and staff. Clinical support groups for nurses that care for patients with HIV infection have been successful in a teaching hospital in New York City.

The AIDS epidemic has raised questions regarding whether the HIV-infected health care worker may safely continue their patient care activities. Universal precautions should be adequate to ensure staff and patient safety in most clinical settings. Nurses who develop symptomatic HIV infection often require support and assistance. Nurse managers need to take the lead in establishing clear employee assistance procedures for all HIV-infected health care workers where they do not already exist. When appropriate procedures are in place, the nurse manager is responsible for assisting the employee in implementing appropriate procedures.

NURSING EDUCATION

The AIDS epidemic has resulted in a compelling need within nursing education to reach students early in the educational and socialization process. Faculty in schools of nursing are challenged to develop a comprehensive approach to HIV infection within the curriculum.

Issues associated with HIV infection span the continuum of care and affect the delivery of nursing care at a variety of content levels. Educational content within schools of nursing will need to reflect this understanding if future nurses are to be prepared adequately for the realities of the work environment. HIV/AIDS care issues should not be limited to advanced adult health nursing courses. These issues are also relevant content for those studying parent-child, mental health, community health, and nursing administration, as well as in courses dealing with ethical and professional issues. A necessary first step within some educational institutions may be the need to update faculty knowledge in the area of HIV infection. If faculty are not knowledgeable or comfortable in the provision of care to HIV-infected persons, students will sense their discomfort. The value of positive faculty role modeling in developing positive attitudes and behaviors toward AIDS care in nursing students cannot be over emphasized.

Without a vaccine or highly effective treatment, the need to care for persons with HIV infection can be expected to increase well into the next century. Nurse educators have a unique opportunity and responsibility to take a leadership role in meaningfully responding to the AIDS epidemic. Research studies need to be designed to examine current interventions and develop and test creative approaches to care. The National Center for Nursing Research has acknowledged the need for nurses to investigate both the physiological and psychosocial aspects of HIV infection. Research needs to be based in the clinical realities of caring for HIV-infected persons and focus on the evaluation of nursing interventions as they relate to client outcomes. Student involvement in research activities can set the stage for further work and interest in the area. The future of nursing lies with the next generation of nurses. It is that future that nurse educators have the chance to influence positively to the benefit of society, the nursing profession, and especially those persons and their families who are at risk for HIV infection.

SUGGESTED READING

Chenitz CW. Living with AIDS. In: Flaskerud JH, Ungvarski PJ, eds. *HIV/AIDS: A guide to nursing care*, 2nd ed. Philadelphia: WB Saunders, 1993;440–459.

Cohen FL, Nehring WM. Foster care of HIV-positive children in the United States. *Public Health Rep* 1994;109:60–67.

Corbin J, Strauss A. *Unending work and care: managing chronic illness at home*. San Francisco: Jossey-Bass, 1988.

Flaskerud JH, Ungvarski PJ. *HIV/AIDS: A guide to nursing care*, 3rd ed. Philadelphia: WB Saunders, 1995.

Hall BA, Allan JD. Self in relation: a prolegomenon for holistic nursing. *Nurs Outlook* 1994:42(4):110–116.

McGaffic CM, Longman AJ. Connecting and disconnecting: bereavement experiences of six gay men. *J Assoc Nurs Aids Care* 1993;4(1):49–57.

McKusick L. Counseling across the spectrum. *HIV Frontline* #8, June, 1992;1–8.

Millstein SG, Moscicki A, Broering J. Female adolescents at high, moderate and low risk of exposure to HIV: difference in knowledge, beliefs, and behavior. *J Adolesc Health* 1993;15:133–142.

Newcombe R, Parry A. The Mersey harm-reduction model: a strategy for dealing with drug users. Paper presentation at the International Conference on Drug Policy Reform, Bethesda, MD, October 22, 1988.

Newshan GT, Wainapel SF. Pain characteristics and their management in persons with AIDS. *J Assoc Nurs Aids Care* 1993;4(2)53–59.

Ragsdale D, Kotarba JA, Morrow JR. Work-related activities to improve quality of life in HIV disease. *J Assoc Nurs Aids Care* 1992;3(1):39–44.

Sowell RL, Lowenstein A. Comprehensive planning for AIDS-related services. *J Nurs Admin* 1988; 18(5):40–44.

Sowell RL, Meadows TM. An integrated case management model: developing standards, evaluation, and outcome criteria. *Nurs Admin Q* 1994;18(2):53–64.

Stein E, Wade K, Smite DG. Clinical support groups that work. *J Assoc Nurs Aids Care* 1991;2:29–36.

Valente SM, Saunders JM, Uman G. Self-care, psychological distress, and HIV disease. *J Assoc Nurs Aids Care* 1993;4(4):15–27.

Subject Index

1-Chloro-2, 4-dinitrobenzene (DNCB)
  alternate therapy use, 384–385
  immunomodulating effects of, 384–385
Chronic inflammatory demyelinating
    polyneuropathy (CIDP), as autoimmune
    disease, 165, 166
Ciprofloxacin (Cipro)
  forms / price, 309, 310
  pharmacology, 309–310
Clarithromycin (Biaxin)
  forms / price, 310
  in MAC infection treatment, 40, 43,
    310–311
  pharmacology, 311
Clindamycin, use in OI treatment, 50, 124, 125
Clofazimine (Lamprene)
  forms / price, 311
  in MAC infections, 311
  pharmacology, 311–312
Clotrimazole (Lotrimin)
  forms / price, 312
  indications, 312
  pharmacology, 312–313
Coccidioides immitis
  clinical manifestations, 44, 45–46, 136–137
  management, 137
  MRI findings in, 177
Cognitive function
  AZT therapy and, 102–103, 281, 285
  in children, 102–103, 112
  nursing role in, 413–414
Colitis
  antibiotic associated, 214
  CMV infection and, 211–212, 217,
    218–219
  therapy, 218–219
Compound Q
  alternate therapy use, 390–391
  in Chinese cucumber root extract, 390–391
Computerized tomography (CT)
  of ADC in children, 158
  in brain biopsy guidance, 152, 154
  of cerebral abscess, 187, 188
  of encephalitis, 144
  of fungal brain lesion, 144
  in *H. influenzae* infection, 147, 148
  of meningitis, 156, 184, 185
  of PML, 144, 181–182
  of thrombocytopenia, 195
  of toxoplasma infection, 144, 153, 172–173,
    174, 193, 194
Contraceptive choices, in HIV-infected women,
    77–78
Counseling
  coping strategies and, 31–32
  as nursing issue, 404, 409
  topics in, 31–32
Creatine phosphokinase (CPK), in HIV-infected

myopathy, 26
Creatinine clearance
  formula for, 297
  variables in, 297–298
Cryptococcus (C.) neoformans infection
  meningitis and, 175–177
  of pulmonary system, 134–135
Cryptosporidial infection, GI dysfunction in,
    207–208, 217
Curcumin, alternate therapy use, 292–293
Cutaneous manifestations
  bacillary epithelial angiomatosis as, 57, 58
  bacterial infections as, 54, 57
  CD4+ counts in, 57
  eosinophilic pustular folliculitis as, 59–60
  fungal infections as, 56, 57
  herpes simplex infection as, 54
  KS as, 54, 55, 237–238
  listing of, 56, 59
  management of, 56
  morbilliform eruptions as, 54, 56
  seborrheic dermatitis as, 58–59, 60
Cysteine
  alternate therapy use, 387–388
  efficacy, 387–388
  NAC and, 387, 388
Cytokines, KS pathogenesis and, 236
Cytomegalovirus (CMV) infection
  chemoprophylaxis, 40, 49, 126, 179,
    218–219, 224
  diagnosis, 179, 215, 217
  fever and, 44–45, 46
  funduscopic appearance, 46
  GI dysfunction in, 211, 212, 217, 224
  of nervous system, 178–179
  oral, 203, 204–205
  pneumonitis, 138
  prevention, 266

D

Dapsone (Alvoslfon)
  forms / price, 313
  in PCP treatment, 40, 41, 95, 124, 313
  pharmacology, 41, 313–314
  in toxoplasmosis, 40, 41
Depression
  antidepressant use in, 362
  pain treatment and, 362, 371–373
Diarrhea
  chronic, 208, 209, 217
  E. bieneusi and, 209, 218
  etiology, 47, 52, 206–209
  giardiasis and, 209
  management, 47–48, 218, 406
  stool volume and, 215, 216
Didanosine (ddI, Videx)
  in ADC, 161
  AZT combination, 292

gender differences and, 70–71
of GI tract, 224
glucocorticoid effects on, 236
of nervous system, 191
of oral cavity, 55, 203, 238, 239
pain and, 360
pathogenesis, 236–237, 242–243
prognostic factors, 240
pulmonary manifestations, 138–139, 239
staging system, 239–240
Kaposi's sarcoma treatment
in advanced stages, 236
AZT in, 235, 241, 242, 282
bleomycin-vincristine combination in, 242
in early stages, 236
factors influencing, 240–241
interferon in, 241
laser use in, 224
local therapies as, 241
radiation in, 241
relapses in, 242
single-agent chemotherapy as, 242
Ketoconazole (Nizoral)
dosage / forms / price, 333
indications, 49, 176, 333
pharmacology, 333–334

L

Lactate dehydrogenase (LDH) levels
in liver dysfunction, 26, 27
in PCP, 120
Lamivudine (3TC)
as antiretroviral agent, 33, 290, 294, 350
AZT combination, 350
dosage / forms / price, 350
pharmacology, 350
Levorphanol, analgesic properties, 367, 368
Liver function, LDH levels and, 26, 27
Lorazepam (Ativan)
dosage / forms / price, 334–335
indications, 335
pharmacology, 335
Lymphadenopathy, in children, 92
Lymphoid interstitial pneumonitis (LIP)
as AIDS defining, 98
in children, 94, 96, 98, 99–100
prognosis, 99–100
Lymphoma
brain, metastatic, 190–192
brain, primary, 189–190, 246, 248–249
Burkitt's, 191–192, 243
clinical characteristics, 189–190, 245–246, 248–249
epidemiology, 244–245
immune features of, 244
incidence, 189, 243
meningeal, 191
non-Hodgkins, 190–191

pathology, 243–244
PCP development and, 247–248
prognosis, 190, 246, 249
staging, 246
T-cell, 244
therapeutic considerations, 246–248, 249
treatment protocols, 190, 247–248, 249, 282

M

Magnetic resonance imaging (MRI)
as complimentary to CT, 145–146
of CNS, 143–148, 172
of PML, 145, 181–182
of toxoplasmosis infection, 172
of white matter pathology, 143, 145, 146
Measles, in children, 93–94
Megesterol acetate (Megace)
as appetite stimulant, 53, 336
dosage / forms / price, 336
pharmacology, 336
Meningitis
bacterial, 187–189
clinical presentation, 167, 175–176, 183, 189
cryptococcal, 175–177
CSF findings in, 148, 176, 185, 189
in mycobacterial infections, 183–186
treatment, 176–177
Meperidine, analgesic properties, 368
Methadone (Dolophine)
dosage / forms / price, 336–337, 368
indications, 337
pharmacology, 337–338, 368
Metronidazole (Flagyl)
dosage / forms / price, 338
indications, 338
pharmacology, 338–339
B_2-Microglobulin, in HIV infection monitoring, 24–25
Microsporidial infection, GI dysfunction in, 209, 210, 215, 217
Mortality, AIDS-related, 9–10
Mucormycosis
clinical presentation, 178
neurologic manifestations, 178
Mucosal immunity, CD4+ cells in, 200
Muscle disease
clinical presentation, 165
management, 165
mitochondrial myopathy as, 169
Mycobacterium avium complex (MAC) infection
of brain, 184
chemoprophylaxis, 21, 40, 43, 51, 68, 96, 219, 310–311
fever and, 44, 45
GI dysfunction in, 212, 213, 215, 217, 219
M. kansasii and, 134, 183
prevention, 42–43

ISBN 0-7817-0304-2

9 780781 703048